Microbiology: A Guide for Medical Practitioners

Microbiology: A Guide for Medical Practitioners

Edited by Erika Tanner

hayle
medical

New York

Hayle Medical,
750 Third Avenue, 9th Floor,
New York, NY 10017, USA

Visit us on the World Wide Web at:
www.haylemedical.com

ISBN: 978-1-63241-658-2

Cataloging-in-Publication Data

Microbiology : a guide for medical practitioners / edited by Erika Tanner.
     p. cm.
Includes bibliographical references and index.
ISBN 978-1-63241-658-2
1. Medical microbiology. 2. Microbiology. 3. Diagnostic microbiology. I. Tanner, Erika.
QR46 .M53 2019
616.904 1--dc23

Table of Contents

Permissions

List of Contributors

Index

Preface

Microbiology is the science of the study of unicellular, acellular and multicellular organisms. Infection with bacteria, virus, fungi, parasites and a protein called prion result in a number of infectious diseases. Some of these are hepatitis C, malaria, typhoid fever, tuberculosis, etc. Studying the characteristics of pathogens, their transmission mechanisms, and processes of infection and growth, provide better insight into human diseases. The subset of microbiology called medical microbiology is concerned with the diagnosis, treatment and prevention of infectious diseases. The diagnosis of an infectious disease is based on a microbial culture, biochemical tests, microscopy and genotyping. When abnormalities arise in the internal physiology due to the growth of an infectious agent, it can be detected using CAT scans, NMR, X-rays and PET scans. Some infections can be dealt with by the immune system of the body. However in case of more serious infections, antimicrobial drugs such as antibacterials, antifungals, antivirals and antiparasitics aid in fighting the infection. While using a line of antibiotics, it is necessary to consider the strain of the microbe and its antibiotic resistance, the toxicity of antimicrobial drugs and the site of the infection. This book elucidates new techniques and applications of microbiology in a multidisciplinary manner. The topics included in this book on the clinical applications of microbiology are of utmost significance and bound to provide incredible insights to readers. As this field is emerging at a rapid pace, the contents of this book will help the readers understand the modern concepts and applications of the subject.

This book unites the global concepts and researches in an organized manner for a comprehensive understanding of the subject. It is a ripe text for all researchers, students, scientists or anyone else who is interested in acquiring a better knowledge of this dynamic field.

I extend my sincere thanks to the contributors for such eloquent research chapters. Finally, I thank my family for being a source of support and help.

Editor

Evidences of the Low Implication of Mosquitoes in the Transmission of *Mycobacterium ulcerans*, the Causative Agent of Buruli Ulcer

Rousseau Djouaka,[1] Francis Zeukeng,[1,2] Jude Daiga Bigoga,[2] David N'golo Coulibaly,[3] Genevieve Tchigossou,[1,4] Romaric Akoton,[1,4] Sylla Aboubacar,[3] Sodjinin Jean-Eudes Tchebe,[4] Clavella Nantcho Nguepdjo,[2] Razack Adeoti,[1] Innocent Djegbe,[1] Manuele Tamo,[1] Wilfred Fon Mbacham,[2] Solange E. Kakou-Ngazoa,[3] and Anthony Ablordey[5]

[1]*AgroEcoHealth Platform, International Institute of Tropical Agriculture (IITA), 08 P.O. Box 0932, Tri-Postal, Cotonou, Benin*
[2]*Faculty of Science, Department of Biochemistry, University of Yaoundé I, P.O. Box 812, Yaoundé, Cameroon*
[3]*Department of Technics and Technology, Platform of Molecular Biology, Pasteur Institute Abidjan, P.O. Box 490 Abidjan 01, Abidjan, Côte d'Ivoire*
[4]*Faculty of Science and Techniques, University of Abomey-Calavi, P.O. Box 526, Abomey-Calavi, Benin*
[5]*Department of Bacteriology, Noguchi Memorial Institute for Medical Research, University of Ghana, P.O. Box 581, Legon, Accra, Ghana*

Correspondence should be addressed to Francis Zeukeng; zeusfranck07@yahoo.com

Academic Editor: Maria De Francesco

Background. Buruli ulcer (BU) continues to be a serious public health threat in wet tropical regions and the mode of transmission of its etiological agent, *Mycobacterium ulcerans (MU)*, remains poorly understood. In this study, mosquito species collected in endemic villages in Benin were screened for the presence of *MU*. In addition, the ability of mosquitoes larvae to pick up *MU* from their environment and remain colonized through the larval developmental stages to the adult stage was investigated. *Methods.* 7,218 adults and larvae mosquitoes were sampled from endemic and nonendemic villages and screened for *MU* DNA targets (*IS2404, IS2606,* and KR-B) using qPCR. *Results. MU* was not detected in any of the field collected samples. Additional studies of artificially infected larvae of *Anopheles kisumu* with *MU* strains revealed that mosquitoes larvae are able to ingest and host *MU* during L1, L2, L3, and L4 developmental stages. However, we noticed an absence of these bacteria at both pupae and adult stages, certainly revealing the low ability of infected or colonized mosquitoes to vertically transmit *MU* to their offspring. *Conclusion.* The overall findings highlight the low implication of mosquitoes as biological vectors in the transmission cycle of *MU* from the risk environments to humans.

1. Introduction

Buruli ulcer (BU) is a neglected emerging disease that has recently been reported in some countries as the second most frequent mycobacterial disease in humans after tuberculosis [1–3]. BU continues to be one of the most debilitating cutaneous diseases causing significant morbidity. The disease is characterized by severe subcutaneous necrotic lesions that lead to chronic opened sores and ulcerations, ultimately affecting the bone in extreme cases [4]. Mycolactone, a secreted exotoxin, is the only virulence factor identified to date for *Mycobacterium ulcerans (MU)* [5].

During the last two decades, there has been a reemergence of BU across diverse regions of the world [3, 6, 7]. Its prevalence has increased and currently is seen in over 33 countries worldwide [8]. Although the distribution of BU is global and affects people of all ages, the burden of this disease is most severe in West and Central Africa, as well as some parts of Australia [1, 9, 10]. More than 30,000 cases of BU have been reported in Africa over the last decade and the West African region accounts for more than 67% of the reported cases [6].

The environmental pathogen *Mycobacterium ulcerans (MU)* is the etiologic agent of Buruli ulcer [11]. Merritt et al. [1] provided a series of hierarchical criteria analogous to Koch's postulates and/or the Bradford Hill guidelines emphasizing epidemiological/ecological association and the use of logical inference for establishing cause and effect in biological disease transmission. They further discussed the application of this process to indictment of insect vectors for transmission of *MU*. However, the mode of transmission of *MU* from the risk environments to humans remains unknown and its reservoirs in the environment are still being uncovered [1]. The direct transmission of *MU* from human-to-human is extremely rare and cases usually occur in proximity to slow moving or stagnant bodies of water and among rural and economically deprived populations [12–18]. Recent studies in Australia have demonstrated that mosquitoes may be potential reservoirs or vectors of BU [7, 19–23]. Similarly, a recent study conducted in an endemic area of Cameroon revealed the presence of *MU* molecular markers in hematophagous families of insects like Culicidae (mosquito's family), Ceratopogonidae, and Psychodidae [24]. However, a similar study in an endemic area of Benin did not detect *MU* molecular markers in mosquito species [25]. An experimental laboratory study conducted by Wallace et al. [26] also failed to confirm the implication of mosquitoes as biological vectors in the transmission of BU. These recent studies highlight controversial concerns whether mosquitoes actually play a role in the transmission dynamics of BU. Mosquitoes are the most important group of insects involved in the spread of human and animal diseases [27]. One hypothesis is that they could transmit *MU* to humans. However, there is no scientific or historic precedent for mosquitoes transmitting a bacterium to host in any disease system, either directly or mechanically [1]. In the vector ecology, they may serve as biological vectors and hosts for pathogen replication, or mechanical vectors carrying organisms from hosts to hosts without serving as a site of replication [26, 27]. This last hypothesis has recently been reinforced by Wallace et al. [28] who reported a biologically plausible mechanical transmission mode of BU via natural or anthropogenic skin punctures (trauma). These authors further highlighted that a significant low quantity of *MU* delivered beneath the skin surface of animal (BALB/C mice) by a minor injury created by mosquitoes might cause BU in return [28]. Previously in 1974, Meyers et al. [29] reported that skin trauma could be an important mode of transmitting *MU* infections or of introducing *MU* into the dermis of subcutaneous tissue from superficially contaminated skin. However, Williamson et al. [30] recently established that abrasions (trauma) of the skin in Guinea pig models and subsequent application of *MU* are not sufficient enough to cause an ulcer. Mosquitoes contamination or colonization by *MU* remains an event which has only been reported in Australia and which could

vary according to mosquito species. As BU infections occur in humid areas of Africa where high densities of mosquito species are recorded, there is a need to further investigate whether they could be involved in the transmission cycle of BU in African settings and more specifically in Benin.

In this study, we tested the hypothesis of the implication of mosquito species in the transmission of *MU* in an endemic area of Sedje-Denou in the Southern Benin. We further evaluated whether mosquitoes could pick *MU* bacteria from water breeding sites during larval developmental stages leading to colonization and whether colonization continues into the adult stage where they become infective to humans (vertical transmission of *MU* by mosquitoes). Based on these assumptions, we screened wild mosquitoes populations collected from three endemic villages found in Sedje-Denou for molecular targets of *MU*. Coupled to this field based activity, we also investigated the potential for vertical transmission of *MU* within mosquitoes populations using the laboratory strain *Anopheles kisumu*.

2. Methods

2.1. Ethical Considerations. This research which was mainly laboratory based received administrative clearance from the International Institute of Tropical Agriculture (IITA). In addition, the community consent was obtained prior to mosquitoes sampling in the three villages of Sedje-Denou.

2.2. Study Area. This study was carried out in three endemic communities (Agbahounsou, Agodenou, and Agongbo) of Sedje-Denou (6°32′N and 2°13′E) in the Southern Benin (Figure 1). One nonendemic village, Tanongou (10°48′N and 1°26′E), in the Northern Benin was selected as a negative control village for data comparison. Sedje-Denou (also named Sedje) is located in the Commune of Ze which is the second most endemic locality in Benin with a reported prevalence of 450 cases of BU per 100,000 inhabitants [14]. The presence of rivers and wetlands make this locality an appropriate environment for BU. According to Wagner et al. [31], drainage basins as well as forest land cover with variable wetness patterns are prolific for the growth of MU and associated with higher BU disease prevalence rates. These patterns could also influence the distribution and abundance of vectors, or mediating vector-human interactions. The climate at Sedje is a subequatorial type with two discontinuous dry and wet seasons. The annual average rainfall measures 1,000 mm with an annual average temperature of 24°C and a mean altitude of 20 m. The population of 5,496 inhabitants are distributed into six different villages. Sedje is a rural area where agricultural works being the predominant occupation could contribute to increased exposure to *MU* due to the close spatial proximity with the risk environments [31].

Tanongou is also a rural locality under the Department of Atakora in Northern Benin (Figure 1). This village is administratively subdivided into two close villages named Tanongou 1 and Tanongou 2. BU epidemiological data in Benin show that this locality is a nonendemic area for the disease. The climate is a wet Sudanese type with one long dry season (November to May) and a short rainy season (June to October). This region

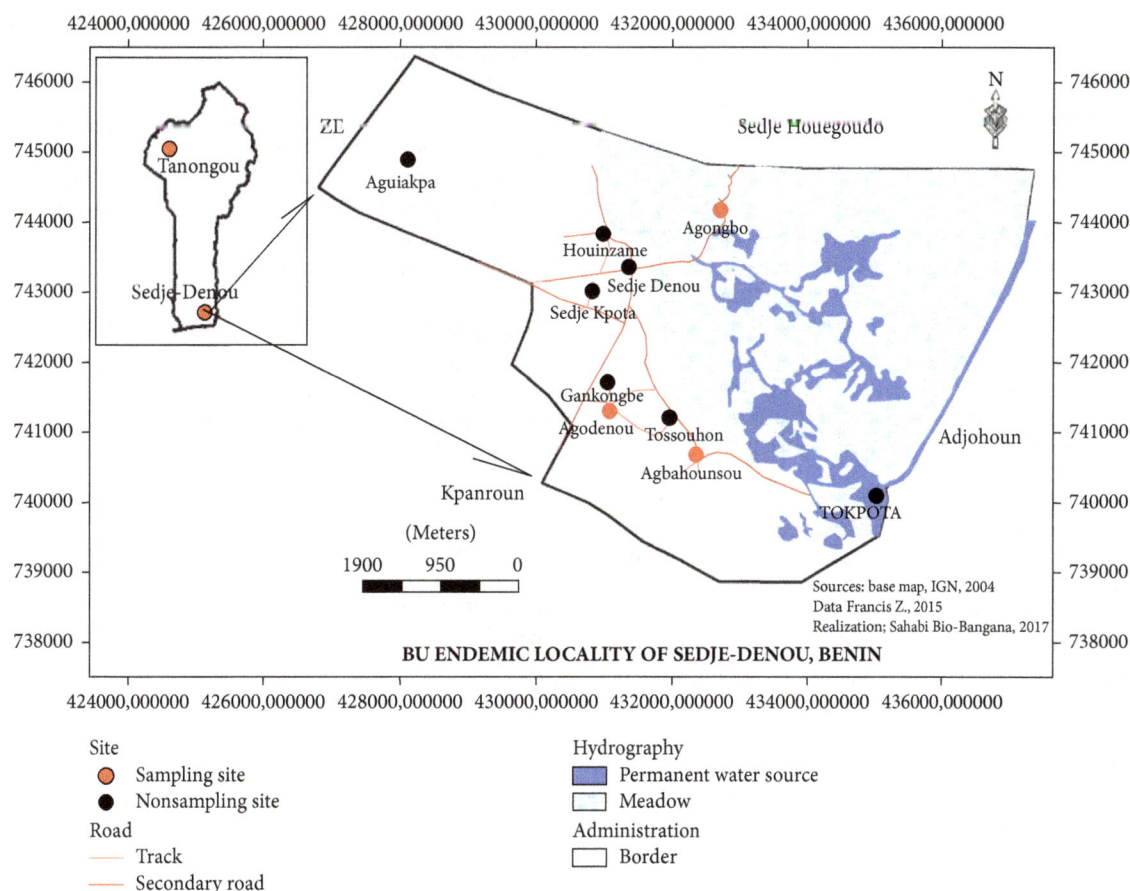

FIGURE 1: Location map of study sites in the Buruli ulcer endemic area in Southern Benin and the nonendemic area in Northern Benin.

is dominated by hills of up to 800 m of altitude and several small water bodies, which makes the region colder and relatively wet. Annual rainfall ranges from 1200 to 1300 mm per year, the vegetation is partially of wet savanna type, and the temperature in this part of the country ranges between 23 and 31°C. Agriculture is the prominent activity of the region.

2.3. Sampling of Mosquito Species in BU Endemic and Nonendemic Areas

2.3.1. Sampling of Adult Mosquitoes. Field surveys for mosquitoes collections were conducted during rainy seasons at the 3 villages of Sedje-Denou from 2014 to 2016. Similarly, mosquitoes samples were collected at Tanongou (Tanongou 1 + Tanongou 2) during rainy seasons as well. Adult mosquitoes were caught indoors using insecticide spraying technique which is one of the effective methods for collecting indoors resting mosquitoes [32]. Mosquitoes were harvested about twenty minutes after house spraying. They were safely transferred into Petri dishes labeled with room/house references and were taken to the laboratory. In the laboratory, each mosquitoes sample was morphologically identified using Edward identification keys [33]. Mosquitoes were identified to genus and to species. No molecular test was performed for mosquito identification. For each identified

species *(Anopheles gambiae s.l., Culex quinquefasciatus, Mansonia africana, and Aedes aegypti)*, pools of 10 mosquitoes each were prepared and kept at −20°C in Eppendorf tubes filled with silica gel. Mosquitoes from Tanongou 1 and Tanongou 2 were pooled and considered as from a single control village of Tanongou.

2.3.2. Sampling of Mosquito Larvae. Mosquito larvae were collected from temporal, semipermanent, and permanent breeding areas using the WHO protocol [34]. Collected larvae were transported to the laboratory where they were morphologically identified and pooled as were the adults. Larvae pools were prepared and stored at −20°C in 70% alcohol.

2.4. Molecular Identification of MU in Mosquitoes Samples

2.4.1. Extraction of Genomic DNA. Genomic DNA was extracted from a total of 721 pools of mosquitoes samples (adult and larvae) using the phenol/chloroform extraction method described by Sambrook and Russell [35]. Several types of controls were put in place to guide against false positive and negative results. To reduce cross-contaminations, extractions were conducted in batches of 10 pools and the 10 pools completely processed (extraction and PCRs) before moving back to a new set of extractions. Negative controls (nuclease-free water, Sigma-Aldrich) were added at a frequency of 10% (1 control per batch of extraction) to monitor potential cross-contaminations. Pooled mosquitoes samples were ground using an electric grinder in sterile 100 μl 1x PBS and the homogenates were suspended in 300 μl preheated lysis buffer made of 5 M NaCl, 0.5 M EDTA, 1 M Tris-HCl (pH 8.0), 10% SDS, and proteinase K (Qiagen, Hilden). The mixture was heated at 60°C for one hour and DNA extracted with phenol/chloroform/isoamyl acid in the ratio 25 : 24 : 1. This was briefly mixed by a pulse vortex and centrifuged for 2 min at 13,000 g. The DNA was precipitated by adding 2 volumes of pure ethanol and the mixture was incubated for 2 hours and centrifuged 10 min at 13,000 g. The DNA was washed by 70% cold ethanol, dried 20 min at room temperature, and eluted in 50 μl of nuclease-free water (Sigma-Aldrich).

2.4.2. Detection of MU DNA in Mosquitoes Samples Using TaqMan qPCRs.

The TaqMan *IS2404* qPCR analysis described by Fyfe et al. [36] was performed on extracted mosquitoes DNA samples to detect *Mycobacterium* DNA in these samples. A total of 404 pools of DNA samples from adult mosquitoes and a total of 317 pools of DNA samples from mosquitoes larvae from the 4 villages (3 endemic villages and one control village) were subjected to PCR analysis for detecting the presence of *MU* in these wild mosquitoes populations. Briefly, 2.5 μl of the DNA extract was amplified in 12.5 μl PCR mixture using the SensiMix buffer system (BioLine). Each reaction mixture contained 7.5 μl SensiMix (2x SensiMix II probe, No-Rox Mix, BioLine), 0.9 μM *IS2404* primer pair, 0.25 μM *IS2404* probe, a reference Rox dye (Rox Passive Reference Dye, Bio-Rad), and sterile nuclease-free water (Sigma-Aldrich). One positive control (*MU* Agy99 DNA) as well as a no-template negative control (nuclease-free water, Sigma-Aldrich) was used to guide this experiment against false positive and negative results. The amplification process was performed in the Mx3500P automate (MxPro Agilent Technologies, Stratagene Mx3500P) under the following cycling conditions: 50°C for 2 min, 95°C for 10 min, 40 cycles of 95°C for 15 s, and 60°C for 1 min. Negative samples to *IS2404* were diluted 1/10 and resubmitted to molecular analyses for the detection of PCR inhibitors. In addition to the screening of the *IS2404* target, other quantitative real time PCR *IS2606/KR* multiplex assays were performed on *IS2404*-positive samples to screen the presence of *Mycobacterium* conservative insertion sequence *2606 (IS2606)* and the Ketoreductase B *(KR-B)* domain of the mycolactone polyketide synthase gene of *MU* plasmid (pMUM001) [36]. QPCR mixtures here contained 1 μl of DNA template, 0.9 μM of each primer, 0.25 μM of each probe, 12.5 μl of the SensiMix buffer system (2x SensiMix II probe, No-Rox Mix, BioLine), and nuclease-free water (Sigma-Aldrich) in a total volume of 25 μl. Amplification and detection conditions were performed as described above.

2.5. Investigations on the Capability of Mosquitoes to Pick and Host MU Bacteria from Larval to Adult Stages (Vertical Transmission of MU in Mosquitoes).

This experiment was carried out in the insectary of the AgroEcoHealth Platform of the International Institute of Tropical Agriculture (IITA-Benin). The laboratory strain *Anopheles gambiae kisumu* and *MU* strain isolates were used in this experiment.

2.5.1. The Mosquitoes Strain Anopheles kisumu.

Anopheles kisumu is a reference laboratory strain originating from the Kisumu region in Western Kenya. This strain is commonly used in standardization experiments and is well maintained in most malaria entomology research laboratories.

2.5.2. The Bacterial Strain Mycobacterium ulcerans Agy99.

Mycobacterium ulcerans Agy99 (*MU* Agy99) is a well-characterized Ghanaian human isolate obtained from the Department of Bacteriology at the Noguchi Memorial Institute for Medical Research (NMIMR, Ghana). Agy99 is a reference *MU* strain with a sequenced genome [37].

2.5.3. Experimental Infection of Mosquitoes Larvae with Mycobacterium ulcerans and Monitoring of Infected Larvae.

Mosquitoes larvae were infected by ingestion of *MU* contaminated Tetramin® Baby Fish Food (Charterhouse Aquatics, London, UK). The infection protocol was adapted from Wallace et al. [26]. Prior to infection, the preserved stock of *MU* strain was diluted in 1X PBS and vortexed 5 min.

(1) Experimental Infection of Mosquitoes Larvae with MU. Six groups (4 tests and 2 controls) of 100 eggs of *An. kisumu* each were distributed for rearing into labeled plastic bowls containing 250 ml sterile water. Prior to introducing eggs into bowls, the breeding/rearing water in test groups received 80 mg of Tetramin Baby Fish Food (Charterhouse Aquatics, London, UK) contaminated with 100 μl of *MU* (2.0 10^5 CFU/ml). The control groups (2 bowls) were prepared in the same way as the test bowls without introducing *MU* contaminated Tetramin Baby Fish Food (Charterhouse Aquatics, London, UK). The mixture (eggs-food-*MU*) was kept in the insectary at 27°C, 75% RH, and 12 : 12 LD for eggs hatching. The first instars larvae progeny (L1) obtained was kept in the contaminated breeding water for ingestion of the bacteria *(MU)* for 24 hours after which the breeding water was completely replaced with a new *MU* free breeding water (water + food only). The L1 larvae were fed with Tetramin and bred till obtaining the second, third, and fourth instars larvae, as well as the pupae and adult mosquitoes. To avoid cross-contaminations during the experiments, all materials and consumables such as rearing bowls, rearing water, and larvae food used for mosquitoes breeding were replaced on daily basis. Rearing waters as well as Tetramin Baby Fish Food were initially tested (qPCR analysis) and confirmed free of *MU* prior to be used in the experiments. Breeding bowls remained covered throughout larval rearing. The entire experiment was repeated thrice to ascertain the accuracy of the data.

(2) Monitoring of Infected Mosquitoes. Pools of 10 individuals per developmental stage (egg, L1, L2, L3, L4, pupae, and adult) were prepared from test and control bowls. These pools of individuals were kept in labeled Eppendorf tubes with 70% ethanol and stored at −20°C for molecular screening of *MU*. In addition, we also harvested from breeding water

TABLE 1: Distribution of field-caught mosquito species in study sites.

Mosquito species	Developmental stages	Study areas				Total
		Agbahounsou	Agongbo	Agodenou	Tanongou	
Anopheles gambiae s.l.	Adult	134	162	119	800	1215
	Larvae	210	110	303	630	1253
Mansonia africana	Adult	190	870	200	140	1400
Culex quinquefasciatus	Adult	320	690	232	90	1332
	Larvae	450	550	354	310	1664
Aedes aegypti	Adult	20	46	25	5	96
Unknown sp.	Pupae	80	65	113	0	258
Total		1404	2493	1346	1975	7218

the cuticles from the different larval molting phases and preserved them for similar molecular analysis. Finally, the third group of stored samples was constituted of small volumes (1 ml) of breeding water collected during the entire larval developmental stages. Collected breeding waters were spun at 14,000 rpm for 5 minutes; then, the condensate was vortexed vigorously and 250 μl was used for DNA extraction. The rationale of preserving cuticles and breeding water is to be certain after analysis that the bacterium was effectively ingested by the larvae and is inside the larvae system and not on its skin (due to cuticle colonization). For example, the presence of the bacterium DNA in larvae and its total absence in the water and the cuticle at a given developmental stage will imply that the bacterium was not on the larva skin (colonization of the skin) but is within/inside the larvae. For this infection monitoring experiment, preserved pools of larvae/adults were screened for 2 MU markers (IS2404 and KR-B which is more specific to MU). A standard curve of the qPCR values (Cts) and the bacterial loads was plotted and this curve was used to determine the bacterial infection rate and to monitor the presence of the bacteria at all larval developmental stages and also at the mosquitoes emergence (the adult stage).

2.6. Statistical Analysis. Statistical analysis of generated data was performed using SPSS 17.0 software (SPSS Inc., Chicago IL, USA). Chi-square test was used to set the difference in proportions (mosquitoes distribution and distribution of MU targets between localities and eggs hatching rates). Nonparametric ANOVA test (Kruskal-Wallis) was used to set the difference in means (bacterial loads and "Ct" values according to mosquitoes developmental stage), whereas the Pearson logistic regression test was used to establish the correlation between MU bacterial loads and the corresponding "Ct" values (Table 5). A pool of mosquitoes (adults or larvae) was defined infected with MU if found positive for the three targets (IS2404, IS2606, and KR-B) for field screened samples and two targets (IS2404 and KR) for laboratory infected samples. Two standard curves were plotted from serial dilutions of MU strain (Agy99) and the Ct values for IS2404 and KR-B genes. Based on these standard curves, the cycle threshold (Ct) cut-off was set at less than 35 cycles for IS2404 and less than 37 cycles for KR-B. Threshold for statistical significance was set at $p < 5\%$.

3. Results

3.1. Distribution of Mosquito' Species Collected in Studied Localities. A total of 4,043 adult mosquitoes were collected during surveyed periods in the three targeted BU endemic villages (Agongbo, Agodenou, and Agbahounsou) and the single BU nonendemic village (Tanongou). 404 pools of 10 adults were generated from sampled mosquitoes which were identified to genus and to species. Pools were grouped by identified species of mosquitoes in each village. Four mosquito species were found in surveyed localities, namely, *Mansonia africana* (34.63%), *Culex quinquefasciatus* (32.95%), *Anopheles gambiae s.l.* (30.05%), and *Aedes aegypti* (2.37%) (Table 1).

In addition to sampled adult mosquitoes, 3,175 mosquitoes larvae were collected from mosquitoes breeding sites found in the endemic villages and the control site. These larvae were used to generate 317 pools of 10 larvae. Larvae identified in the endemic sites included 60.6% of *Culex quinquefasciatus*, 27.86% of *Anopheles gambiae s.l.*, and 11.54% of the pupal stage of an *unknown species (unknown sp.).* In the nonendemic control site only two larvae of two genera were detected, *Anopheles gambiae s.l.* (67.02%) and *Culex quinquefasciatus* (32.98%) (Table 1).

3.2. Screening of IS2404, IS2606, and KR-B Targets in Wild Populations of Mosquitoes from Endemic and Nonendemic Localities

3.2.1. Screening of IS2404. Out of 301 pools of adult mosquitoes (3,010 mosquitoes) from endemic villages subjected to real time quantitative PCR analysis, 26 pools (8.63%) were found positive to IS2404 target (Table 2). At Agbahounsou, 8 pools (12.12%) of mosquitoes were found positive to IS2404, 12 pools (6.82%) at Agongbo, and 6 pools (10.17%) at Agodenou for this same molecular marker. Unexpectedly, we recorded an identical trend of positive number of pools (10/103, 9.7%) in samples from the nonendemic control site (Table 2).

Out of 223 pools of collected mosquitoes larvae (2,235 mosquitoes larvae) from endemic villages subjected to qPCR analysis, 39 pools (17.49%) were found positive to IS2404 target with 10 pools (13.51%) at Agbahounsou, 24 pools (32.88%) at Agongbo, and 5 pools (6.58%) at Agodenou. At Tanongou

TABLE 2: Distribution of *MU* targets in field-caught adult mosquitoes.

Study sites		Pools of 10 adult mosquitoes analyzed	IS2404-qPCR		KR-qPCR		IS2606-qPCR		MU distribution
			Positive	P (%)	Positive	P (%)	Positive	P (%)	
BU endemic villages	Agbahounsou	66	8	12.12	1	12.5	0	—	Absent
	Agongbo	176	12	6.82	0	—	0	—	Absent
	Agodenou	59	6	10.17	0	—	0	—	Absent
Total		301	26	8.63	1	12.5	0	—	Absent
BU nonendemic village	Tanongou	103	10	9.7	0	—	0	—	Absent

P: percentage of targets distribution. No statistical difference was found in the distribution of *IS2404* target between the endemic and nonendemic localities ($p = 0.601$).

TABLE 3: Distribution of *MU* targets in field collected mosquitoes larvae.

Study sites		Pools of 10 mosquito larvae analyzed	IS2404-qPCR		KR-qPCR		IS2606-qPCR		MU distribution
			Positive	P (%)	Positive	P (%)	Positive	P (%)	
BU endemic villages	Agbahounsou	74	10	13.51	0	—	2	16.67	Absent
	Agongbo	73	24	32.88	0	—	1	5.26	Absent
	Agodenou	76	5	6.58	0	—	0	—	Absent
Total		223	39	17.49	0	—	0	—	Absent
BU nonendemic village	Tanongou	94	11	11.70	0	—	0	—	Absent

P: percentage of targets distribution. No statistical difference was found in the distribution of *IS2404* target between the endemic and nonendemic localities ($p = 0.347$).

the control site, 11 pools (11.70%) out of 94 tested from 940 mosquitoes larvae were found positive to *IS2404* target (Table 3). No statistical difference was found in the distribution of this target between the test and control localities in both adult and larval mosquitoes ($p > 0.05$).

3.2.2. Screening of IS2606. Out of 26 pools of adult mosquitoes tested positive to *IS2404* target in the three endemic villages (Agongbo, Agodenou, and Agbahounsou), none was found to be positive for the *IS2606* target. The same finding was observed after real time quantitative PCR analysis of the 10 pools of mosquitoes tested positive to *IS2404* in the control site. No sample was found positive to *IS2606* in the nonendemic site (Table 2).

However, the *IS2606* target was detected in 3/39 (7.7%) pools of larvae which were positive to *IS2404* target in the endemic sites (Table 3). None of the *IS2404* positive mosquitoes larvae (positive pools) from one endemic site (Agodenou) or the control site were positive for the *IS2606* target (Table 3).

3.2.3. Screening of KR-B. Only one pool (3.84%) out of 26 pools of adult mosquitoes tested positive to *IS2404* target was found positive for the *KR-B* target in samples from the endemic villages. This single KR-B positive pool of mosquitoes belonged to the genus *Anopheles* caught at Agbahounsou. However, it is worth indicating that this unique KR-B (*MU* plasmid marker) positive pool was not found positive to the *IS2606*. None of the 10 pools of *IS2404* positive mosquitoes from the control site tested positive for the *KR-B* target (Table 2).

In addition, none of the mosquitoes larvae that tested positive to *IS2404* target was found to be positive for the *KR-B* in both the endemic and the nonendemic areas (Table 3).

3.2.4. Summary of Results from the Screening of the 3 Targets Related to the Presence of MU in Analyzed Wild Populations of Mosquitoes. None of the adult and larvae pools was found to contain the three *MU* targets (*IS2404*, *IS2606*, and *KR-B*). This demonstrated the absence of MU in the wild mosquitoes populations in the endemic region surveyed. Although the *IS2404* target was detected in mosquitoes caught in the nonendemic village, these samples also lacked the three targets related to the presence of *MU* and most likely represent the presence of other environmental mycobacterial species (Tables 2 and 3).

3.3. Analysis of the Low Capability of Mosquitoes to Pick and Host MU from Larval to Adult Stages. Following the inoculation of *Anopheles kisumu* eggs in simulated laboratory breeding experiment (bowls containing water, larvae food) fed with *MU*, we recorded an average hatching rate of 94.010 ± 1.289% in the 4 bowls which served as "test bowls" (water + food + MU + eggs of *An. kisumu*) and an average hatching rate of 93.87 ± 0.546% in the 2 bowls serving as "control bowls" (water + food + eggs of *An. kisumu*). Overall, the bacterial load decreased throughout the experiment from the young (1st instars larvae) to the old (pupae and adult stages) developmental stages of *An. kisumu* (Figure 2). No significance difference was observed in the decrease of the bacterial loads throughout the mosquitoes developmental stages in mosquitoes samples ($p = 0.220$), cuticles ($p = 0.199$), and breeding waters ($p = 0.092$).

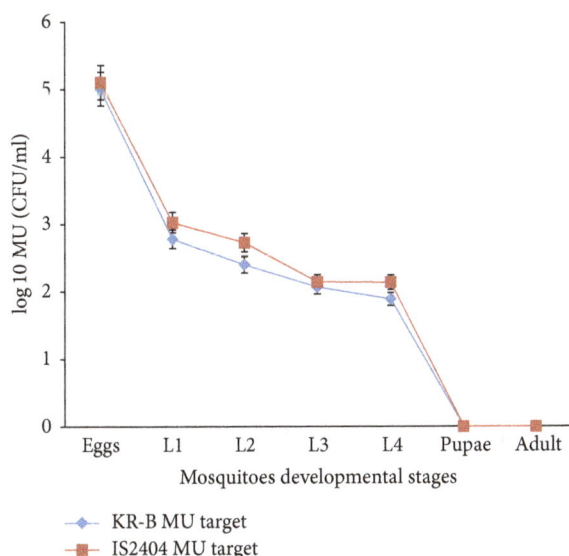

FIGURE 2: Distribution of average bacterial load during mosquito developmental stages. L1, L2, L3, and L4 correspond to first, second, third, and fourth instars larvae, respectively. Values are given with error bars at 5%.

3.3.1. Distribution of MU in First Instars Larvae (L1) of Anopheles kisumu. Randomly selected L1 larvae from the 4 "test" bowls (1 pool of 10 L1 larvae per bowl, making a total of 4 pools for the 4 bowls) showed after qPCR analysis that all 4 pools of L1 mosquitoes larvae were infected/colonized by *MU*. Real time PCR analysis targeting the KR-B domain of *MU* revealed a mean Ct value of 31.592 ± 3.151 cycles which corresponds to a mean bacterial load of $E + 2.779 \pm E + 0.817$ CFU/ml in L1 larvae. The analysis of cuticles (1 pool of 10 cuticles from each bowl, making a total of 4 pools of cuticles from test bowls) released from the metamorphosis of L1 larvae revealed the presence of *MU* in all the 4 pools from "test" bowls (100% infection rate with *MU*, 4/4 pools). The mean Ct value of 36.516 ± 2.096 cycles corresponding to the mean bacterial load of $E + 1.503 \pm E + 0.523$ CFU/ml was from L1 released cuticles. When the breeding water was analyzed during L1 larval development, the mean planktonic bacterial load in the water was $E + 3.034 \pm E + 1.024$ CFU/ml, corresponding to a mean Ct value of 30.610 ± 2.801 cycles. As observed with larvae and cuticles, *MU* was also detected in all breeding waters (4/4) during the L1 developmental stage of *An. kisumu*. *MU* was not found in L1 larvae, cuticles, or breeding water collected from the 2 bowls constituting the "control group" (Table 4).

3.3.2. Distribution of MU in Second Instars Larvae (L2) of Anopheles kisumu. Randomly selected L2 larvae pools from the "test" bowls and controls were collected as was the case for the L1 larval stages. All 4 test pools of L2 mosquitoes larvae were infected or colonized by *MU*. Real time PCR of the *MU* KR-B domain of *MU* yielded a mean Ct value of 33.063 ± 2.984 cycles equivalents to a mean bacterial load of $E + 2.399 \pm E + 0.773$ CFU/ml. Cuticles released from the metamorphosis of L2 larvae had *MU* in 3/4 (75% infection/colonization rate)

pools from "test" bowls. The mean Ct value of 36.823 ± 1.652 cycles equivalent to a mean bacterial load of $E + 1.424 \pm E + 0.428$ CFU/ml was recorded. When the breeding water was analyzed during L2 larval development, the estimated mean planktonic bacterial load found in the water was $E + 2.705 \pm E + 0.680$ CFU/ml. Bacteria was found in all 4 tests during the L2 developmental stage of *An. kisumu*. Traces of bacteria were not found in L2 larvae, cuticles, or breeding water in the "control group" (Table 4).

3.3.3. Distribution of MU in Third Instars Larvae (L3) of Anopheles kisumu. Randomly selected L3 larvae pools as previously described for L1 and L2 showed that all 4 pools of L3 mosquitoes larvae were infected or colonized by *MU* and had mean Ct values to the KR-B region of 34.33 ± 3.349 cycles equivalent to a mean bacterial load of $E + 2.070 \pm E + 0.031$ CFU/ml in L3. The analysis of cuticles only showed the presence of *MU* in 1/4 (25%) pools from "test" bowls. The breeding water during L3 larval development had an estimated mean planktonic bacterial load of $E + 2.277 \pm E + 0.023$ CFU/ml. MU was not detected in any of the control group samples (Table 4).

3.3.4. Distribution of MU in Fourth Instars Larvae (L4) of Anopheles kisumu. Randomly selected L4 larvae from the 4 "test" bowls showed that only 3/4 (75%) pools of L4 mosquitoes larvae were infected or colonized by *MU*. The mean Ct value of 35.03 ± 1.177 cycles equivalent to a mean bacterial load of $E + 1.88 \pm E + 0.441$ CFU/ml was recorded in L4. *MU* was not detected in samples of cuticles released from the metamorphosis of L4 larvae. Breeding water samples had estimated mean planktonic bacterial loads of $E + 1.652 \pm E + 0.019$ CFU/ml. Three out of 4 (75%) breeding water samples were contaminated with the bacteria during the L4 developmental stage. *MU* was not detected in any of the samples from the L4 control group samples (Table 4).

3.3.5. Distribution of MU in Pupae Stages of Anopheles kisumu. MU was not detected from the randomly selected pupae from the 4 "test" bowls. In addition, *MU* was not detected in the cuticles released from the emergence of adult mosquitoes from pupae. Only one out of 4 (25%) breeding water samples was contaminated with the bacteria *MU* during pupae developmental stage, with a KR-B Ct value of 35.47 cycles. As above, *MU* was not detected in samples constituting the control group (Table 4).

3.3.6. Distribution of MU in Adult Stages of Anopheles kisumu. Overall, *MU* was not detected in any of adult stage samples or their controls (Table 4).

4. Discussion

4.1. Wild Populations of Mosquitoes Are Unlikely to Be MU Reservoirs in Sedje-Denou. According to WHO, a reservoir is any person, animal, arthropod, plant, soil, or substance, or a combination of these, in which an infectious agent lives and multiplies and where it reproduces itself in such a manner that it can be transmitted to a susceptible host [38]. Difficulties to cultivate *Mycobacterium ulcerans (MU)* from

TABLE 4: MU distribution among mosquitoes developmental stages, cuticles, and breeding waters.

Nature of the samples	Mosquitoes developmental stages	Distribution of MU targets		Pool positive/pool tested	Presence of MU
		Mean Cts (IS2404)	Mean Cts (KR-B)		
Mosquito*	Eggs	19 ± 1.79	21 ± 2.22	4/4	Yes
	L1	27.67 ± 2.66	31.59 ± 3.15	4/4	Yes
	L2	29.92 ± 2.58	33.06 ± 2.98	4/4	Yes
	L3	31.36 ± 2.98	34.33 ± 3.34	4/4	Yes
	L4	31.38 ± 2.20	35.03 ± 1.17	3/4	Yes
	Pupae	NoCt	NoCt	0/4	No
	Adults	37.89	NoCt	0/4	No
Mosquito cuticles*	Eggs	NA	NA	NA	NA
	L1	30.72 ± 1.78	36.51 ± 2.09	4/4	Yes
	L2	34.25 ± 2.83	36.82 ± 1.65	3/4	Yes
	L3	34.13	39.53	1/4	Yes
	L4	NoCt	NoCt	0/4	No
	Pupae	38	NoCt	0/4	No
	Adults	NA	NA	NA	NA
Mosquito breeding waters*	Eggs	18.43 ± 2.03	21.49 ± 1.63	4/4	Yes
	L1	23.04 ± 3.19	30.61 ± 2.80	4/4	Yes
	L2	22.71 ± 2.59	31.88 ± 2.60	4/4	Yes
	L3	28.4 ± 2.86	33.53 ± 3.00	4/4	Yes
	L4	32.00 ± 2.64	35.94 ± 1.04	3/4	Yes
	Pupae	33.65	35.47	1/4	Yes
	Adults	NA	NA	NA	NA

L1, 2, 3, and 4 correspond to first, second, third, and fourth instars larvae, respectively. Yes or no corresponds to the presence or the absence of the bacteria in analyzed samples. NA stands for not applicable. *The bacterial loads did not vary significantly among the developmental stages ($p < 0.05$).

TABLE 5: Characteristics of the standard curves linking "Ct" values of MU targets and corresponding bacterial loads (MU Agy99 serial dilutions).

MU targets	Regression coefficient (R^2)	Regression equation (95% CI)	p value
IS2404	0.9955	$Y = 9.6569 - 0.2396X$	0.000008
KR-B	0.9968	$Y = 10.9682 - 0.2592X$	0.000004

Independent variable, Ct values (cycle threshold); dependent variable, log10 MU (CFU/ml).

contaminated environmental samples remains the main challenge in the identification of reproductive reservoir(s) for this *Mycobacterium* as well as the understanding of its transmission mode(s) from the MU contaminated environment to humans. Most environmental samples that have been identified with MU have been classified as "potential reservoirs" [1, 39]. Aquatic water bugs have been shown to replicate MU in their salivary glands [40] and MU has been successfully recovered by culture from theses insects [11], and thus, the "reservoir" capacity of other "suspected organisms" remains unclear. The aquatic environment has been identified as the most predominant source of MU contamination [12–18, 31, 41–45]. This research was conducted in the wet agroecosystem of Sedje-Denou region and more specifically in three endemic villages which served as test sites for this study. From the three thousand and ten adult mosquitoes subjected to real time PCR, twenty-six pools (8.64%) were positive to the insertion sequence IS2404, which is not specific enough to infer the presence of MU. We recorded the presence of this insertion (IS2404) in mosquitoes samples collected from nonendemic location (Tanongou in the Northern Benin). These results further highlight the nonspecificity of this marker for MU detection from environmental samples [4, 36, 45]. The use of two additional targets (IS2606 and KR) to increase the specificity of MU detection in our study showed that none of the mosquitoes tested to be simultaneously positive for all three targets. These results certainly confirm the low capability of wild mosquitoes populations to carry MU as previously described by others in this same Southern region of Benin [25]. However, our data seems to contradict works conducted in Australia which detected MU in mosquitoes samples [7, 19–23, 26]. Johnson et al. [22] described the contamination of mosquito species by MU as a consequence of resting and feeding or breeding in storm water drains, whereas Wallace et al. [26], in an experimental study, suggested an unlikely role for mosquitoes as BU biological vectors. In their study using mice and both natural and anthropogenic forms of inoculation, they emphasized that reducing exposure to insect bites and destroying mosquitoes breeding sites around households would break the chain of BU transmission [28]. These series of studies on the role of mosquitoes in the transmission of MU show the need of further investigations whether mosquitoes can act as both reservoir and vector of MU. In this current study, none of the 2,235 mosquitoes larvae collected from both endemic and nonendemic areas for BU were found to be positive for MU, suggesting that mosquitoes larvae in the wild were unlikely to be reservoirs for MU. Although our results generated from wild mosquitoes populations are in favor of previous studies conducted in Benin which revealed the inability of

mosquitoes to be involved in MU transmission [25], a laboratory designed experimental model was designed to better understand the poor implication of mosquitoes in increased number of BU cases in West and Central Africa [1, 6].

4.2. Inability of An. kisumu Larvae to Pick Up MU from Their Environment and Remain Colonized through the Larval Developmental Stages to the Adult Stage. Mosquitoes (Culicidae) development, as characteristic of all holometabolous insects, proceeds through embryonic, larval, pupal, and adult stages that reflect considerable morphological and physiological differences [34]. These stages exhibit distinct niches; larvae and pupae are aquatic while adults are free-flying and terrestrial. In mosquitoes vectors, vertical transmission has been demonstrated for certain pathogens which include yellow fever virus, dengue virus, St. Louis encephalitis virus, Japanese encephalitis virus, and West Nile virus (WNV) [46]. Vertical transmission involves the transmission of pathogens from female mosquitoes to their offspring. The laboratory experimental model showed that mosquitoes larvae readily ingested MU and that MU colonized the larval stages through the pupal stage. However, at the pupae series of high energy demanding [47], metabolism taking place in the mosquitoes certainly affects MU development leading to the clearing of MU colonization by the end of pupation and at the adult stage (Figure 2). Our research demonstrated the total absence of MU at both pupae and adult stages as reported by Wallace et al. [28] and, thus, highlights the inability of these biting dipterans to act as a good vector/host of MU in an endemic environment. Results from this laboratory based experiment are consistent with those obtained from the analysis of thousands of wild populations of mosquitoes collected in the endemic locations which did not show any MU colonization through molecular testing. Data published by Wallace et al. [26] suggested that MU is unlikely to persist in the mosquito's body system, a behavior which stands as a natural protective mechanism of mosquitoes to bacterial infections. According to Hoxmeier et al. [48], the contamination of *Anopheles gambiae* mosquitoes with MU resulted in disruptions to phospholipid metabolic pathways in the mosquitoes, especially the use of glycolipid molecules. Moreover, glycolipids are actively involved in signaling and are mediators in cellular and immune processes [49]. The disruption of synthesis of this molecule probably has a negative impact on the various interactions between MU cells and *Anopheles* and the poor capability of mosquitoes to serve as biological vectors for MU [45]. Instead of acting as biological vectors for MU as described in this study, mosquitoes might act as mechanical vectors as recently described in an experimental study with *Aedes notoscriptus* and BALB/C mice [28]. However, mechanical transmission of *MU* seems to happen only after skin trauma either by an insect bite or by any other environmental stress (e.g., a thorn, penetrating wood splinters, and scorpion stings) [29]. The traumatized skin should initially be colonized by *MU*, a phenomenon that could naturally happen during repetitive contacts with the risk environments such as water bodies or contaminated biofilms [1, 17, 28]. Furthermore, in behavioral study with *Aedes aegypti*, Sanders et al. [50] suggested that if a biofilm of *MU* was on a person, the bacteria may be attracting mosquitoes which in return would lead to a puncture insertion of *MU* as recently reported by Wallace et al. [28]. Although mechanical transmission of *MU* stands as a common mechanism that could correlate transmission studies from both Africa and Australia, Williamson et al. [30] recently established that abrasions (trauma) of the skin in Guinea pig models and subsequent application of *MU* are not sufficient enough to cause an ulcer. Further laboratory and epidemiological studies are therefore required to understand the extent of the mechanical transmission of *MU* and how frequent animals including humans can carry and remain colonized with *MU* on their skin to facilitate such transmission mode. *MU* could be traced from the risk environments to humans or animals directly after they had contact with colonized environments. In such hypothetical situations and for preventive measures, individuals from endemic areas should remain aware and avoid frequent contacts with mosquito's bites by sleeping under mosquitoes bed nets, wearing protective clothing while farming or using clean water for bathing and cleaning [1, 7, 15, 17, 19, 28].

Mosquitoes larvae breeding in an *MU* contaminated water body are capable of ingesting this bacterium as shown by Hoxmeier et al. [48] and Wallace et al. [26] in *Aedes aegypti*, *Aedes albopictus*, *Culex restuans*, and *Ochlerotatus triseriatus* larvae. Although several experimental studies have established the potential of predaceous aquatic insects to temporally maintain *MU* during their developmental stages in water [37, 40], our findings in addition to confirming these previous results also show that *MU* colonization of mosquitoes larvae is very temporal as larvae system is capable of clearing the bacterial load during pupae and adult developmental stages. The vertical transmission of *MU* therefore seems not to be effective in mosquitoes populations as documented with several viruses. The noncontamination/colonization of field-caught mosquito species by *MU* as found in this study might suggest that mosquitoes are unable to move *MU* from one source to another in endemic areas in Benin.

5. Conclusion

This study revealed the absence of *MU* in hematophagous mosquitoes trapped in households in BU endemic locations in the Sedje-Denou division in Benin. Using an experimental model, we also showed the inability of laboratory infected or colonized *An. kisumu* larvae to transfer the bacteria to their pupae and the emerging adults. This low ability of mosquitoes to vertically transmit *MU* pathogens to their offspring coupled with the absence of *MU* in field-caught mosquitoes further highlights the low probability of these biting insects as biological vectors for *MU* in endemic villages

in Benin. Mosquitoes may therefore not be involved in the dissemination of this pathogen from the risk environments to humans in investigated areas. However, further studies should be performed to evaluate their mechanical implication, before completely excluding whether they are involved or not in the transmission cycle of this emerging disease.

Authors' Contributions

Rousseau Djouaka, Francis Zeukeng, Jude Daiga Bigoga, Wilfred Fon Mbacham, Solange E. Kakou-Ngazoa, and Anthony Ablordey conceived and designed the experiments. Rousseau Djouaka, Francis Zeukeng, Genevieve Tchigossou, Sylla Aboubacar, Romaric Akoton, David N'golo Coulibaly, Sodjinin Jean-Eudes Tchebe, Clavella Nantcho Nguepdjo, Romaric Akoton, Innocent Djegbe, and Solange E. Kakou-Ngazoa participated in collection and analyses of the data. Rousseau Djouaka, Francis Zeukeng, Razack Adeoti, Sodjinin Jean-Eudes Tchebe, and Innocent Djegbe performed the experimental study on the vertical transmission of *M. ulcerans* in mosquitoes. Jude Daiga Bigoga, Wilfred Fon Mbacham, Solange E. Kakou-Ngazoa, Manuele Tamo, and Anthony Ablordey supervised the experiments. Rousseau Djouaka and Francis Zeukeng performed the statistical analysis of the data. Rousseau Djouaka and Francis Zeukeng drafted the manuscript. Anthony Ablordey, Solange E. Kakou-Ngazoa, and Manuele Tamo made critical revisions of the manuscript. All authors read and approved the final manuscript.

Acknowledgments

This work was supported in part by a research grant from the International Society for Infectious Diseases (ISID, United States) attributed to Francis Zeukeng and the AgroEco-Health Platform of the International Institute of Tropical Agriculture (IITA-Benin). The authors express their gratitude to household heads and community health workers of the Sedje-Denou and Tanongou localities for their assistance during sample collections. They also extend their gratitude to Professor Dorothy Yeboah-Manu and Dr. Anthony Ablordey for providing the bacterial strain used in this study, their assistance, and the supervision of Francis Zeukeng internships in the Bacteriology Department of Noguchi Memorial Institute for Medical Research (NMIMR) in Accra, Ghana.

References

[1] R. W. Merritt, E. D. Walker, P. L. C. Small et al., "Ecology and transmission of Buruli ulcer disease: a systematic review," *PLoS Neglected Tropical Diseases*, vol. 4, no. 12, p. e911, 2010.

[2] G. E. Sopoh, R. C. Johnson, A. Chauty et al., "Buruli ulcer surveillance, Benin, 2003–2005," *Emerging Infectious Diseases*, vol. 13, no. 9, pp. 1374–1376, 2007.

[3] M. Debacker, J. Aguiar, C. Steunou et al., "*Mycobacterium ulcerans* disease (Buruli ulcer) in rural hospital, southern Benin,

1997–2001," *Emerging Infectious Diseases*, vol. 10, no. 8, pp. 1391–1398, 2004.

[4] World Health Organization, *Laboratory Diagnosis of Buruli Ulcer: A Manual for Health Care Providers*, WHO, Geneva, Switzerland, 2014.

[5] K. M. George, D. Chatterjee, G. Gunawardana et al., "Mycolactone: a polyketide toxin from *Mycobacterium ulcerans* required for virulence," *Science*, vol. 283, no. 5403, pp. 854–857, 1999.

[6] World Health Organization, *Buruli ulcer: Number of New Cases of Buruli Ulcer Reported (Per Year)*, WHO, Geneva, Switzerland, 2011, http://apps.who.int/neglected_diseases/ntd-data/buruli/buruli.html.

[7] T. Y. J. Quek, E. Athan, M. J. Henry et al., "Risk factors for *Mycobacterium ulcerans* infection, southeastern Australia," *Emerging Infectious Diseases*, vol. 13, no. 11, pp. 1661–1666, 2007.

[8] World Health Organization, *Buruli ulcer (Mycobacterium ulcerans infection)*, WHO Media centre, 2015, http://www.who.int/mediacentre/factsheets/fs199/en/.

[9] H. R. Williamson, M. E. Benbow, L. P. Campbell et al., "Detection of *Mycobacterium ulcerans* in the environment predicts prevalence of Buruli ulcer in Benin," *PLoS Neglected Tropical Diseases*, vol. 6, no. 1, Article ID e1506, 2012.

[10] G. Francis, M. Whitby, and M. Woods, "*Mycobacterium ulcerans* infection: a rediscovered focus in the Capricorn Coast region of central Queensland," *Medical Journal of Australia*, vol. 185, no. 3, pp. 179-180, 2006.

[11] F. Portaels, W. M. Meyers, A. Ablordey et al., "First cultivation and characterization of *Mycobacterium ulcerans* from the environment," *PLoS Neglected Tropical Diseases*, vol. 2, no. 3, article no. e178, 2008.

[12] M. W. Bratschi, M. T. Ruf, A. Andreoli et al., "*Mycobacterium ulcerans* persistence at a village water source of Buruli ulcer patients," *PLoS Neglected Tropical Diseases*, vol. 8, no. 3, Article ID e2756, 2014.

[13] J. Landier, J. Gaudart, K. Carolan et al., "Spatio-temporal patterns and landscape-associated risk of buruli ulcer in Akonolinga, Cameroon," *PLoS Neglected Tropical Diseases*, vol. 8, no. 9, p. e3123, 2014.

[14] G. E. Sopoh, Y. T. Barogui, R. C. Johnson et al., "Family relationship, water contact and occurrence of buruli ulcer in Benin," *PLoS Neglected Tropical Diseases*, vol. 4, no. 7, article e746, 2010.

[15] M. Debacker, F. Portaels, J. Aguiar et al., "Risk factors for buruli ulcer, Benin," *Emerging Infectious Diseases*, vol. 12, no. 9, pp. 1325–1331, 2006.

[16] R. W. Merritt, M. E. Benbow, and P. L. C. Small, "Unraveling an emerging disease associated with disturbed aquatic environments: the case of Buruli ulcer," *Frontiers in Ecology and the Environment*, vol. 3, no. 6, pp. 323–331, 2005.

[17] H. Aiga, T. Amano, S. Cairncross, J. A. Domako, O.-K. Nanas, and S. Coleman, "Assessing water-related risk factors for Buruli ulcer: a case-control study in Ghana," *American Journal of Tropical Medicine and Hygiene*, vol. 71, no. 4, pp. 387–392, 2004.

[18] L. Marsollier, J. Aubry, J.-P. Saint-André et al., "Ecology and transmission of *Mycobacterium ulcerans*," *Pathologie Biologie*, vol. 51, no. 8-9, pp. 490–495, 2003.

[19] C. J. Lavender, J. A. M. Fyfe, J. Azuolas et al., "Risk of Buruli ulcer and detection of Mycobacterium ulcerans in mosquitoes in Southeastern Australia," *PLoS Neglected Tropical Diseases*, vol. 5, no. 9, Article ID e1305, 2011.

[20] P. D. R. Johnson and C. J. Lavender, "Correlation between buruli Ulcer and vector-borne notifiable diseases, Victoria, Australia," *Emerging Infectious Diseases*, vol. 15, no. 4, pp. 614-615, 2009.

[21] T. Y. J. Quek, J. M. Henry, A. J. Pasco et al., "*Mycobacterium ulcerans* infection: factors influencing diagnostic delay," *Medical Journal of Australia*, vol. 187, pp. 561–563, 2007.

[22] P. D. R. Johnson, J. Azuolas, C. J. Lavender et al., "*Mycobacterium ulcerans* in mosquitoes captured during outbreak of Buruli ulcer, southeastern Australia," *Emerging Infectious Diseases*, vol. 13, no. 11, pp. 1653–1660, 2007.

[23] P. D. R. Johnson, T. Stinear, and P. L. C. Small, "Buruli ulcer (*M. ulcerans* infection): new insights, new hope for disease control," *PLoS Medicine*, vol. 2, no. 4, article e108, 2005.

[24] P. Le Gall, J. Landier, J. De Matha Ndengue et al., *Detection of Mycobacterium ulcerans in domestic arthropods in a Buruli ulcer endemic site, Akonolinga, Cameroon*, World Health Organization, Geneva, Switzerland, 2015.

[25] B. Zogo, A. Djenontin, K. Carolan et al., "A field study in Benin to investigate the role of mosquitoes and other flying insects in the ecology of mycobacterium ulcerans," *PLoS Neglected Tropical Diseases*, vol. 9, no. 7, Article ID e0003941, 2015.

[26] J. R. Wallace, M. C. Gordon, L. Hartsell et al., "Interaction of *Mycobacterium ulcerans* with mosquito species: implications for transmission and trophic relationships," *Applied and Environmental Microbiology*, vol. 76, no. 18, pp. 6215–6222, 2010.

[27] B. F. Eldridge, "Mosquitoes, the culicidae," in *Biology of disease vectors*, W. C. Marquardt, Ed., p. 108, Elsevier Academic Press, New York, NY, USA, 2005.

[28] J. R. Wallace, K. M. Mangas, J. L. Porter et al., "*Mycobacterium ulcerans* low infectious dose and mechanical transmission support insect bites and puncturing injuries in the spread of Buruli ulcer," *PLOS Neglected Tropical Diseases*, vol. 11, no. 4, p. e0005553, 2017.

[29] W. M. Meyers, W. M. Shelly, D. H. Connor, and E. K. Meyers, "Human *Mycobacterium ulcerans* infections developing at sites of trauma to skin," *American Journal of Tropical Medicine and Hygiene*, vol. 23, no. 5, pp. 919–923, 1974.

[30] H. R. Williamson, L. Mosi, R. Donnell, M. Aqqad, R. W. Merritt, and P. L. C. Small, "*Mycobacterium ulcerans* fails to infect through skin abrasions in a guinea pig infection model: implications for transmission," *PLoS Neglected Tropical Diseases*, vol. 8, no. 4, Article ID e2770, 2014.

[31] T. Wagner, M. E. Benbow, T. O. Brenden, J. Qi, and R. C. Johnson, "Buruli ulcer disease prevalence in Benin, West Africa: associations with land use/cover and the identification of disease clusters," *International Journal of Health Geographics*, vol. 7, article 25, 2008.

[32] World Health Organization, *Guidelines for Testing Mosquito Adulticides for Indoor Residual Spraying and Treatment of Mosquito Nets*, WHO, Geneva, Switzerland, 2006.

[33] F. Edwards, "Mosquitoes of the Ethiopian Region III," in *Culicine adults and pupae*, B. M. N. Hist, Ed., London, UK, 1941.

[34] World Health Organization, *Entomologie Du Paludisme Et Contrôle Des Vecteurs, Guide Du Stagiaire*, vol. 1, part 1, WHO, Geneva, Switzerland, 2003.

[35] J. Sambrook and D. W. Russell, "Purification of nucleic acids by extraction with phenol: chloroform," in *Commonly Used Techniques in Molecular Cloning*, J. Sambrook and D. W. Russell, Eds., vol. 3, appendix 8, Cold Spring Harbor Laboratory Press, Cold Spring Harbor, NY, USA, 3rd edition, 2001.

[36] J. A. M. Fyfe, C. J. Lavender, P. D. R. Johnson et al., "Development and application of two multiplex real-time PCR assays for the detection of *Mycobacterium ulcerans* in clinical and environmental samples," *Applied and Environmental Microbiology*, vol. 73, no. 15, pp. 4733–4740, 2007.

[37] T. P. Stinear, T. Seemann, S. Pidot et al., "Reductive evolution and niche adaptation inferred from the genome of *Mycobacterium ulcerans*, the causative agent of Buruli ulcer," *Genome Research*, vol. 17, no. 2, pp. 192–200, 2007.

[38] World Health Organization, *Yellow Fever*, WHO, Geneva, Switzerland, 1998, http://www.who.ch/gpv-documents/.

[39] S. Gryseels, D. Amissah, L. Durnez et al., "Amoebae as potential environmental hosts for *Mycobacterium ulcerans* and other mycobacteria, but doubtful actors in buruli ulcer epidemiology," *PLoS Neglected Tropical Diseases*, vol. 6, no. 8, Article ID e1764, 2012.

[40] L. Marsollier, R. Robert, J. Aubry et al., "Aquatic insects as a vector for *Mycobacterium ulcerans*," *Applied and Environmental Microbiology*, vol. 68, no. 9, pp. 4623–4628, 2002.

[41] J. Hayman, "Postulated epidemiology of *Mycobacterium ulcerans* infection," *International Journal of Epidemiology*, vol. 20, no. 4, pp. 1093–1098, 1991.

[42] K. Kibadi, M. Panda, J.-J. M. Tamfum et al., "New foci of buruli ulcer, Angola and Democratic Republic of Congo," *Emerging Infectious Diseases*, vol. 14, no. 11, pp. 1790–1792, 2008.

[43] A. A. Duker, F. Portaels, and M. Hale, "Pathways of *Mycobacterium ulcerans* infection: a review," *Environment International*, vol. 32, no. 4, pp. 567–573, 2006.

[44] F. Portaels, K. Chemlal, P. Elsen et al., "*Mycobacterium ulcerans* in wild animals," *Revue Scientifique et Technique de l'OIE*, vol. 20, no. 1, pp. 252–264, 2001.

[45] A. L. Morris, J.-F. Guegan, D. Andreou et al., "Deforestation-driven food-web collapse linked to emerging tropical infectious disease, *Mycobacterium ulcerans*," *Science Advances*, vol. 2, no. 12, p. e1600387, 2016.

[46] I. Unlu, A. J. MacKay, A. Roy, M. M. Yates, and L. D. Foil, "Evidence of vertical transmission of West Nile virus in field-collected mosquitoes," *Journal of Vector Ecology*, vol. 35, no. 1, pp. 95–99, 2010.

[47] B. W. Harker, S. K. Behura, B. S. Debruyn et al., "Stage-specific transcription during development of Aedes aegypti," *BMC Developmental Biology*, vol. 13, no. 1, article 29, 2013.

[48] J. C. Hoxmeier, B. D. Thompson, C. D. Broeckling et al., "Analysis of the metabolome of *Anopheles gambiae* mosquito after exposure to *Mycobacterium ulcerans*," *Scientific Reports*, vol. 5, article 9242, 2015.

[49] G. C. Atella and M. Shahabuddin, "Differential partitioning of maternal fatty acid and phospholipid in neonate mosquito larvae," *Journal of Experimental Biology*, vol. 205, no. 23, pp. 3623–3630, 2002.

[50] M. L. Sanders, H. R. Jordan, C. Serewis-Pond et al., "*Mycobacterium ulcerans* toxin, mycolactone may enhance host-seeking and oviposition behaviour by *Aedes aegypti* (L.) (Diptera: Culicidae)," *Environmental Microbiology*, vol. 19, no. 5, pp. 1750–1760, 2017.

Diarrheagenic *Escherichia coli* Associated with Acute Gastroenteritis in Children from Soriano, Uruguay

Vivian Peirano,[1,2] **María Noel Bianco,**[1] **Armando Navarro,**[3] **Felipe Schelotto** (iD),[1] **and Gustavo Varela** (iD)[1]

[1]*Bacteriology and Virology Department, Hygiene Institute, Medicine Faculty, Universidad de la República, Uruguay*
[2]*Mercedes Hospital Laboratory, State Health Services Administration (ASSE), Uruguay*
[3]*Public Health Department, Medicine Faculty, UNAM (Universidad Nacional Autónoma de Mexico), Mexico City, Mexico*

Correspondence should be addressed to Felipe Schelotto; felipe@higiene.edu.uy

Academic Editor: Cinzia Marianelli

Introduction. Acute diarrheal disease still deserves worldwide attention due to its high morbidity and mortality, especially in developing countries. While etiologic determination is not mandatory for management of all individual cases, it is needed for generating useful epidemiologic knowledge. Diarrheagenic *Escherichia coli* (DEC) are relevant enteropathogens, and their investigation requires specific procedures to which resources and training should be dedicated in reference laboratories. *Methodology.* Following the hypothesis that enteric pathogens affecting children in towns located in the interior of Uruguay may be different from those found in Montevideo, we conducted a diagnostic survey on acute diarrheal disease in 83 children under 5 years of age from populations in the south of the country. *Results.* DEC pathotypes were the only bacterial pathogens found in diarrheal feces (20.48%), followed by rotavirus (14.45%) and enteric adenovirus (4.81%). Atypical EPEC (aEPEC) was the most frequent DEC pathotype identified, and unexpectedly, it was associated with bloody diarrheal cases. These patients were of concern and provided with early consultation, as were children who presented with vomiting, which occurred most frequently in rotavirus infections. aEPEC serotypes were diverse and different from those previously reported in Montevideo children within the same age group and different from serotypes identified in regional and international studies. Enteroinvasive (EIEC) O96 : H19, associated with large outbreaks in Europe, was also isolated from two patients. Antibiotic susceptibility of pathogenic bacteria identified in this study was higher than that observed in previous national studies, which had been mainly carried out in children from Montevideo. *Conclusion.* The reduced number of detected species, the marked prevalence of aEPEC, the scarce resistance traits, and the diverse range of serotypes in the virulent DEC identified in this study confirm that differences exist between enteropathogens affecting children from interior towns of Uruguay and those circulating among children in Montevideo.

1. Introduction

Infectious diarrhea causes almost 500,000 deaths per year, especially among children up to five years of age from Asia, Africa, and Latin America [1, 2]. Incidence varies between countries and regions, due to a number of recognized factors, such as the socioeconomic group, nutritional status, access to safe water sources, wastewater disposal, food safety, electricity supply, refrigeration of food, and close contact with animal reservoirs of potential pathogens. Infectious

diarrheal diseases are particularly prevalent in younger children from low income homes [3–5].

Diarrheal disease is very important due to its high morbidity and mortality. Attention must also be given to its links with malnutrition and to the high cost of medical attention that impacts an already burdened health system in many developing countries [6]. Severe cases and related complications often require specialized care, which includes diarrheal diseases characterized by severe dehydration (found in cholera cases), bloody diarrhea caused by *Shigella*, haemolytic-uremic syndrome (HUS) associated with infection by Shiga toxin-producing *E. coli* (STEC), Guillain–Barré Syndrome (GBS) linked to *Campylobacter,* and invasive illness by *Salmonella* or acute abdominal pain due to mesenteric adenitis and *Yersinia enterocolitica* [7, 8].

Laboratory investigation of all potential diarrheal agents presently involves complicated and expensive procedures, and it is not usually required or performed to manage individual cases [9, 10]. However, control measures to combat acute diarrheal disease of children in primary care settings cannot be adequately oriented if predisposing conditions, etiologic agents, and their epidemiologic-spread profile are not fully known and available to health care decision-makers [2, 5].

Diarrheagenic *E. coli* (DEC) is a group of strains that do not form part of the human intestinal microbiota but can be transmitted from food or infected humans to susceptible children and adults resulting in a range of disease that can be very serious and frequent. Several overlapping virulent types that are capable of gene transfer include enterotoxigenic *E. coli* (ETEC), enteropathogenic *E. coli* (EPEC), enteroaggregative *E. coli* (EAEC), Shiga-toxin-producing *E. coli* (STEC), and enteroinvasive *E. coli* (EIEC). Diffuse-adherent *E. coli* DAEC or adherent-invasive *E. coli* AIEC is also a potential member of DEC that requires further study [11, 12].

For many years, our workgroup has participated in the surveillance of acute diarrheal disease in Uruguayan children [13–16], and we confirmed that EPEC is the most prevalent DEC pathotype locally. Shiga toxin-producing *Escherichia coli* (STEC), mainly non-O157, EAEC, and ETEC were also identified as being present locally, and EIEC was confirmed but less frequently [13, 14].

Most Uruguayan DEC studies (and more general studies concerning diarrheal disease and pertinent agents) have been conducted in urban Montevideo [13–16] and have provided useful information. However, these studies need to be complemented with studies from smaller towns and rural areas where the epidemiology, spread, distribution, and characteristics of enteropathogenic microorganisms can vary [17].

This study deals with the etiology of acute diarrhea in children and intends to overcome the mentioned weaknesses of existing knowledge, by focusing on DEC detection in children from small towns in the interior regions of Uruguay and on characterization of isolates.

2. Materials and Methods

The study period ran from October 2012 to March 2015.

2.1. Approvals and Consent. The study was approved by the Ethics Bureau of Medicine Faculty, UdelaR, and by the Mercedes Hospital Committee. An informed consent was obtained from each child´s parent, following the explanation of the study and procedures.

2.2. Sampling and Data Recording. We examined stool samples (n = 83) from children up to 5 years of age who suffered acute community diarrhea, defined as three or more

discharges within 12 hours, or just one liquid or semiliquid stool including mucus, pus, or blood. The children were brought to the attention of health services of small- or medium-sized towns; most of them in Mercedes, Soriano. Children with persistent diarrhea, patients receiving antibiotics, or those who had been hospitalized within 30 days prior to the onset of diarrhea were excluded.

A single stool sample was obtained from each child through spontaneous defecation and was collected in a sterile, wide-mouth plastic container. Part of the sample was transferred with a sterile swab to a tube of semisolid Cary–Blair transport medium (C-B) (HIMEDIA®Laboratories).

Data regarding the symptoms of the disease, macroscopic stool aspect, nutritional and hydration status, therapy administered, and potential infected contacts, were collected for each patient as carefully as possible.

2.3. Microbiological Analysis of Stools. The detection of rotavirus and adenovirus antigens was performed in the Mercedes Hospital Laboratory by the immunochromatographic technique, according to the manufacturers´ instructions (RIDA Quick Norovirus and RIDA Quick Rotavirus/Adenovirus Combi-Biopharm AG, Darmstadt, Germany). Both parts of the sample (with and without C-B transport medium) were immediately sent to the Bacteriology and Virology Department, at the Institute of Hygiene. Identification of enteric pathogens was conducted there as previously described [13, 14].

Following macroscopic observation to identify abnormal components (blood, pus, or mucus), two slide smears were prepared from feces without the transport medium: one stained with methylene blue for detection and gross quantification of fecal leucocytes, and the other one stained with the modified Gram technique (Ziehl's fuchsin diluted 1/10 instead of Safranin as counterstain) to discover spiral forms, suggestive of *Campylobacter.*

Enrichment broths for STEC, *Salmonella, Yersinia,* and selective-differential plate media for isolation of *Salmonella, Shigella, Yersinia enterocolitica, Campylobacter,* and *E. coli* pathotypes were inoculated from both parts of the stool sample (with and without C-B transport medium) to optimize pathogen recovery. Dense feces were diluted in saline solution.

The enrichment broths used were Tetrathionate broth (TT) for *Salmonella,* cefixime-tellurite trypticase Soy Broth (CT-TSB) for STEC, and peptone sorbitol bile broth (PSB) for *Yersinia.* Plating media were MacConkey Lactose and Sorbitol MacConkey (SMAC), mainly employed for the isolation of DEC, *Salmonella-Shigella* agar (SS), and Skirrow selective medium for *Campylobacter. Yersinia enterocolitica* was selected on MacConkey agar or cefsulodin-irgasan-novobiocin (CIN) agar. The commercial sources for most of the culture media were Difco®, Becton-Dickinson, and Oxoid® Ltd., Basingstoke, Hampshire, UK, while Sigma-Aldrich® and bioMérieux®, Marcy l'Etoile, France, provided added chemical or antimicrobial mixes.

One gram or 1 ml stools were inoculated in 10 ml liquid enrichment broths. Subculture from CT-TSB was performed on SMAC before 18 hours incubation, after 24 hours from TT to SS for *Salmonella* and after 21 days incubation at 4°C–8°C on MacConkey or CIN media from PSB. Incubation was kept at 35°C–37°C for most media, at 28°C for *Yersinia*, at 43°C for TT broth, and for Skirrow plates included in microaerophilic environment.

Classical phenotypic tests were employed to identify *Salmonella, Shigella, Yersinia*, and *Campylobacter*. Occasionally, it was necessary to use the API 20E system (bio-Mérieux®, Marcy l'Etoile, France) or Vitek 2 and MicroScan/AutoScan® equipment for completing the identification of isolates.

2.4. Investigation of DEC Pathotypes. Suspected *E. coli* colonies on MacConkey or SMAC plates were studied by PCR screening [14, 16, 18] following a two-step process:

(a) Firstly, gene-specific PCR assays were performed to detect DEC pathotypes (Table 1) in DNA extracted from the confluent growth zone of spread plates and from several 10-colony pools taken from primary or subculture plates. The pools included sorbitol negative, sorbitol positive, and lactose-positive bacteria. Individual colonies were kept at 4°C for further studies.

(b) A confirmation step followed to amplify sequences of DNA extracted from slant cultures obtained from individual colonies of positive pools. This was not always possible, due to loss of viability of some saved colonies.

For DNA extraction, bacterial cultures suspended in Milli-Q® water and heated in boiling water for 5 minutes. After 10 min at 4°C, they were centrifuged at 13,000 rpm for 10 min, and the supernatant containing released DNA was kept at −20°C until use.

Amplifications were performed in reaction volumes of 25 μL containing 0.2 mM dNTPs, 0.2 μM primers (SBS Genetech Co, Ltd), 10 mM Tris-HCl, 2 mM MgCl$_2$, 1.5 U Taq polymerase (HybriPol Bioline, UK), and 2.5 μL crude template DNA. The thermocycler used was a GeneAmp 2700 (Applied Biosystems®, California, US).

Conditions were similar for all reactions, consisting of 94°C initial denaturation for 5 minutes, followed by 30 cycles of 1 min at 94°C followed by different annealing temperatures for 1 min and a further 1 min at 72°C. The final extension period was set at 72°C for 10 min. PCR products were visualized with ethidium bromide staining after electrophoresis in 2% agarose gels in 0.5X TBE buffer.

The first PCR screenings were performed with *stx*1/*stx*2 and *eae* primers focusing on the selection of STEC or EPEC DEC. DNA yielding positive *eae* and negative *stx*1/*stx*2 PCR results was then examined with *bfp* primers to differentiate tEPEC from aEPEC. Negative *eae* and *stx*1/*stx*2 extracts were examined with pCVD432 primers for plasmidic EAEC sequences, *ipa*H primers for detecting genes coding the invasion plasmid antigen of EIEC (and *Shigella)*, and with PCR tests for *eltA* and *estA* genes of ETEC labile and stable enterotoxins.

The primer sequences, annealing temperatures, expected sizes of PCR products, and information sources can be seen in Table 1 [16–22].

Isolates selected as presumptive DEC were biochemically tested to confirm that they belonged to the *E. coli* species. Serotyping and antimicrobial susceptibility assays were performed. Pathotypes were confirmed, and data were added to strains identification.

Serotypes were determined at the Universidad Nacional Autónoma de Mexico, using Ørskov and Ørskov's agglutination assay, 96-well microtiter plates, and rabbit serum (SERUNAM) obtained against 187 somatic antigens and 53 flagellar antigens of *E. coli.*

The disc diffusion method was employed as recommended by Clinical Laboratory Standards Institute (CLSI standards) for determining antimicrobial susceptibility of all confirmed DEC isolates [23]. Employed discs (Oxoid® Ltd., Basingstoke, Hampshire, UK) contained ampicillin, cefradine, cefoxitin, cefuroxime, ceftriaxone, ceftazidime, sulbactam-ampicillin, imipenem, meropenem, ciprofloxacin, trimethoprim-sulfamethoxazole, nalidixic acid, gentamicin, and amikacin. Vitek® or MicroScan® systems were used for confirmation when required.

2.5. Data Analysis. Statistical analysis was performed by Epi-Info 2000 software developed by PAHO (Pan American Health Organization). When comparing relative frequencies, the chi-square test was used for establishing or discarding a link between qualitative variables. Fisher's exact test was used if sample sizes were small. A *p* value <0.05 was regarded as statistically significant.

3. Results

Forty female and 43 male infants (*n* = 83) were studied, aged from 20 days to 5 years; the average age was 10 months.

All children showed an adequate nutritional status and hydration level upon onset of acute diarrhea. Other basic clinical data of the children with diarrhea caused by a single enteropathogen are shown in Table 2. Ongoing diarrhea was watery in 24 children (28.91%), semiliquid in 28 (33.75 %), mucoid in 26 (31.32 %), and blood-stained in five (6.02 %).

Cases occurred throughout the year, with higher frequency in late spring and summer.

3.1. Number and Types of Detected Enteropathogens. One or more potentially pathogenic enteric agents were identified in 30 of the 83 children (36.14%).

There were 33 enteropathogens identified: DEC, 17 (20.48 %); rotavirus, 12 (14.45%); and adenovirus, 4 (4.81%). DEC distribution was as follows: aEPEC (*eae+, bfp-, and stx-*) in 13 children, EIEC (*ipa*H+) in 3, and STEC (*eae+, stx*2+) in one child. Neither ETEC nor EAEC sequences were detected. Three children showed coinfections: aEPEC and rotavirus in two cases and aEPEC and adenovirus in one. Viruses were found as single diarrhea-associated pathogens in 13 children and DEC in 14 cases.

TABLE 1: Primers employed for DEC detection.

Gene	Primer	Sequence 5′-3′	Amplicon Size (bp)	Annealing temperature (°C)	Reference
eae	EAE 1 EAE 2	GAGAATGAAATAGAAGTCGT GCGGTATCTTTCGCGTAATCGCC	775	55	[18]
bfp	EP1 EP2	AATGGTGCTTGCGCTTGCTGC GCCGCTTTATCCAACCTGGTA	324	55	[19]
stx1	VT1-A VT1-B	GAAGAGTCCGTGGGATTACG AGCGATGCAGCTATTAATAA	131	55	[20]
stx2	VT2 a VT2 b	TTAACCACACCCCACCGGGCAGT GCTCTGGATGCATCTCTGGT	348	55	[20]
ipaH	EI1 EI2	GTTCCTTGACCGCCTTTCCGATACCGTC GCCGGTCAGCCACCCTCTGAGAGTAC	620	55	[21]
pCDV 432	EAEC1 EAEC2	CTGGCGAAAGACTGTATCAT CAATGTATAGAAATCCGCTGTT	630	60	[16]
eltA	LT-A-1 LT-A-2	GGCGACAGATTATACCGTGC CCGAATTCTGTTATATATGTC	332	55	[16]
estA	STA-1 STA-2	ATTTTTATTTCTGTATTGTCTTT GGATTACAACACAGTTCACAGCAG	147	48	[16]

TABLE 2: Clinical findings as related to etiology of diarrhea.

	Children with single identified pathogen[1] ($n = 27$)				Children without identified pathogen[1] ($n = 53$)
	aEPEC ($n = 10$)	EIEC ($n = 3$)	STEC ($n = 1$)	Virus[2] ($n = 13$)	
Children with					
Watery diarrhea	6 (60%)	—	—	10 (76, 9%)	7 (13.2%)
Semiliquid diarrhea	—	—	—	—	28 (52.8%)
Bloody diarrhea	3 (30%)	1 (33.3%)	1 (100%)		—
Mucoid stools	1 (10%)	2 (66.6%)	—	3 (23.1%)	18 (34%)
Abdominal pain	4 (40%)	2 (66.6%)	1 (100%)	6 (46.2%)	6 (11.3%)
Fever	2 (20%)	2 (66.6%)	1 (100%)	5 (35.5%)	5 (9.4%)
Vomiting	1 (10%)	—	—	6 (46.2%)	7 (13.2%)
Fecal leucocytes[3]	1 (10%)	2 (66.6%)	—	—	—

[1]No child was vaccinated against rotavirus at the time of entering to the study; [2]considering together: rotavirus in 10 children and adenovirus in 3; [3]significant presence of fecal leucocytes (++ or +++). —, no child showed those conditions.

Individual colonies were available for further studies in 13 of the 17 samples in which PCR yielded positive results for DEC. This could not be done with the 4 other DEC suspected plates. Table 3 shows the pathotypes and serotypes of recovered DEC isolates.

Recovered EIEC isolates ($n = 2$) were lactose and lysine-decarboxylase positive, motile, and indol negative. API 20E identification code was the same for both (5104572).

No *Salmonella, Yersinia enterocolitica, Shigella,* or *Campylobacter* isolates were recovered. Significant presence of fecal leucocytes (++ or +++) was only observed in smears from 3 children: 2 with presumptive EIEC and one with confirmed aEPEC. Microscopic examination did not show any spiral bacteria suggestive of *Campylobacter.*

Clinical presentation of cases as related to etiology is shown in Table 2. Diarrhea was more frequently liquid in children from which a pathogen could be identified (16/27 = 59.3% vs 7/53 = 13.2%). Bloody diarrhea was significantly associated with aEPEC etiology: 3 out of 5 children with bloody feces (4, 16, and 35 months old) were aEPEC positive, as compared with 10 of 78 with nonbloody diarrhea ($p < 0.05$). In those 3 cases, there was no virus coinfection.

TABLE 3: Pathotypes and serotypes of recovered DEC isolates in Soriano, Uruguay.

Sample	Serotype	Pathotype	Lactose utilization	Resistant to*
V4[1]	O166:H21	aEPEC	+	A
V20[1]	O137:H6	aEPEC	+	—
V23	O165:H8	aEPEC	+	—
V30	O184:H8	aEPEC	+	A, SAM, CE
V49	O118:H5	aEPEC	+	—
V54	O63: HNT[2]	aEPEC	+	CE
V56	O184:H4	aEPEC	+	A, CE, SxT
V61[1]	ONT:H−[3]	aEPEC	+	A, SxT
V66	O127:H−	aEPEC	+	CE
V74	ONT:H8[3]	aEPEC	+	CE
V18[1]	O145:H−	STEC	+	A
V48	O96:H19	EIEC	+	—
V73[1]	O96:H19	EIEC	+	—

*A, ampicillin; CE, cefradine; SAM, sulbactam-ampicillin; SxT, trimethoprim-sulfamethoxazole; —, no resistance traits. [1]Isolates recovered from children with bloody diarrhea. [2]HNT, H-nontypable; [3]ONT, O-nontypable.

Rotavirus-infected children presented with vomiting more frequently (46.2%) than aEPEC-positive patients (10%), as shown in Table 2. This difference was not significant ($p > 0.05$). Regarding rotavirus vaccine status, none of the children had been vaccinated at the time of entering the study.

3.2. Antimicrobial Susceptibility. Most aEPEC studied strains showed some antibiotic resistance, with ampicillin, cefradine, sulbactam-ampicillin, and trimethoprim-sulfamethoxazole resistance being detected, as shown in Table 3. Two strains were resistant to three mentioned compounds, and 1 to two of them. Both EIEC strains and the single STEC isolate were susceptible to all assayed antimicrobials.

4. Discussion

The main observation in this study was that DEC, and especially aEPEC, were the most frequent pathogens found in this group of children, who lived in small towns of southern Uruguay. Rotaviruses were also frequently detected.

All recovered EPEC isolates were classified as atypical, due to the lack of *bfp* plasmidic genes as revealed by negative PCR results [24]. Atypical EPEC had been thought to be less virulent than tEPEC strains; however, it has not been proven that they are less pathogenic. In addition to virulence factors coded in LEE, intimin, Esp (*E. coli* secreted proteins), Tir (translocated intimin receptor), and T3SS (type 3 secretion system), they can express EAST1 (enteroaggregative heat stable toxin 1), E-hly (EHEC-enterohemolysin), Afa (afimbrial adhesin), and many others. Variants of intimin and other components are usually different between tEPEC and aEPEC subtypes, as are O and H antigens defining serotypes. aEPEC is a heterogeneous group of strains with diverse virulence profiles that may have acquired LEE through horizontal transfer or may have come from tEPEC that have lost the EAF plasmid [25–27]. Some strains seem to show more genetic similarity with STEC cell lines than with tEPEC. An aEPEC strain can be a STEC bacterium that has lost phages that code Shiga toxins. STEC and aEPEC have other antigenic and virulence traits in common, for which their relationships deserve attention and analysis in terms of molecular epidemiology. However, clinical isolates of aEPEC from patients in Australia and New Zealand [26] did not seem to derive from STEC or from tEPEC, and their study suggested that type I fimbriae or other adherence structures that are similar in function to bfp may contribute to their virulence.

Fecal leucocytes are seldom found in EPEC infections. However, more sensitive approaches may disclose intestinal inflammatory features or blood contents in diarrheal episodes associated with EPEC [28, 29]. In our study, a significant association was seen between aEPEC infection and bloody diarrhea; aEPEC were present in feces of 3 out of 5 children with bloody diarrhea, a clinical presentation causing concern for parents and health workers. Two of those three strains could be serotyped: O137 : H6, which was reported as an aEPEC isolate from children's feces in Denmark some years ago [30] and O166 : H21 serotype that

was previously isolated by other workers as a STEC pathotype strain [31]. Our O166 : H21 isolate was obtained from a child who underwent surgery due to intestinal intussusception, a condition not easily distinguishable from HUS. This is noteworthy because STEC bacteria can lose phages-coding Shiga toxins even during laboratory subcultures and are defined as EHEC-LST [32, 33]. Complete sequencing of these and other aEPEC isolates recovered from children with bloody diarrhea may eventually disclose their genetic relation with STEC strains.

Atypical EPEC have been recovered from children's diarrhea in countries and population groups of middle to high socioeconomic level [34, 35]. Typical EPEC strains are still prevalent in poor regions of sub-Saharan Africa [36], but in other developing areas, aEPEC predominates as seen in developed countries [37]. In America, tEPEC (as defined through classic serogroup determination) was prevalent some decades ago, mainly in developing regions [13, 15, 38]. More recent surveillance work has revealed that aEPEC are more frequent than tEPEC in high-income and also in low income populations and regions [39–45].

In Uruguay, tEPEC and aEPEC still cocirculated 15 years ago among poor children [16], but aEPEC are prevalent in recent years both in children of high and low socioeconomic groups, as shown in this study and in another study performed using identical methods, that included children from high-income households [14].

It is important to highlight the great diversity of serotypes identified in this study that are also different from those found in the aforementioned local studies, and from aEPEC serotypes reported in other countries or regions [42, 46, 47]. However, most of the isolated serotypes and serogroups in this study have been reported as aEPEC or STEC present in animals or food of animal origin that are potential sources of human infection, except those from the O184 serogroup, that may represent a novel finding of diarrhea-associated *E. coli* bacteria that deserves further analysis [30, 31].

Atypical EPEC can have an animal reservoir, are adapted to human and animal hosts, and require particular attention, as well as STEC, when food-borne infection is suspected [24, 30, 48, 49].

Only one O145 STEC strain was identified. STEC isolates are not common in Uruguayan children, even in bloody diarrheal disease [50]. They seem to occur more frequently in children from high or middle-high socioeconomic groups and in small towns outside Montevideo [7, 14, 17, 51, 52]. Non-O157 STEC (O26, O145, and others) are the STEC groups usually found in our children, despite the geographical closeness with Argentina, where the O157 : H7 serotype is prevalent [53]. However, O157 : H7 has been found in Uruguay in a single case of HUS [17], in urinary tract infections of two older patients who did not develop HUS [51] and in multiple food samples [54].

It should be noted that an O96 : H19 EIEC serotype was isolated from two cases without an obvious epidemiological link; this serotype is described as being particularly virulent [55]. Our isolates seemed to be identical, but they require further molecular analysis and comparison with previous regional isolates and with European strains [55–58].

ETEC or EAEC pathotype strains were not found in this group of patients, although they were usually recognized in previous groups of children from Montevideo [13, 14, 16]. In general, ETEC strains are recovered from children who are hospitalized with acute diarrhea and severe dehydration and live in areas with a significant lack of basic services [59]. It does not seem to be the case in our current study. With regard to EAEC, we cannot rule out the participation of atypical strains that do not carry the high molecular weight plasmid (pCVD432). To establish the true role of EAEC strains in diarrheal episodes, we should have performed a screening using the HEp-2 adherence assay or a multiplex PCR targeting plasmid and chromosomal genes. To date, all our EAEC recognized isolates using pCVD432 PCR screening were lysine-decarboxylase positive, which raises doubts about their capacity to cause diarrhea [14, 60].

Antimicrobial treatment is not generally recommended for treatment of diarrheal diseases, with few exceptions. Susceptibility of enteric bacteria should be monitored because resistant genes selected in enteric pathogens or the microbiota can remain undisclosed and be transferred to highly pathogenic microorganisms.

Resistance to the antimicrobial agents was scarce in the DEC isolated in our study, as compared with that observed in previous studies focused on poor children in Montevideo [13]. This fact may result from a general tendency of enteric bacteria in Uruguay towards susceptibility or may simply confirm that the resistance level of bacterial pathogens recovered from towns in the interior of the country is usually lower than that found in the Capital city, where antimicrobial treatment is more widely available and prescribed, contributing to the selection of resistant variants.

Rotavirus infection was observed to be more frequent (14.45%) in the group of children reported here than in another previously studied group (5%) for which vaccination was available [14]. However, groups of children were also different in terms of social parameters and location. Rotavirus vaccine is effective [61] and has been employed in some health services in Uruguay, following WHO recommendation.

The overall proportion of positive etiologic diagnosis was lower (36.14%) in this study than that obtained in a recent similar study (51%) [14], and a limited variety of pathogens was identified. Despite using identical microbiological methods in both studies, delay or difficulties in the sample transport, differences between studied populations, influence of non-declared previous antibiotic treatment, or other factors may provide additional support to explain a reduced frequency in etiologic diagnosis. However, if appropriate resources and laboratory conditions had been available, investigation of norovirus, usage of CIN for all *Yersinia* cultures, added primers for EAEC PCR, or molecular methods directly applied to feces could have identified a higher proportion and diversity of involved pathogens [11, 62].

5. Conclusions

DEC and especially aEPEC are frequently associated with childhood diarrhea in Uruguay.

Atypical EPEC is a presently prevalent pathotype that includes strains closely related to STEC cell lines. Comparative characterization of these bacteria and their molecular relationship or evolution must be performed to provide additional information and data to help support prevention and control.

Animal reservoirs of aEPEC deserve particular attention and further research, considering the close relationship of suburban and rural population with production animals, and taking into account that production and export of food is frequently animal in origin is the main economic activity and income source for Uruguay.

Rotavirus infection is frequent in children throughout the country. Vaccination against this pathogen is an effective health measure that should be extended to all children.

Acknowledgments

Thanks to Delia Licona, Luis Antonio León, and Gabriel Pérez (Medicine Faculty, UNAM) for their technical assistance in the laboratory. Thanks to CSIC (Scientific Research Committee of Universidad de la República, Uruguay) for funding through the Research Groups support program.

References

[1] C. L. Fischer Walker, J. Perin, M. J. Aryee, C. Boschi-Pinto, and R. E. Black, "Diarrhea incidence in low and middle-income countries in 1990 and 2010: a systematic review," *BMC Public Health*, vol. 12, no. 1, p. 220, 2012.

[2] J. Liu, J. A. Platts-Mills, J. Juma et al., "Use of quantitative molecular diagnostic methods to identify causes of diarrhoea in children: a reanalysis of the GEMS case-control study," *The Lancet*, vol. 388, no. 10051, pp. 1291–1301, 2016.

[3] World Health Organization, *Diarrhoeal Disease Fact Sheet 2013*, World Health Organization, Geneva, Switzerland, 2013.

[4] K. L. Kotloff, J. P. Nataro, W. C. Blackwelder et al., "Burden and aetiology of diarrhoeal disease in infants and young children in developing countries (the global enteric multi-center study, GEMS): a prospective, case-control study," *The Lancet*, vol. 382, no. 9888, pp. 209–222, 2013.

[5] N. Bulled, M. Singer, and R. Dillinghama, "The syndemics of childhood diarrhoea: a biosocial perspective on efforts to combat global inequities in diarrhoea-related morbidity and mortality," *Global Public Health*, vol. 9, no. 7, pp. 841–853, 2014.

[6] F. Ngabo, M. Mvundura, L. Gazley et al., "The economic burden attributable to a child's inpatient admission for diarrheal disease in Rwanda," *PLoS One*, vol. 11, no. 2, Article ID e0149805, 2016.

[7] L. Pérez, L. Apezteguía, C. Piñeyrúa et al., "Hemolytic uremic syndrome with mild renal involvement due to Shiga toxin-

producing *Escherichia coli* (STEC) O145 strain," *Revista Argentina de Microbiología*, vol. 46, no. 2, pp. 103–106, 2014.

[8] L. Pardo, M. I. Mota, G. Giachetto, M. Parada, C. Pírez, and G. Varela, "Adenitis mesentérica por *Yersinia enterocolitica*," *Revista Médica del Uruguay*, vol. 23, pp. 265–268, 2007.

[9] R. M. Humphries and A. J. Linscott, "Laboratory diagnosis of bacterial gastroenteritis," *Clinical Microbiology Reviews*, vol. 28, no. 1, pp. 3–31, 2015.

[10] M. L. Cooke, "Causes and management of diarrhoea in children in a clinical setting," *South African Journal of Clinical Nutrition*, vol. 23, no. 1, pp. S42–S46, 2010.

[11] E. Miliwebsky, F. Schelotto, G. Varela, D. Luz, I. Chinen, and R. M. F. Piazza, "Human diarrheal infections: diagnosis of diarrheagenic *Escherichia coli* pathotypes. Chapter 15," in *Escherichia coli in the Americas*, A. G. Torres, Ed., pp. 343–369, Springer, Switzerland, 2016.

[12] M. A. Croxen, R. J. Law, R. Scholz, K. M. Keeney, M. Wlodarska, and B. B. Finlay, "Recent advances in understanding enteric pathogenic *Escherichia coli*," *Clinical Microbiology Reviews*, vol. 26, no. 4, pp. 822–880, 2013.

[13] M. E. Torres, M. C. Pírez, F. Schelotto et al., "Etiology of children's diarrhea in Montevideo, Uruguay: associated pathogens and unusual isolates," *Journal of Clinical Microbiology*, vol. 39, no. 6, pp. 2134–2139, 2001.

[14] G. Varela, L. Batthyány, M. N. Bianco et al., "Enteropathogens associated with community-acquired acute diarrhea in children from households with high socio-economic level," *International Journal of Microbiology*, vol. 2015, Article ID 592953, 8 pages, 2015.

[15] F. Alvarez, C. E. Hormaeche, R. Demarco, C. Alía, and F Schelotto, "Consideraciones clínico-bacteriológicas de diarrea aguda de lactantes hospitalizados. (Clinical-Bacteriological considerations about acute diarrhea of hospitalized infants)," *Archivos de Pediatría del Uruguay*, vol. 45, pp. 210–221, 1974.

[16] G. Varela, C. Jazisnky, P. Gadea et al., "Classic Enteropathogenic *Escherichia coli* (EPEC) associated with diarrhea in children users of the Hospital Pereira Rossell. Clinical aspects and characteristics of involved strains," *Revista Medica del Uruguay*, vol. 23, pp. 153–163, 2007.

[17] M. Gadea, G. Varela, M. Bernadá et al., "Primer aislamiento en Uruguay de *Escherichia coli* productora de toxina Shiga del serotipo O157:H7 en una niña con síndrome urémico hemolítico. (First uruguayan isolate of O157:H7 STEC from a girl undergoing HUS)," *Revista Medica del Uruguay*, vol. 20, pp. 79–81, 2004.

[18] M. Rivas, I. Chinen, G. Leotta, and G. Chillemi, "Manual de Procedimientos. Diagnóstico y caracterización de *Escherichia coli* productor de toxina Shiga O157 y no-O157 a partir de especímenes clínicos. (Diagnostic procedures for investigation of STEC from clinical samples)," *OPS-Pan American Health Organization. Servicio Fisiopatogenia, Depto. de Bacteriologia INEI- ANLIS "Carlos G. Malbrán" Argentina*, no. 1, pp. 14-15, 2011.

[19] S. T. Gunzburg, N. G. Tornieporth, and L. W. Riley, "Identification of enteropathogenic *Escherichia coli* by PCR-based detection of the bundle-forming pilus gene," *J Clin Microbiol*, vol. 33, pp. 1375–1377, 1995.

[20] D. R. Pollard, W. M. Johnson, H. Lior, S. D. Tyler, and K. R. Rozee, "Rapid and specific detection of verotoxin genes in *Escherichia coli* by the polymerase chain reaction," *Journal of Clinical Microbiology*, vol. 28, no. 3, pp. 540–545, 1990.

[21] O. Sethabutr, M. Venkatesan, G. S. Murphy, B. Eampokalap, C. W. Hoge, and P. Echeverria, "Detection of Shigellae and enteroinvasive *Escherichia coli* by amplification of the invasion plasmid antigen H DNA sequence in patients with dysentery," *Journal of Infectious Diseases*, vol. 167, no. 2, pp. 458–461, 1993.

[22] M. Blanco, J. E. Blanco, A. Mora et al., "Serotypes, virulence genes, and intimin types of Shiga toxin (verotoxin)-producing *Escherichia coli* isolates from healthy sheep in Spain," *Journal of Clinical Microbiology*, vol. 41, no. 4, pp. 1351–1356, 2003.

[23] Clinical and Laboratory Standards Institute, *Performance Standards for Antimicrobial Susceptibility Testing: 21th Informational Supplement M100-S21*, CLSI, Wayne, Pa, USA, 2011.

[24] L. R. Trabulsi, R. Keller, and T. A. Tardelli-Gomes, "Typical and atypical enteropathogenic *Escherichia coli*," *Emerging Infectious Diseases*, vol. 8, no. 5, pp. 508–513, 2002.

[25] J. E. Afset, E. Anderssen, G. Bruant, J. Harel, L. Wieler, and K. Bergh, "Phylogenetic backgrounds and virulence profiles of atypical enteropathogenic *Escherichia coli* strains from a case-control study using multilocus sequence typing and DNA microarray analysis," *Journal of Clinical Microbiology*, vol. 46, no. 7, pp. 2280–2290, 2008.

[26] S. M. Tennant, M. Tauschek, K. Azzopardi et al., "Characterization of atypical enteropathogenic *E. coli* strains of clinical origin," *BMC Microbiology*, vol. 9, no. 1, pp. 117–121, 2009.

[27] V. Bueris, J. Huerta-Cantillo, F. Navarro-Garcia, R. M. Ruiz, A. M. Cianciarullo, and W. P. Elias, "Late establishment of the attaching and effacing lesion caused by atypical enteropathogenic *Escherichia coli* depends on protein expression regulated by Per," *Infect Immun*, vol. 83, no. 1, pp. 379–388, 2015.

[28] V. C. Pacheco, D. Yamamoto, C. M. Abe et al., "Invasion of differentiated intestinal Caco-2 cells is a sporadic property among atypical enteropathogenic *Escherichia coli* strains carrying common intimin subtypes," *Pathogens and Disease*, vol. 70, no. 2, pp. 167–175, 2014.

[29] J. Hu and A. G. Torres, "Enteropathogenic *Escherichia coli*: foe or innocent bystander?," *Clinical Microbiology and Infection*, vol. 21, no. 8, pp. 729–734, 2015.

[30] C. Jensen, S. Ethelberg, B. Olesen et al., "Attaching and effacing *Escherichia coli* isolates from Danish children: clinical significance and microbiological characteristics," *Clinical Microbiology and Infection*, vol. 13, no. 9, pp. 863–872, 2007.

[31] C. García-Aljaro, M. Muniesa, J. E. Blanco et al., "Characterization of Shiga toxin-producing *Escherichia coli* isolated from aquatic environments," *FEMS Microbiology Letters*, vol. 246, no. 1, pp. 55–65, 2005.

[32] M. Bielaszewska, R. Köck, A. W. Friedrich et al., "Shiga toxin-mediated hemolytic uremic syndrome: time to change the diagnostic paradigm?," *PLoS One*, vol. 2, no. 10, Article ID e1024, 2007.

[33] M. Bielaszewska, B. Middendorf, R. Köck et al., "Shiga toxin-negative attaching and effacing *Escherichia coli*: distinct clinical associations with bacterial phylogeny and virulence traits and inferred in-host pathogen evolution," *Clinical Infectious Diseases*, vol. 47, no. 2, pp. 208–217, 2008.

[34] S. Scotland, H. Smith, T. Cheasty et al., "Use of gene probes and adhesion test to caracterize *Escherichia coli* belonging to enteropathogenic serogroups isolated in United Kingdom," *Journal of Medical Microbiology*, vol. 44, no. 6, pp. 438–443, 1996.

[35] J. Tobias, E. Kassem, U. Rubinstein et al., "Involvement of main diarrheagenic *Escherichia coli*, with emphasis on enteroaggregative *E. coli*, in severe non-epidemic pediatric

diarrhea in a high-income country," *BMC Infectious Diseases*, vol. 15, no. 1, p. 79, 2015.

[36] J. Sumbana, E. Taviani, A. Manjate, B. Paglietti, A. Santona, and M. M. Colombo, "Genetic determinants of pathogenicity of *Escherichia coli* isolated from children with acute diarrhea in Maputo, Mozambique," *Journal of Infection in Developing Countries*, vol. 9, no. 6, pp. 661–664, 2015.

[37] T. V. Nguyen, P. Le Van, C. Huy, K. Nguyen Gia, and A. Weintraub, "Detection and characterization of diarrheagenic *Escherichia coli* from young children in Hanoi, Vietnam," *Journal of Clinical Microbiology*, vol. 43, no. 2, pp. 755–760, 2005.

[38] M. R. Toledo, M. C. Alvariza, J. Murahovschi, S. R. Ramos, and L. R. Trabulsi, "Enteropathogenic *Escherichia coli* serotypes and endemic diarrhea in infants," *Infection and Immunity*, vol. 39, no. 2, pp. 586–589, 1983.

[39] F. E. A. Assis, S. Wolf, M. Surek et al., "Impact of *Aeromonas* and diarrheagenic *Escherichia coli* screening in patients with diarrhea in Paraná, southern Brazil," *Journal of Infection in Developing Countries*, vol. 8, no. 12, pp. 1609–1614, 2014.

[40] V. Bueris, M. Palma Sircili, C. Romano Taddei et al., "Detection of diarrheagenic *Escherichia coli* from children with and without diarrhea in salvador, Bahia, Brazil," *Memórias do Instituto Oswaldo Cruz*, vol. 102, no. 7, pp. 839–844, 2007.

[41] S. N. Buss, A. Leber, K. Chapin et al., "Multicenter evaluation of the BioFire FilmArray gastrointestinal panel for etiologic diagnosis of infectious gastroenteritis," *Journal of Clinical Microbiology*, vol. 53, no. 3, pp. 915–925, 2015.

[42] M. A. Foster, J. Iqbal, C. Zhang et al., "Enteropathogenic and enteroaggregative *E. coli* in stools of children with acute gastroenteritis in Davidson County, Tennessee," *Diagnostic Microbiology and Infectious Disease*, vol. 83, no. 3, pp. 319–324, 2015.

[43] O. G. Gómez-Duarte, O. Arzuza, D. Urbina et al., "Detection of *Escherichia coli* enteropathogens by multiplex polymerase chain reaction from children's diarrheal stools in two caribbean–colombian cities," *Foodborne Pathogens and Disease*, vol. 7, no. 2, pp. 199–206, 2010.

[44] D. M. Lozer, T. B. Souza, M. V. Monfardini et al., "Genotypic and phenotypic analysis of diarrheagenic *Escherichia coli* strains isolated from Brazilian children living in low socioeconomic level communities," *BMC Infectious Diseases*, vol. 13, no. 1, p. 418, 2013.

[45] T. J. Ochoa and C. A. Contreras, "Enteropathogenic *Escherichia coli* infection in children," *Current Opinion in Infectious Diseases*, vol. 24, no. 5, pp. 478–483, 2011.

[46] M. A. Vieira, T. A. T. Gomes, C. H. Camargo et al., "Atypical enteropathogenic *Escherichia coli* as etiologic agents of sporadic and outbreak-associated diarrhea in Brazil," *Journal of Medical Microbiology*, vol. 65, no. 9, pp. 998–1006, 2016.

[47] R. M. Robins-Browne, A. M. Bordun, M. Tauschek et al., "*Escherichia coli* and community-acquired gastroenteritis, Melbourne, Australia," *Emerging Infectious Diseases*, vol. 10, no. 10, pp. 1797–1805, 2004.

[48] F. H. Martins, B. E. C. Guth, R. M. F. Piazza et al., "Lambs are an important source of atypical enteropathogenic *Escherichia coli* in southern Brazil," *Veterinary Microbiology*, vol. 196, pp. 72–77, 2016.

[49] R. Comery, A. Thanabalasuriar, P. Garneau et al., "Identification of potentially diarrheagenic atypical enteropathogenic *Escherichia coli* strains present in Canadian food animals at slaughter and in retail meats," *Applied and Environmental Microbiology*, vol. 79, no. 12, pp. 3892–3896, 2013.

[50] M. I. Mota, M. P. Gadea, S. González et al., "Bacterial pathogens associated with bloody diarrhea in Uruguayan children," *Revista Argentina de microbiología*, vol. 42, no. 2, pp. 114–117, 2010.

[51] M. P. Gadea, N. Deza, M. I. Mota et al., "Two cases of urinary tract infection caused by Shiga toxin-producing *Escherichia coli* O157:H7 strains," *Revista Argentina de microbiología*, vol. 44, no. 2, pp. 94–96, 2012.

[52] G. Varela and F. Schelotto, "Síndrome Urémico hemolítico en Uruguay. Aspectos microbiológicos y clínicos, aportes para su conocimiento regional. (Haemolytic-Uremic-Syndrome in Uruguay. Microbiological and clinical aspects; contribution to its regional knowledge)," *Revista Facultad de Ciencias de la Salud UDES*, vol. 2, no. 1, pp. 25–30, 2015.

[53] L. Pianciola, B. A. D'Astek, M. Mazzeo, I. Chinen, M. Masana, and M. Rivas, "Genetic features of human and bovine *Escherichia coli* O157:H7 strains isolated in Argentina," *International Journal of Medical Microbiology*, vol. 306, no. 2, pp. 123–130, 2016.

[54] G. Varela, Chinen, P. Gadea et al., "Detection and characterization of Shiga toxin-producing *Escherichia coli* from clinical cases and food in Uruguay," *Revista Argentina de microbiología*, vol. 40, no. 2, pp. 93–100, 2008.

[55] M. Escher, G. Scavia, S. Morabito et al., "A severe foodborne outbreak of diarrhoea linked to a canteen in Italy caused by enteroinvasive *Escherichia coli*, an uncommon agent," *Epidemiology and Infection*, vol. 142, no. 12, pp. 2559–2566, 2014.

[56] S. Newitt, V. MacGregor, V. Robbins et al., "Two linked enteroinvasive *Escherichia coli* outbreaks, Nottingham, UK, june 2014," *Emerging Infectious Diseases*, vol. 22, no. 7, pp. 1178–1184, 2016.

[57] M. R. Toledo and L. R. Trabulsi, "Correlation between biochemical and serological characteristics of *Escherichia coli* and results of the Sérény test," *Journal of Clinical Microbiology*, vol. 17, no. 3, pp. 419–421, 1983.

[58] I. Chinen, M. Rivas, M. I. Caffer, R. O. Cinto, and N. Binsztein, "Diagnosis of Entero-Invasive *Escherichia coli* associated with diarrhea," *Revista Argentina de microbiología*, vol. 25, no. 1, pp. 27–35, 1993.

[59] T. J. Ochoa, E. H. Mercado, D. Durand et al., "Frequency and pathotypes of diarrheagenic *Escherichia coli* in Peruvian children with and without diarrhea," *Revista Peruana de Medicina Experimental y Salud Pública*, vol. 28, no. 1, pp. 13–20, 2011.

[60] A. Weintraub, "Enteroaggregative *Escherichia coli*: epidemiology, virulence and detection," *Journal of Medical Microbiology*, vol. 56, no. 1, pp. 4–8, 2007.

[61] WHO, "Rotavirus vaccines. WHO position paper—January (2013)," *Weekly Epidemiological Record No. 5*, vol. 88, no. 5, pp. 49–64, 2013.

[62] Å. Sjölinga, L. Sadeghipoorjahromi, D. Novak, and J. Tobias, "Detection of major diarrheagenic bacterial pathogens by multiplex PCR panels," *Microbiological Research*, vol. 172, pp. 34–40, 2015.

"Ticking Bomb": The Impact of Climate Change on the Incidence of Lyme Disease

Igor Dumic (ID)[1,2] **and Edson Severnini** (ID)[3]

[1]*Mayo Clinic College of Medicine and Science, Rochester, MN, USA*
[2]*Division of Hospital Medicine, Mayo Clinic Health System, Eau Claire, WI, USA*
[3]*Carnegie Mellon University, Heinz College, 4800 Forbes Ave., Pittsburgh, PA, USA*

Correspondence should be addressed to Igor Dumic; dumic.igor@mayo.edu

Academic Editor: Paola Di Carlo

Lyme disease (LD) is the most common tick-borne disease in North America. It is caused by *Borrelia burgdorferi* and transmitted to humans by blacklegged ticks, *Ixodes scapularis*. The life cycle of the LD vector, *I. scapularis*, usually takes two to three years to complete and goes through three stages, all of which are dependent on environmental factors. Increases in daily average temperatures, a manifestation of climate change, might have contributed to an increase in tick abundance via higher rates of tick survival. Additionally, these environmental changes might have contributed to better host availability, which is necessary for tick feeding and life cycle completion. In fact, it has been shown that both tick activity and survival depend on temperature and humidity. In this study, we have examined the relationship between those climatic variables and the reported incidence of LD in 15 states that contribute to more than 95% of reported cases within the Unites States. Using fixed effects analysis for a panel of 468 U.S. counties from those high-incidence states with annual data available for the period 2000–2016, we have found sizable impacts of temperature on the incidence of LD. Those impacts can be described approximately by an inverted U-shaped relationship, consistent with patterns of tick survival and host-seeking behavior. Assuming a 2°C increase in annual average temperature—in line with mid-century (2036–2065) projections from the latest U.S. National Climate Assessment (NCA4)—we have predicted that the number of LD cases in the United States will increase by over 20 percent in the coming decades. These findings may help improving preparedness and response by clinicians, public health professionals, and policy makers, as well as raising public awareness of the importance of being cautious when engaging in outdoor activities.

1. Introduction

Lyme disease (LD) is the most common reportable vector-borne zoonosis in the United States, and its incidence has sharply increased over the last decade. The causative pathogen, spirochete *B. burgdorferi*, is transmitted to humans by a tick vector. The main vector of LD is *I. scapularis* in the northeastern and midwestern Unites States, and *Ixodes pacificus* in the Pacific Northwest [1].

The first evidence of Lyme disease dates back to 1883, when a German physician described acrodermatitis chronica atrophycans, which was later recognized as the late dermatological manifestation of LD [2, 3]. Later on, other seemingly unassociated manifestations were reported such as erythema chronicum migrans in 1913 by Lipschutz [4]. In 1930 Hellstrom associated neurological symptoms with dermatologic manifestations of the disease [5]. Nevertheless, it was not until 1976, when an outbreak of juvenile arthritis and skin rash occurred in Connecticut's city of Lyme, that LD was described [6]. Several years after, in 1982, the American entomologist Willy Burgdorfer described the causative agent of LD, a spirochete, named after him *B. burgdorferi* [7].

If not treated, LD progresses through three stages. The first stage—early localized disease—manifests by erythema migrans, which is an erythematous macule or papule that occurs one to two weeks following the tick bite and subsequently enlarges [1]. This rash can be uniformly erythematous or might have central clearing ("bull's eye") with a median diameter around 15 cm [8]. Left untreated, *B. burgdorferi* disseminates from the site of the bite, and the disease progresses to the early disseminated stage. In this stage, which occurs three to five weeks following the initial bite, multiple (secondary) erythema migrans occur. These lesions tend to be similar to the primary erythema migrans but are usually smaller [8]. Cardiac and neurologic manifestations are also seen in the early disseminated stage, with atrioventricular heart block being the most common cardiac manifestation. Peripheral nerve palsy (particularly facial nerve) and meningitis are the most common neurological manifestations of this stage of LD. In the United States, the most common manifestation of the late disseminated stage of LD is Lyme arthritis [1, 8]. Lyme arthritis is usually mono or oligoarticular, affects large joints (knee, most commonly), and occurs weeks to months after the bite. Unlike in Europe, neurological manifestations of late LD are rare in the United States [8].

The major reservoirs for *B. burgdorferi* are birds and small mammals such as mice and chipmunks [1, 9]. While deer are not competent hosts for *B. burgdorferi*, they are essential for the *I. scapularis* life cycle. The tick *I. scapularis* has three stages of development: larva, nymph, and adult tick [1]. In North America, the life cycle of *I. scapularis* takes approximately two years to complete [9]. Egg laying usually begins in May; hence, larvae are the most abundant during the summer. These larvae feed on small mammals such as the white footed mouse during summer, at which point transmission of *B. burgdorferi* occurs. As the winter approaches, the tick larvae enter a dormant stage in which they stay throughout the winter. In the beginning of the spring of the second year, the larvae that survived the winter mold into the next stage of tick development—nymph. During the spring/summer of the second year those nymphs seek suitable hosts for feeding, including humans. Following a bloody meal, the nymphs mold into adults. If an adult tick survives the winter, it will seek another host (usually a large mammal such as deer) on which it will feed and be able to lay eggs. At that point the two year life cycle is completed [8, 9].

Nymphs are usually responsible for the majority of the infection transmission to humans. They are abundant during the spring and summer months when humans' outdoor activities are at the peak. Their small size (only few millimeters in diameter unlike common dog ticks) and the secretion of bradykininases (enzymes that break bradykinins—enzymes of inflammation) contribute to the fact that the majority of patients do not remember the tick bite [8, 10]. The risk of infection transmission from the infected tick depends on the duration of feeding. The ticks are most likely to transmit infection after a prolonged period of feeding, such as 36 hours or more. Yet, infection can be transmitted even after as little as 24 hours of feeding [10].

There is a growing body of evidence showing that climate change may affect the incidence and prevalence of certain vector-borne diseases such as malaria, dengue, West Nile fever, and LD. Unlike weather, which defines a condition of the atmosphere over a short period of time, climate represents atmospheric "behavior" over a relatively long period

of time [11]. Climate change, therefore, refers to changes in long-term averages of daily weather including temperature, humidity, air pressure, and precipitation. The incidence of tick-born zoonoses such as LD is particularly likely to be affected by climate change because ticks spend the majority of their life cycle outside the host in an environment where temperature and humidity directly affect their development, activity, survival, and host-seeking behavior [12]. The number of annually reported cases of LD in the United States has sharply increased over the last three decades, from about 10,000 in 1991 to about 28,000 annually in recent years [13]. Not only did the incidence of the disease increase, but also its geographical distribution. While climate change might significantly contribute to the emergence of new infections, it is interesting to contrast this change in the incidence of tick-borne diseases in the United States with the changes happening in Europe. There, during the 9 years prior to 2015, the growth of the cases of louse-born relapsing fever (due to *B. recurrentis*) has been associated to the increase in refugees [14–16]. Furthermore, in the last few decades, newly recognized tick-borne rickettsioses have been shown to be present. *R. conorii* sub sp. *Israelensis* has been detected in human cases in Sicily and Sardinia in Italy and in different regions of Portugal [17].

This emergence of Lyme disease in the United States is at least partially attributed to climate change [12]. However, the magnitude of impact is still unclear. In this study, we investigate the effect of climatic variables on the incidence of LD in 15 U.S. states with the highest incidence of the disease. Those states contribute to 95 percent of reported cases.

2. Materials and Methods

We merged two types of data to conduct the fixed effects analysis in this study: annual county-level epidemiological data on LD cases from the Centers for Disease Control and Prevention (CDC) and meteorological data from the National Oceanic and Atmospheric Administration (NOAA). Both databases are publicly available.

2.1. Epidemiological Data. LD cases have been voluntarily reported to the CDC since 1991 by state and territorial health departments as part of the National Notifiable Disease Surveillance System (NNDSS). The annual county-level number of cases for the period 2000–2016 is publicly available at http://.cdc.gov/lyme/stats/ and is the main input for our analysis. A total of 482,297 cases were reported during that period (see the evolution of the number of cases in annual maps elaborated by the CDC, also available at http://.cdc.gov/lyme/stats/). Until 2007, a case of LD was defined as either (1) a physician-diagnosed erythema migrans rash of more than 5 cm in diameter or (2) at least one objective late manifestation (i.e., musculoskeletal, cardiovascular, or neurologic) with laboratory evidence of infection with *B. burgdorferi* (CDC 1997). The national surveillance case definition was revised in 2008 to include probable cases. State or local health departments are responsible for ensuring that cases reported to the CDC meet the case definition, and state health officials have used various methods to ascertain cases including provider-initiated passive surveillance, laboratory-based surveillance, and enhanced or active surveillance [18]. Over 95 percent of LD cases in the United States occurred in 15 states during our study period, primarily in the Northeast and Upper Midwest (Connecticut, Delaware, Maine, Maryland, Massachusetts, Minnesota, New Hampshire, New Jersey, New York, Pennsylvania, Rhode Island, Vermont, Virginia, West Virginia, and Wisconsin). These are the "high-incidence states," where the average incidence was at least 10 confirmed cases per 100,000 persons in the previous three reporting years (see http://.cdc.gov/lyme/stats/tables.html). We focus our analysis on counties from those states and present results for the incidence of LD—cases per 100,000 population—including all cases reported during our period of analysis. Because the case definition changed in 2008, we also provide estimates based on the LD incidence reported before and after 2008. Annual population data used to calculate the LD incidence is publicly available from the U.S. Bureau of Economic Analysis (http://.bea.gov/itable/index_regional.cfm).

2.2. Meteorological Data.

For meteorological data, we used daily measurements of maximum and minimum temperature as well as total precipitation from NOAA, publicly available at http://.ncdc.noaa.gov/cdo-web/datasets. This dataset provides detailed weather measurements at over 20,000 weather stations across the country. Daily average temperature was calculated as the arithmetic average of daily maximum and minimum temperatures, in degree Celsius (°C). Annual average temperature for the period 2000–2016 was obtained by averaging all daily observations throughout the year. For counties with no weather stations, we imputed annual average temperature by computing a weighted average of that variable from the counties within 50 miles of the original county centroid using inverse distance weights. With measures of annual county-level average temperatures in hand, indicator variables for bins of annual average temperature were generated straightforwardly. Each indicator variable takes the value one if the annual average temperature for a county is in the prespecified range, and zero otherwise. We created indicators for the following ranges: below 5, 5–7, 7–9, 9–11, 11–13, 13–15, and above 15°C. The shares of observations in each bin are reported in Table 1. Annual total precipitation for the period 2000–2016 was obtained by summing all daily precipitation for a county, in centimeters (cm). Imputation for counties with no weather stations was done as described for temperature. Indicator variables for bins of annual total precipitation were generated in a fashion similar to temperature for the following ranges: below 70, 70–120, 120–170, 170–220, 220–270, and above 270 cm. Again, the shares of observations in each bin are reported in Table 1. The average annual total precipitation for the counties in our sample is approximately 174 cm. For reference, the average annual rainfall is 20 cm in Phoenix (Arizona), 87 cm in Madison (Wisconsin), 120 cm in Providence (Rhode Island), 157 cm in Miami (Florida), and 300 cm in Mt. Rainier (Washington).

TABLE 1: Summary statistics from our sample.

Variable	Obs.	Mean	Std. dev.	Min.	Max.
Incidence of Lyme disease	7,956	41.75	76.24	0	1581.15
Avg. temp.: below 5°C	7,956	0.07	0.25	0	1
Avg. temp.: 5–7°C	7,956	0.16	0.36	0	1
Avg. temp.: 7–9°C	7,956	0.26	0.44	0	1
Avg. temp.: 9–11°C	7,956	0.19	0.39	0	1
Avg. temp.: 11–13°C	7,956	0.18	0.38	0	1
Avg. temp.: 13–15°C	7,956	0.11	0.31	0	1
Avg. temp.: above 15°C	7,956	0.03	0.18	0	1
Total prcp.: below 70 cm	7,956	0.05	0.22	0	1
Total prcp.: 70–120 cm	7,956	0.20	0.40	0	1
Total prcp.: 120–170 cm	7,956	0.27	0.44	0	1
Total prcp.: 170–220 cm	7,956	0.22	0.42	0	1
Total prcp.: 220–270 cm	7,956	0.15	0.35	0	1
Total prcp.: above 270 cm	7,956	0.10	0.31	0	1
Connecticut	7,956	0.01	0.12	0	1
Delaware	7,956	0.01	0.08	0	1
Maine	7,956	0.03	0.18	0	1
Maryland	7,956	0.04	0.19	0	1
Massachusetts	7,956	0.03	0.17	0	1
Minnesota	7,956	0.17	0.37	0	1
New Hampshire	7,956	0.02	0.14	0	1
New Jersey	7,956	0.04	0.20	0	1
New York	7,956	0.12	0.32	0	1
Pennsylvania	7,956	0.12	0.33	0	1
Rhode Island	7,956	0.01	0.09	0	1
Vermont	7,956	0.03	0.17	0	1
Virginia	7,956	0.12	0.33	0	1
West Virginia	7,956	0.10	0.29	0	1
Wisconsin	7,956	0.15	0.35	0	1

Note: this table presents the summary statistics regarding the sample used in our, not or analysis. Our sample contains 7,956 observations from 468 counties over 17 years (2000–2016). Those counties are from the 15 states considered by the CDC as the states with the highest incidence of LD (over 95 percent of all cases in the United States). All variables with the exception of the incidence of LD are indicator variables taking the value of one if the statement on the far left is valid, and zero otherwise. Hence, the means for those indicator variables represent shares of the total number of observations. For example, 26 percent of the county-year observations have annual average temperature between 7 and 9°C, and 17 percent of the county-year observations come from Minnesota.

Once we merged the information of LD cases with climatic variables, our sample contained a balanced panel of 468 U.S. counties over the period 2000–2016. Figure 1 displays the counties in our sample in the map of the United States, with color code based on the incidence of LD. Table 1 reports the summary statistics of our sample. Observe that most of the counties used in our sample come from Minnesota, Wisconsin, New York, Pennsylvania, Virginia, and West Virginia. Also, notice that the temperature bins with the highest shares of observations cover the range 7–13°C and the precipitation bins with the largest shares cover the range 70–220 cm.

2.3. Empirical Strategy.

Using standard longitudinal or fixed effects methods [19–21], the typical panel regression model to examine the impact of climatic variables C—in our case,

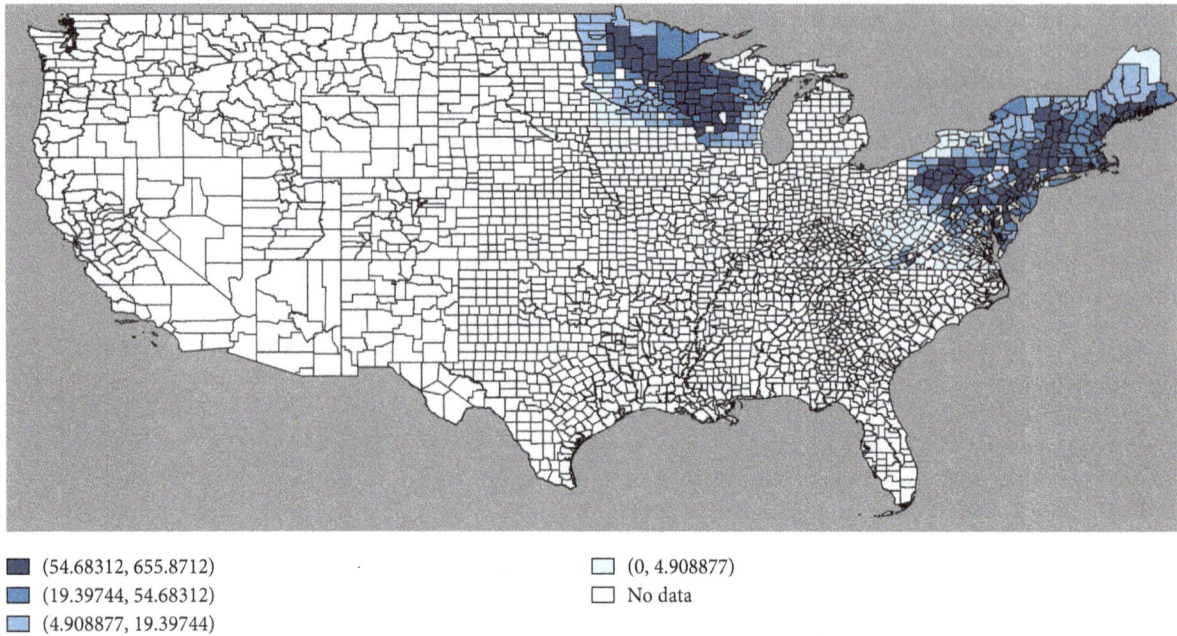

■ (54.68312, 655.8712)
■ (19.39744, 54.68312)
□ (4.908877, 19.39744)
□ (0, 4.908877)
□ No data

FIGURE 1: Map of the United States with highlighted counties from our Sample. Note: this map displays our sample of 468 counties in the 15 states considered by CDC as the states with the highest incidence of LD (over 95 percent of all cases in the United States). Darker blue colors represent higher incidence of the disease—cases per 100,000 population.

annual average temperature and annual total precipitation—on an outcome of interest y—in our case, the incidence of LD (cases per 100,000 population)—takes the form

$$y_{it} = \beta C_{it} + \gamma Z_{it} + \mu_i + \theta_t + \lambda_s f(t) + \varepsilon_{it}, \quad (1)$$

where i indexes different geographic areas (in our case, counties), t indexes time (in our case, years), and s indexes a larger geographical area (in our case, states) [22]. The additional explanatory variables will be explained below, but the error process ε is typically modeled using robust standard errors, allowing for arbitrary correlation over time and space in the covariance matrix by clustering at the county level.

Noting that C varies plausibly randomly over time—i.e., "weather" draws from the county "climate" distribution—this approach resembles an experimental design and, therefore, β identifies the causal effect of weather shocks on the incidence of LD [22]. The fixed effects for county, μ_i, absorb fixed spatial characteristics, whether observed or unobserved, disentangling the shock from many possible sources of omitted variable bias, such as geographic features (e.g., elevation and ruggedness) and county baseline economic characteristics (e.g., GDP, population, and number of hospital beds and number of physicians per 100,000 population) that are likely to be correlated to climatic variables. Time-fixed effects, θ_t, further neutralize any common trends and thus help ensure that the relationships of interest are identified from idiosyncratic local shocks. State-specific time trends, $\lambda_s f(t)$, are added to allow for differential trends in subsamples of the data, controlling for a number of observed and unobserved factors affecting the outcome of interest that vary over time at the state level, such

as state health expenditures and state public awareness campaigns regarding the incidence of particular diseases. In our preferred specification of Equation (1), $f(t)$ is a quadratic function of time, that is, it includes state-specific quadratic time trends, as will be explained in more details in Results and Discussion.

It is imperative to explain the choice of temperature and precipitation as our climatic variables. One can assume that the incidence of LD might be related to tick activity. In fact, laboratory studies indicate that temperature determines whether or not, and to what extent, *I. scapularis* can move to seek hosts, whereas humidity determines how high ticks quest above ground level, where their resource for rehydration exists, and for how long they can remain actively host-seeking before retreating to rehydrate [23–25]. We use precipitation instead of the ideal measure of relative humidity because the latter is only available for half of our county-year observations. Nevertheless, in unreported analysis available upon request, we find similar results when using the subsample with information on relative humidity. Besides the biological effects of climate on tick vector abundance and activity, there may be behavioral impacts of climate on human exposure to ticks. Previous studies have found that individuals spend more time outdoors as temperature rises, up to a point where being outside becomes undesirable due to the excessive heat [26, 27]. Additionally, individuals may engage in adaptive responses to avoid exposure to ticks such as the use of deer-baiting devices to kill ticks [28].

A fundamental issue in Equation (1) is regarding the functional form of C. Following previous studies [29–32], we use indicator variables for bins of annual average temperature and for bins of annual total precipitation. These bins are listed in Table 1 and were described in the data section. Thus, the only functional form restriction is that the impact of the annual average temperature on the incidence of LD is constant within 2°C intervals. The choice of narrow temperature bins represents an effort to allow the data, rather than parametric assumptions, to determine the incidence-temperature relationship, while also obtaining estimates that are precise enough that they have empirical content [29–32]. This degree of flexibility and freedom from parametric assumptions is only feasible because we are using 16 years of data from a large area of the United States. Similarly, we use simple indicator variables for precipitation based on annual rainfall in county i in year t. Each indicator corresponds to a 50-cm bin, ranging from less than 70 cm to more than 270 cm.

Another important methodological decision to make when implementing panel regression models concerns the inclusion of other time-varying observables, Z_{it}. Including Z_{it} may absorb residual variation, hence producing more precise estimates. However, adding more controls will not necessarily produce an estimate of β that is closer to the true β. If the Z's are themselves an outcome of C, which may well be the case for controls such as GDP, institutional measures, and population, including them will induce an "over-controlling problem" (in the language of the model, if Z is in fact $Z(C)$, then Equation (1) would instead be written as $y = f(C), Z(C))$ and estimating an equation that included both Z and C would not capture the true net effect of C on y (again, see Dell et al. [22]). For example, suppose that poorer counties in the United States tend to be both hot and have low-quality institutions. If hot climates were to cause low-quality institutions, which in turn cause low income, then controlling for institutions in Equation (1) can have the effect of partially eliminating the explanatory power of climate, even if climate is the underlying fundamental cause. Therefore, if the incidence of LD is the outcome of interest, for example, then controlling for changes in health personnel or infrastructure would be problematic if the climatic variables influence those changes, directly or indirectly. Our preferred specification of Equation (1) does not include additional time-varying explanatory variables, but we also report separate estimates for counties above and below the U.S. median per capita income. This variable should reflect patterns of development across the nation.

3. Results and Discussion

Tick-borne diseases are an important public health concern and the incidence of these infections is increasing in the Unites States and worldwide [33]. Complex interactions between humans and climate change are contributing to the emergence of new diseases and the spread of already known ones to regions where they were unable to exist before. Environmental factors such as temperature and humidity have been shown to influence tick abundance, availability of hosts, their survival, and disease transmission. LD is a classic example of linkage between environmental factors and disease occurrence and spread (the U.S. Environmental Protection Agency (EPA) is actually using the number of LD cases as

a climate change indicator (http://.epa.gov/climate-indicators/climate-change-indicators-lyme-disease)). For a region to be suitable for LD occurrence and transmission, the climate needs to allow the survival of both ticks and mammalian hosts necessary for completion of tick life cycle [25]. The emergence of LD in the northeast of the Unites States in 1970 was thought to be due to the expansion of the tick population associated with reforestation and expansion of the key host for tick life cycle—deer [34]. However, a recent study from Canada demonstrated the expansion of *I. scapularis* population despite deforestation [35]. Previous studies, both empirical and simulation-based, have demonstrated that a warming climate has a positive effect on the expansion of the tick population through an increase in tick survival and improved access to hosts necessary for feeding [36, 37]. Our study aimed to determine the influence of temperature and humidity on the incidence of LD within 15 U.S. states that account for the majority of reported cases.

Our estimated impacts of climatic variables on the incidence of LD—cases per 100,000 population—are reported on Table 2. Recall that the main sample contains only counties from those 15 U.S. states with the highest incidence of LD cases according to CDC. In column 1, we controlled for observed and unobserved time-varying factors affecting all sample counties equally in each year such as macroeconomic conditions and changes in health law and health expenditure at the federal level, and for observed and unobserved time-invariant factors affecting each county over the sample period such as county geographical features and historical (baseline) health infrastructure. In column 2, we added state-specific linear time trend to control for observed and unobserved changes in state variables affecting the health outcomes such as expansion of Medicaid, campaigns to raise awareness of healthy behaviors, etc. For our preferred specification in column 3, we allowed those state-specific time trends to reverse direction over time by adding quadratic terms. For example, we are controlling for observed and unobserved increases in state health expenditures in a number of years as well as decreases afterwards, or decreases in funds for campaigns raising awareness of LD, and increases in funding once more cases are confirmed. Column 3 is our preferred specification not only because the increase in the R-squared relative to previous columns indicates an improvement in the goodness-of-fit of our econometric model, but also because it takes into account important controls. In fact, the similarity in the increase in the R-squared and in the adjusted R-squared indicates that the additional explanatory variables are indeed relevant to explain the incidence of LD. Otherwise, the adjusted R-squared would have penalized our column-3 econometric specification. Both the R-squared and the adjusted R-squared reveal that our model explains over 70 percent of the variation in the incidence of LD in the United States over the period 2000–2016.

We now describe the results from our preferred specification (Table 2, column 3). Relative to counties with annual average temperature above 15°C, counties with annual average temperature below 5°C have 1.6 additional cases of LD per 100,000 population, but this estimate is not statistically

TABLE 2: The impacts of temperature and precipitation on the incidence of LD.

Dep. var.: LD incidence	Main results		
	(1)	(2)	(3)
Avg. temp.: below 5°C	7.9101 (6.1820)	4.9673 (5.9583)	1.6156 (5.7073)
Avg. temp.: 5–7°C	17.2713*** (5.6208)	13.3615** (5.4461)	10.7294** (5.0919)
Avg. temp.: 7–9°C	21.3359*** (5.2593)	16.2189*** (5.2152)	15.1306*** (4.8862)
Avg. temp.: 9–11°C	19.9290*** (4.3244)	15.4690*** (4.5382)	14.4033*** (4.2444)
Avg. temp.: 11–13°C	9.7629*** (2.9059)	6.5636** (3.1989)	5.3232* (2.9025)
Avg. temp.: 13–15°C	6.6229*** (2.0306)	4.7761** (2.1972)	3.8847** (1.9730)
Reference: above 15°C	0	0	0
Total prcp.: below 70 cm	13.0452** (5.4358)	13.5556*** (4.5898)	4.6664 (4.5738)
Total prcp.: 70–120 cm	10.7113** (4.7829)	11.8325*** (4.0619)	4.2597 (3.9230)
Total prcp.: 120–170 cm	8.1580** (4.1505)	10.4118*** (3.6474)	5.3288 (3.4688)
Total prcp.: 170–220 cm	3.7551 (3.1761)	6.3591** (2.8603)	3.6003 (2.6573)
Total prcp.: 220–270 cm	1.8596 (2.8608)	2.3633 (2.8913)	1.2022 (2.8126)
Reference: above 270 cm	0	0	0
Year fixed effects	Yes	Yes	Yes
County fixed effects	Yes	Yes	Yes
Linear trend by state		Yes	Yes
Quadratic trend by state			Yes
Observations	7,956	7,956	7,956
R^2	0.6771	0.7068	0.7226
Adjusted R^2	0.656	0.687	0.703

Note: this table presents the estimated impacts of climatic variables on the incidence of LD–cases per 100,000 population. Avg. temp. is annual average temperature, and total prcp. is annual total precipitation. Robust standard errors clustered at the county level are reported in parentheses. ***Significance at 1 percent; **significance at 5 percent; *significance at 10 percent.

significant (not distinguishable from zero, or alternatively not distinguishable from the reference group). That estimate jumped to 10.7 cases per 100,000 population for counties with annual average temperature between 5 and 7°C, and to 15.1 for counties with annual average temperature between 7 and 9°C. Then, it stabilized for counties with annual average temperature between 9 and 11°C—14.4 cases per 100,000 population—but dropped to 5.3 and 3.9 for counties with annual average temperature between 11 and 13°C, and 13 and 15°C, respectively. We display these estimates more clearly in Figure 2, where we can see the approximately concave or inverted-U shape of the incidence of LD response to temperature.

Three features of these results are worth discussing. First, the sharp increase in the number of LD cases per 100,000 population happens in the 5–7 and 7–9°C annual average temperature bins. This might be associated with tick activity (Schulze et al. provided suggestive evidence that precipitation and temperature played a limited role in predicting the abundance of I. scapularis nymphs at an LD-endemic area over the period 1998–2005. Thus, we focus on tick activity in understanding our findings, as in Burtis et al.). Indeed, Duffy and Campbell [38] used flagging samples of adults I. scapularis through the winter to infer a minimum temperature threshold for activity of approximately 4°C. Clark [23] used laboratory experiments to determine a minimum temperature threshold for activity by adult I. scapularis of 9–11°C, but some individual nymphs were capable of movement and coordinated movement at much lower temperatures, 4.2 and 6.3°C, respectively. (Notice that, by definition, annual average temperature includes a range of observed temperatures throughout the

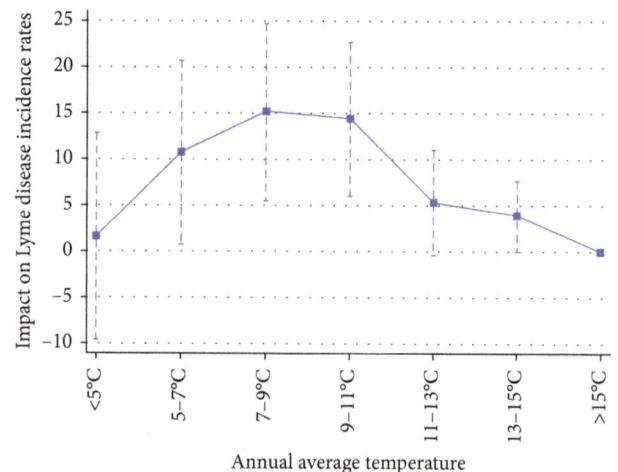

FIGURE 2: The impact of temperature on the incidence of LD. Note: this figure presents the estimated impacts of temperature on the incidence of LD—cases per 100,000 population—reported in the last column of Table 2 and represented here by blue squares. The vertical dashed lines around each blue square represent the 95 percent confidence interval.

year. Therefore, our temperature bins do not have to match precisely the thresholds highlighted in those studies. It is remarkable, however, that the correspondence is approximately accurate.) Second, the similarity of estimates for the ranges of annual average temperature 11–13°C, 13–15°C, and above 15°C. In fact, Vail and Smith [24] found no significant difference in the mean distance moved or time spent in questing posture for I. scapularis nymphs held at 10 versus 15 or 20°C. Third, the concave or inverted-U shape of the LD incidence response to temperature. Vail and Smith [24, 39] and Ogden et al. [25] found laboratory and field evidence that tick survival and activity peaked at certain temperatures, and then decreased, with peak temperatures varying considerably depending on the outcome of interest. The inverted U-shaped relationship between temperature and LD incidence is also consistent with the pattern of human exposure to ticks. In fact, temperature has been shown to have nonlinear impacts on the time adults and children allocate to outdoor activities. As temperature rises, individuals engage in more outdoor activities, but after it reaches a maximum tolerable temperature, they decrease the time spent outdoors [26, 27]. Similarly, as temperature rises, society may engage in adaptive actions to avoid exposure to ticks such as the deployment of deer-baiting devices called four-posters to kill ticks [28]. Feeder stations that resemble four-poster beds lure deers with corn. Rollers soaked with the pesticide permethrin rub the animals' necks as they eat the corn, killing ticks. As an example, this year, dozens of those devices were installed in Shelter and Fire Islands, NY, as part of a $1.2 million tick-removal effort.

While temperature is supposed to influence the extent to which *I. scapularis* can move to seek hosts, humidity is supposed to affect how high ticks quest above ground level, where resources and rehydration are available, and for how long they can remain actively host-seeking [23–25]. In our longitudinal analysis, we included bins of total precipitation during the year as a proxy for humidity. As we can see in our preferred specification (column 3) in Table 2, there was no statistical difference in the incidence of LD between counties with more than 270 cm of total precipitation—the reference group—and counties with less rainfall. This result seems to be consistent with laboratory evidence provided by Vail and Smith [39] who found no difference in the time in questing posture across any levels of relative humidity, and no difference in questing height at levels of relative humidity below 100 percent. Berger et al. [40] also found that mean weekly daytime relative humidity did not significantly predict tick activity in the field. Given such findings, we have focused on the relationship between temperature and LDs cases per 100,000 population in our discussion (it is worth mentioning that although our findings are consistent with laboratory and field evidence on tick activity and survival, and corroborate Subak's [9] findings of a weak relationship between the incidence of LD and a same-year moisture index for seven northeastern U.S. states during 1993–2001, they are different from the results found by McCabe and Bunnell; using data for seven northeastern U.S. states during the 1992–2002 period, those authors found that late spring/early summer precipitation was a significant climate factor affecting the occurrence of LD, but that temperature did not seem to explain the variability in LD reports).

Table 3 reports the impacts of climatic variables on the incidence of LD for counties above and below the U.S. median income per capita, and for cases reported before and after 2008. Although richer counties might have more resources to deal with clinical and public health issues, we did not find any statistical difference between our estimates in richer versus poorer counties. With respect to post-2008,

when probable cases of LD were included along with confirmed cases, we noticed a much noisier relationship between temperature and LD incidence. This is not surprising because attenuation bias from measurement error is usually exacerbated in panel data regressions.

Our results imply that climate change will have a sizable impact on the number of cases of LD in the United States in the coming decades. Using the estimated impacts of temperature on the incidence of the disease in Table 2, column 3, and the distribution of county-year observations in each bin of annual average temperature from Table 1, we have predicted an increase of 8.6 cases of LD per 100,000 population per county-year, an increase of about 21 percent relative to the average incidence of the disease over the period 2000–2016. This was done by assuming a 2°C increase in annual average temperature in the northern area of the United States by mid-century (2036–2065). (The 2°C increase in annual average temperature implies that the share of counties in one 2°C bin in Table 1 would show up in the following 2°C bin. For example, the 26 percent of counties in the 7–9°C temperature bin in Table 1 would show up in the 9–11°C bin. The calculation of the impact of that increase in annual average temperature then used the estimates reported in Table 2, column 3, and the shift up of the shares presented in Table 1.) This temperature increase is assumed to be an approximation for the change the region we focus on might experience in the future. In fact, it is slightly below the mid-century (2036–2065) projections for the Northeast (2.21°C or 3.98°F) and Midwest (2.34°C or 4.21°F) from the Fourth National Climate Assessment (NCA4) (USGCRP 2017). This is under the more conservative Representative Concentration Pathway (RCP) 4.5, which assumes global annual greenhouse gas emissions peaking around 2040, then declining. Under the RCP 8.5, which assumes that emissions will continue to rise throughout the twenty-first century, those mid-century (2036–2065) predicted increases in annual average temperature would be 2.83°C (5.09°F) for the Northeast and 2.94°C (5.29°F) for the Midwest (see definition of the NCA4 regions at scenarios.globalchange. gov/regions_nca4).

Given the increase of 8.6 cases of LD per 100,000 population per county-year associated with a 2°C increase in temperature and the average population for a county-year in our sample of 149,606 persons, we have predicted an increase in the number of LD cases by approximately 6,040 per year in the counties in our sample (again, they represent over 95 percent of the cases in the entire country). Because the average annual number of LD cases in United States over the period 2000–2016 was 28,370, that amount translates into an increase of roughly 21 percent in the number of LD cases in the coming decades.

4. Conclusion

In this study, we have shown that a sizable increase in the incidence of LD cases in endemic areas of the United States due to climate change is imminent. These findings should alert public health agencies, physicians, and patients. On the one hand, better education and increased awareness among

TABLE 3: The impact of climatic variables by income per capita and before vs. after 2008.

Dep. var.: LD incidence	Heterogeneity			
	<PCI median (1)	≥PCI median (2)	<2008 (3)	≥2008 (4)
Avg. temp.: below 5°C	9.8421 (7.2752)	6.5755 (8.5056)	−0.0423 (4.9830)	−6.0330 (6.8374)
Avg. temp.: 5–7°C	16.1789*** (6.1200)	12.2321 (7.7779)	5.9658 (3.9566)	3.3523 (5.7814)
Avg. temp.: 7–9°C	20.0468*** (7.2075)	12.3422 (7.5295)	6.7271* (3.9568)	2.3292 (4.9421)
Avg. temp.: 9–11°C	17.6905*** (6.2141)	15.5235** (7.2675)	5.3618** (2.5961)	6.0453 (4.2411)
Avg. temp.: 11–13°C	7.5071** (3.0650)	8.2686 (5.6081)	2.7109 (1.8782)	−0.6243 (2.5552)
Avg. temp.: 13–15°C	6.1809** (2.3800)	5.3997 (3.3455)	2.7591** (1.2852)	−0.8361 (2.2234)
Reference: above 15°C	0	0	0	0
Total prcp.: below 70 cm	1.8066 (7.2816)	11.1090 (7.5837)	−5.7405 (5.5240)	−2.8211 (7.2106)
Total prcp.: 70–120 cm	0.0188 (6.8925)	9.6526 (6.5876)	−6.3607 (5.3531)	−3.5179 (6.2751)
Total prcp.: 120–170 cm	1.7949 (6.0951)	8.7628 (5.8681)	−2.0996 (4.7471)	−5.4875 (5.2265)
Total prcp.: 170–220 cm	−0.4551 (4.4063)	8.0211* (4.4954)	−3.3351 (4.2346)	−5.8981 (3.8901)
Total prcp.: 220–270 cm	−2.3741 (3.0281)	6.2257 (3.8928)	−1.5489 (2.9620)	−4.7632 (3.4002)
Reference: above 270 cm	0	0	0	0
Year fixed effects	Yes	Yes	Yes	Yes
County fixed effects	Yes	Yes	Yes	Yes
Linear trend by state	Yes	Yes	Yes	Yes
Quadratic trend by state	Yes	Yes	Yes	Yes
Observations	3,978	3,978	3,744	4,212
R^2	0.7804	0.7658	0.8565	0.8237
Adjusted R^2	0.750	0.738	0.830	0.795

Note: this table presents the estimated impacts of climatic variables on the incidence of LD—cases per 100,000 population—by counties above and below the U.S. per capita income (PCI), and by cases before and after 2008, when probable cases of LD were included in the total number of cases in each county. Avg. temp. is annual average temperature, and total prcp. is annual total precipitation. Robust standard errors clustered at the county level are reported in parentheses. ***Significance at 1 percent; **significance at 5 percent; *significance at 10 percent.

patients and physicians is important because early recognition and treatment are usually highly effective in preventing debilitating consequences of untreated Lyme disease and the potential post-Lyme syndrome. On the other hand, public health authorities should be alert to work on strategies to limit tick and host population and consequently decrease the incidence of LD not only in endemic areas, but also in neighboring locations where the disease has only been sporadically reported, or not reported at all. In fact, climate change may make those areas suitable for the establishment of tick and host populations.

Our study has a number of limitations. First, because of data limitations, we have used annual data to examine the relationship between the incidence of LD and climatic variables. Thus, we were unable to address the seasonality of LD cases throughout the year, as highlighted by Moore et al. [41] and the climate change influences on the annual onset of LD, as studied by Monaghan et al. [42]. Second, we have focused our analysis on counties from the highest incidence states, regardless of the spatial distribution of blacklegged ticks. Hence, we cannot comment on whether these reported cases were autochthone—most likely the vast majority of the cases—or imported. In an ongoing research project, we are examining the climate-LD incidence relationship over U.S. counties with established tick population versus counties with ticks reported, but not yet established. Third, although we have overcome a number of omitted variable bias issues with the fixed effects analysis, we have not scaled our results relative to areas with few LD cases. In work still in progress, we are using a border approach to compare our estimates for

the places with high incidence of LD with estimates for their corresponding neighboring areas.

References

[1] E. D. Shapiro, "Clinical practice. Lyme disease," *New England Journal of Medicine*, vol. 370, no. 18, pp. 1724–1731, 2014.

[2] C. Bhate and R. A. Schwartz, "Lyme disease: part I. Advances and perspectives," *Journal of the American Academy of Dermatology*, vol. 64, no. 4, pp. 619–636, 2011.

[3] A. Buchwald, "Ein fall von diffuser idiopathischer Haut-Atrophie," *Vierteljahresschrift für Dermatologie und Syphilis*, vol. 10, no. 1, pp. 553–556, 1883.

[4] B. Lipschutz, "Uber eine saltine Erythemaform (Erythema chronicum migrans)," *Archiv für Dermatologie und Syphilis*, vol. 118, no. 1, pp. 349–356, 1913.

[5] S. Hellestrom, "Erythema chronicum migrans Afzelii," *Acta Dermato-Venereologica*, vol. 11, pp. 315–321, 1930.

[6] A. C. Steere and S. E. Malawista, "Lyme arthritis: an epidemic of oligoarthritis in children and adults in three Connecticut's communities," *Arthritis & Rheumatism*, vol. 20, no. 1, pp. 7–17, 1977.

[7] W. Burgdorfer, A. G. Barbour, S. F. Hayes, J. L. Benach, E. Grunwaldth, and J. P. Davis, "Lyme disease-a tick borne spirochetosis?," *Science*, vol. 216, no. 4552, pp. 1317–1319, 1982.

[8] E. Shapiro and M. Gerber, "Lyme disease," *Clinical Infectious Disease*, vol. 31, no. 2, pp. 2533–2542, 2000.

[9] S. Subak, "Effects of climate on variability in Lyme disease incidence in the northeastern United States," *American Journal of Epidemiology*, vol. 157, no. 6, pp. 531–538, 2003.

[10] R. L. Bratton, J. W. Whiteside, M. J. Hovan, R. L. Engle, and F. D. Edwards, "Diagnosis and treatment of Lyme disease," *Mayo Clinic Proceedings*, vol. 83, no. 5, pp. 566–571, 2008.

[11] https://www.nasa.gov/mission_pages/noaa-n/climate/climate_weather.html.

[12] R. J. Eisen, L. Eisen, N. H. Ogden, and C. B. Beard, "Linkages of weather and climate with *Ixodes scapularis* and *Ixodes pacificus* (Acari: ixodidae), enzootic transmission of *Borrelia burgdorferi*, and Lyme disease in north America," *Journal of Medical Entomology*, vol. 53, no. 2, pp. 250–261, 2016.

[13] https://www.cdc.gov/lyme/stats/tables.html.

[14] C. Colomba, F. Scarlata, P. Di Carlo et al., "Fourth case of louse-borne relapsing fever in Young Migrant, Sicily, Italy, December 2015. Mini review article," *Public Health*, vol. 139, pp. 22–26, 2016.

[15] A. Ciervo, F. Mancini, F. Di Bernardo et al., "Louseborne relapsing fever in Young Migrants, Sicily, Italy, July–September 2015," *Emerging Infectious Diseases*, vol. 22, no. 1, pp. 152-153, 2016.

[16] T. Fasciana, C. Calà, C. Colomba et al., "A New Case of Louse-Borne Relapsing Fever in Sicily: Case Report and Mini Review," *Pharmacologyonline*, vol. 1, pp. 62–66, 2017.

[17] C. Colomba, M. Trizzino, A. Giammanco et al., "Israeli spotted fever in Sicily. Description of two cases and mini review," *International Journal of Infectious Diseases*, vol. 61, pp. 7–12, 2017.

[18] R. M. Bacon, K. J. Kugeler, and P. S. Mead, "Surveillance for LD–United States, 1992-2006," *MMWR Surveillance Summaries*, vol. 57, pp. 1–9, 2008.

[19] G. Chamberlain, "Panel data," in *Handbook of Econometrics*, Z. Griliches and M. D. Intriligator, Eds., vol. 2, pp. 1247–1318, North Holland, Amsterdam, Netherlands, 1984.

[20] J. M. Wooldridge, *Econometric Analysis of Cross Section and Panel Data*, The MIT Press, Cambridge, MA, USA, 2010.

[21] FI. Gunasekara, K. Richardson, K. Carter, and T. Blakely, "Fixed effects analysis of repeated measures data," *International Journal of Epidemiology*, vol. 43, no. 1, pp. 264–269, 2014.

[22] M. Dell, B. F. Jones, and B. A. Olken, "What do we learn from the weather? The new climate-economy literature," *Journal of Economic Literature*, vol. 52, no. 3, pp. 740–798, 2014.

[23] D. D. Clark, "Lower temperature limits for activity of several ixodid ticks (Acari: ixodidae): effects of body size and rate of temperature change," *Journal of Medical Entomology*, vol. 32, no. 4, pp. 449–452, 1995.

[24] S. G. Vail and G. Smith, "Air temperature and relative humidity effects on behavioral activity of blacklegged tick (Acari: ixodidae) nymphs in New Jersey," *Journal of Medical Entomology*, vol. 35, no. 6, pp. 1025–1028, 1998.

[25] N. H. Ogden, L. R. Lindsay, G. Beauchamp et al., "Investigation of relationships between temperature and developmental rates of tick *Ixodes scapularis* (Acari: ixodidae) in the laboratory and field," *Journal of Medical Entomology*, vol. 41, no. 4, pp. 622–633, 2004.

[26] J. Graff-Zivin and M. Neidell, "Temperature and the allocation of time: implications for climate change," *Journal of Labor Economics*, vol. 32, no. 1, pp. 1–26, 2014.

[27] H. Nguyen, L. T. Huong, and L. B. Connelly, *Weather and Children's Time Allocation*, Mimeo, New York, NY, USA, 2018.

[28] T. J. Wong, P. J. Schramm, E. Foster et al., *The Effectiveness and Implementation of 4-Poster Deer Self-Treatment Devices for Tickborne Disease Prevention: A Potential Component of an Integrated Tick Management Program. Climate and Health Technical Report Series–Climate and Health Program*, Centers for Disease Control and Prevention (CS263538-A), Atlanta, GA, USA, 2017, https://www.cdc.gov/climateandhealth/docs/4postertickbornedisease.pdf.

[29] O. Deschenes and M. Greenstone, "Climate change, mortality, and adaptation: evidence from annual fluctuations in weather in the US," *American Economic Journal: Applied Economics*, vol. 3, no. 4, pp. 152–185, 2011.

[30] A. Barreca, K. Clay, O. Deschenes, M. Greenstone, and J. S. Shapiro, "Adapting to climate change: the remarkable decline in the US temperature-mortality relationship over the twentieth century," *Journal of Political Economy*, vol. 124, no. 1, pp. 105–159, 2016.

[31] W. Schlenker and M. J. Roberts, "Nonlinear temperature effects indicate severe damages to U.S. crop yields under climate change," *Proceeding of the National Academy of Sciences (PNAS)*, vol. 106, no. 37, pp. 15594–15598, 2009.

[32] A. Missirian and W. Schlenker, "Asylum applications respond to temperature fluctuations," *Science*, vol. 358, no. 6370, pp. 1610–1614, 2017.

[33] S. J. Robinson, D. F. Neitzel, R. A. Moen et al., "Disease risk in a dynamic environment: the spread of tick-borne pathogens in Minnesota, USA," *Ecohealth*, vol. 12, no. 1, pp. 152–163, 2015.

[34] C. L. Wood and K. D. Lafferty, "Biodiversity and disease: a synthesis of ecological perspectives on Lyme disease transmission," *Trends in Ecology & Evolution*, vol. 28, no. 4, pp. 239–247, 2013.

[35] M. McPherson, A. García-García, F. J. Cuesta-Valero et al., "Expansion of the Lyme disease vector *Ixodes scapularis* in Canada inferred from CMIP5 climate projections," *Environmental Health Perspectives*, vol. 125, no. 5, article 057008, 2017.

[36] K. M. Pepin, R. J. Eisen, and P. S. Mead, "Geographic variation in the relationship between human Lyme disease incidence and density of infected host-seeking *Ixodes scapularis* nymphs in the Eastern United States," *American Journal of Tropical Medicine and Hygiene*, vol. 86, no. 6, pp. 1062–1071, 2012.

[37] N. H. Ogden, M. Bigras-Poulin, and C. J. O'Callaghan, "A dynamic population model to investigate effects of climate on geographic range and seasonality of the tick *Ixodes scapularis*," *International Journal for Parasitology*, vol. 35, no. 4, pp. 375–389, 2005.

[38] D. C. Duffy and S. R. Campbell, "Ambient air temperature as a predictor of activity of adult *Ixodes scapularis* (Acari: ixodidae)," *Journal of Medical Entomology*, vol. 31, no. 1, pp. 178–180, 1994.

[39] S. G. Vail and G. Smith, "Vertical movement and posture of blacklegged tick (Acari: ixodidae) nymphs as a function of temperature and relative humidity in laboratory experiments," *Journal of Medical Entomology*, vol. 39, no. 6, pp. 842–846, 2002.

[40] K. A. Berger, H. S. Ginsberg, L. Gonzalez, and T. N. Mather, "Relative humidity and activity patterns of *Ixodes scapularis*

(Acari: ixodidae)," *Journal of Medical Entomology*, vol. 51, no. 4, pp. 769–776, 2014.

[41] S. M. Moore, R. J. Eisen, A. Monaghan, and M. Paul, "Meteorological influences on the seasonality of LD in the United States," *American Journal of Tropical Medicine and Hygiene*, vol. 90, no. 3, pp. 486–496, 2014.

[42] A. J. Monaghan, S. M. Moore, K. M. Sampson, C. B. Beard, and R. J. Eisen, "Climate change influences on the annual onset of LD in the United States," *Ticks and Tick-Borne Diseases*, vol. 6, no. 5, pp. 615–622, 2015.

4

Molecular Identification of *Mycobacterium* Species of Public Health and Veterinary Importance from Cattle in the South State of México

Adrian Zaragoza Bastida,[1,2] Nallely Rivero Pérez,[2]
Benjamín Valladares Carranza,[3] Keila Isaac-Olivé,[1] Pablo Moreno Pérez,[1]
Horacio Sandoval Trujillo,[4] and Ninfa Ramírez Durán[1]

[1]*Facultad de Medicina, Universidad Autónoma del Estado de México, Paseo Tollocan/Jesús Carranza s/n, 50180 Toluca, MEX, Mexico*
[2]*Área Académica de Medicina Veterinaria y Zootecnia, Instituto de Ciencias Agropecuaria,*
 Universidad Autónoma del Estado de Hidalgo, Av. Universidad Km 1, Ex-Hda. de Aquetzalpa, 43600 Tulancingo, HGO, Mexico
[3]*Centro de Investigación y Estudios Avanzados en Salud Animal, Facultad de Medicina Veterinaria y Zootecnia,*
 Universidad Autónoma del Estado de México, Km 15.5 Carretera Panamericana Toluca-Atlacomulco, 50200 Toluca, MEX, Mexico
[4]*Departamento de Sistemas Biológicos, Universidad Autónoma Metropolitana-Xochimilco, Calzada del Hueso 1100,*
 04960 Ciudad de México, Mexico

Correspondence should be addressed to Ninfa Ramírez Durán; nramirezd@uaemex.mx

Academic Editor: Nahuel Fittipaldi

Mycobacterium genus causes a variety of zoonotic diseases. The best known example is the zoonotic tuberculosis due to *M. bovis*. Much less is known about "nontuberculous mycobacteria (NTM)," which are also associated with infections in humans. The Mexican standard NOM-ZOO-031-1995 regulates the presence of *M. bovis* in cattle; however, no regulation exists for the NTM species. The objective of this study was to isolate and identify nontuberculous mycobacteria species from cattle of local herds in the south region of the State of Mexico through the identification and detection of the 100 bp molecular marker in the 23S rRNA gene with subsequent sequencing of the 16S rRNA gene. Milk samples (35) and nasal exudate samples (68) were collected. From the 108 strains isolated, 39 were selected for identification. Thirteen strains isolated from nasal exudates amplified the 100 bp molecular marker and were identified as *M. neoaurum* (six strains), *M. parafortuitum* (four strains), *M. moriokaense* (two strains), and *M. confluentis* (one strain). Except *M. parafortuitum*, the other species identified are of public health and veterinary concern because they are pathogenic to humans, especially those with underlying medical conditions.

1. Introduction

The genus *Mycobacterium* causes a wide variety of zoonotic diseases. The best known example is zoonotic tuberculosis due to *M. bovis*, for which cattle is the main reservoir. *M. bovis* is part of the "tuberculosis complex," which also includes the species *M. tuberculosis, M. africanum, M. caprae*, and *M. microti* [1].

Within the mycobacterial group are the "nontuberculous mycobacteria (NTM)," which are also associated with infections in humans. The NTM are found in various environmental sources such as soil, water, vegetation, animals, dairy products, and feces and may be transmitted inadvertently by inhalation, ingestion, or skin penetration [2].

The Mexican standard NOM-ZOO-031-1995 regulates the presence of *M. bovis* in cattle to control and eradicate bovine tuberculosis (bTB); however, no regulation exists for the NTM species. The official diagnosis of bovine tuberculosis due to the presence of *M. bovis* at the field level is based on the intradermal test using a purified protein derivative (tuberculin) [3]. Although used for several years, this test does not provide good sensitivity and specificity. Approximately 20% of the animals with tuberculosis do not react to the test [4], and the presence of other mycobacterial species, both tuberculosis complex and NTM species, causes interference that leads to false-positive and false-negative diagnoses.

Although Mexico has a regulatory standard, bTB prevalence in excess of 2% is reported in some areas [5]. Given the poor specificity and sensitivity of the tuberculin test, the actual presence of *M. bovis* is likely to be lower and the infection rate of cattle by other mycobacteria is likely to be higher, respectively. Thus, cattle breeders, veterinarians, technicians, and employees working in the livestock industry might be occupationally exposed to infections by *M. bovis* and NTM. Very little is known about occupational exposure to zoonoses due to NTM species because the identification of these species was a rather difficult task prior to the development of identification techniques based on molecular biology.

Currently, the molecular biology techniques most commonly used for the diagnosis of diseases caused by mycobacteria are restriction fragment length polymorphism (RFLP) for the diagnosis of *M. tuberculosis* [6], spoligotyping for the diagnosis of *M. bovis* [7], and the detection of a 100-base pair (bp) "specific insertion" located on the 23S rRNA gene characteristic of Gram-positive bacteria with a high guanine-cytosine (HGC) content, which is considered a molecular marker for this group of bacteria [8, 9], followed by sequence analysis of the 16S rRNA gene for the identification of bacteria at the species level [10].

Among the NTM species identified by the aforementioned techniques are *M. balnei, M. marinum,* and *M. platypoecilus,* which have caused superficial and deep skin lesions [11]; *M. kansasii* from lung lesions [12]; *M. simiae* from generalized infections [13]; *M. scrofulaceum* from infections of the skin and internal organs [14]; *M. szulgai* associated with pulmonary infections, osteomyelitis, tenosynovitis, and lymphadenitis [15]; *M. ulcerans* associated with subcutaneous granulomas [16]; *M. fortuitum* and *M. chelonae* associated with vasculitis, endocarditis, osteomyelitis, mediastinitis, meningitis, keratitis, and hepatitis [17]; *M. abscessus,* associated with erythematous lesions that progressed to ulcerated nodules [18]; and other species.

The largest percentage of the state inventory for heads of cattle in the State of Mexico in Mexico is concentrated in the southern region, and one of the main economic activities is cattle ranching [19]. The Mexican regulation for cattle control NOM-ZOO-031-1995 only focuses on the tuberculin test for the diagnosis of *M. bovis*. Little is known about the presence of NTM in the cattle of the region. Given the possibility of identifying species of actinobacteria by detection of the 100-base pair molecular marker on the 23S rRNA gene and the subsequent sequencing of the 16S rRNA gene, it is possible to identify the aforementioned NTM species.

The objective of the present study was to isolate and identify NTM species from cattle of the south region of the State of Mexico. The *Mycobacterium* species were isolated from samples of nasal exudate and bovine milk and identified by detecting the 100-base pair molecular marker in the 23S rRNA gene with subsequent sequencing of the 16S rRNA gene.

2. Materials and Methods

2.1. Sampling. A sampling was performed based on the spatial distribution of herds positive for bovine tuberculosis in the state of Mexico conducted by Zaragoza et al. 2015 [20]. Four herds of cattle were selected in the south region of the State of Mexico, one herd belonging to the Municipality of Temascaltepec and three herds belonging to the municipality of Zacazonapan. A total of 103 samples, 35 milk samples and 68 samples of nasal exudate, were collected. The distribution of the number and type of samples collected in each herd is shown in Table 1.

2.2. Obtaining Samples of Milk and Nasal Exudate. The udder and nipples were cleansed with purified water and soap and then dried with paper towels, and nipple asepsis was subsequently performed using swabs soaked in 70% alcohol. Five milliliters of milk was collected directly from the nipple in sterile 20 mL vessels, discarding the initial flow. Nasal exudate was collected directly from the inside of the nasal orifice using a 10 cm long sterile swab, which was then submerged in an isotonic saline solution (0.85%). Samples of milk and nasal exudate were stored at 4°C until processing.

2.3. Sample Processing

2.3.1. Isolation of Mycobacteria. The milk samples were centrifuged at 2500 revolutions per minute (rpm) for 10 minutes. The pellets from the milk and nasal exudate samples were inoculated into the following culture medium selective for mycobacteria: Stonebrink (BD BBL 220504), Middlebrook (BD BBL 254521), and Middlebrook (BD BBL 254521) supplemented with 6 g of sodium pyruvate per liter (Middlebrook-P). The inoculated media were incubated at 37°C for 8 weeks and were assessed every 3 days.

2.3.2. Classification of Isolated Strains. The isolated strains were distributed in groups according to the following characteristics: colony pigmentation, growth time, and colony characteristics (shape, consistency, texture, and pigment production). Isolated strains were stained with Ziehl-Neelsen to confirm the presence of acid-fast bacilli (AFB) [21].

2.4. DNA Extraction. Strains with microscopic characteristics similar to mycobacteria (acid-fast positivity) and two representative strains of each group were selected for identification. To obtain biomass, the strains were inoculated into 30 mL of Middlebrook liquid culture medium (BD BBL 254521) in 125 mL flasks and incubated at 37°C for 7 days. The liquid medium was transferred to sterile 15 mL Falcon tubes and centrifuged for 15 minutes at 14,000 rpm. Then, the supernatant was removed and the pellet was transferred to 1.5 mL Eppendorf tubes; the tubes were then centrifuged at 14,000 rpm × 5 minutes, and the supernatant was discarded. DNA extraction was performed on the resulting pellet using the Wizard Genomic DNA Purification kit (Promega A1120).

TABLE 1: Samples collected in cattle herds in the south region of the State of Mexico.

Characteristic	Herd 1	Herd 2	Herd 3	Herd 4	Total
Municipality	Temascaltepec	Zacazonapan	Zacazonapan	Zacazonapan	
Breed	F1 Swiss-Cebu	Holstein Friesian	Holstein Friesian	Holstein Friesian	
Geographic location	La-19°03'13.7"Lo-100°13'36.7"	La-19°03'39.5"Lo-100°16'30.9"	La-19°04'0.4"Lo-100°15'11.5"	La-19°03'41"Lo-100°16'06"	
History of bTB	Prevalence 0.2%*	Prevalence 0.2%*	Prevalence 0.2%*	Prevalence 0.2%*	
Samples obtained					
Milk	15	20	0	0	35
Nasal exudate	0	18	23	27	68
					103

La: latitude; Lo: longitude; bTB: bovine tuberculosis. *Information obtained from the Committee on the Promotion and Protection of Livestock of the State of Mexico.

2.5. Detection of the Molecular Marker in the 23S rRNA Gene.
The 100 bp molecular marker located on the 23S rRNA gene was amplified according to the methodology described by Roller et al. (1992) using the following primers [8]:

23S InsF, 5′-(AC)A(AGT)GCGTAG(AGCT)CG-A(AT)GG-3′, and 23S InsR, 5′-GTG(AT)CGGTT-T(AGCT)(GCT)GGTA-3′.

The reaction was conducted using a commercial Taq DNA polymerase (Promega M1661). The following thermal cycle conditions were used: a predenaturation step for 5 minutes (94°C); 29 cycles of denaturation for 30 seconds (94°C), hybridization for 45 seconds (46°C), and elongation for 50 seconds (72°C); and, finally, a postelongation cycle of 5 minutes (72°C). The amplified fragments were confirmed on a 2% agarose gel stained with ethidium bromide (SIGMA 46065).

2.6. Amplification of the 16S rRNA Gene. Strains that amplified the 100 bp phylogenetic marker were selected for 16S rRNA sequencing analysis. The following primers were used for the amplification:

8f: AGAGTTTGATCMTGGCTCAG and 1492r: TAC-GGYTACCTTGTTACGACTT.

The reaction was conducted using a commercial Taq DNA polymerase (Promega M1661). The following thermal cycle conditions were used: one predenaturation step for 5 minutes (94°C); 34 cycles of denaturation for 30 seconds (94°C), hybridization for 20 seconds (52°C), and elongation for 1 minute 30 seconds (72°C); and, finally, a postelongation cycle of 7 minutes (72°C).

The amplified fragments were confirmed on a 1% agarose gel stained with ethidium bromide (SIGMA 46065). The products of this amplification were purified using the Amicon Ultra Filter® kit (Millipore UFC901008) and confirmed on a 1% agarose gel to verify their presence and quality.

2.7. Identification of Mycobacterium Species. The amplified products of the 16S rRNA gene were sent to the Macrogen Sequencing Service, Maryland, USA. The obtained sequences were analyzed and corrected using the BioEdit program [22]. Consensus sequences were constructed from the forward and reverse fragments, which were compared with sequences deposited previously in GenBank of the National Center for Biotechnology Information (NCBI) using the BLAST program [23] and EzTaxon 2.1 [24].

2.8. Phylogenetic Analysis. Sequences of the 16S rRNA gene were obtained for the following mycobacterial species from the American Type Culture Collection (ATCC) and the German Collection of Microorganisms and Cell Cultures (DSM): *M. neoaurum* ATCC[25795], *M. parafortuitum* DSM[43528], *M. moriokaense* DSM[44221T], and *M. confluentis* DSM[44017T]. The sequences of the collection strains and those of the strains isolated in the present investigation were aligned with the BioEdit program [22]. Phylogenetic analysis was performed using the maximum parsimony method in MEGA software version 4 [25]. To form the root of the cladogram, the sequence of *Pantoea agglomerans* DSM 3493 was used.

3. Results

The 108 strains isolated from the 103 collected samples were distributed in 13 groups according to their macroscopic and microscopic morphological characteristics (Table 2). Groups 11 and 12, particularly, were composed of acid-fast strains.

For identification at the species level, 39 strains were chosen: 10 of them belonged to group 11 and 7 to group 12. Two strains from each one of the remaining 11 groups were selected to complete the 39 strains. The 100 bp molecular marker was found in the 33% (13/39) of the selected strains. For them, the 16S rRNA gene was amplified for sequencing and identification at the species level.

The overall prevalence of NTM on the collected samples was 12.6% (13/103) considering both milk and nasal exudate samples. However, the specific prevalence for nasal exudate samples was 19.1% (13/68).

According to the sequence comparison, four NTM species of the genus *Mycobacterium* were identified; 64% (6/13) of the strains had 98% and 99% of similarities with *M. neoaurum*, while 31% (4/13) had 99% similarity with *M. parafortuitum*, 15% (2/13) had similarities of 98% and 99% with

TABLE 2: Isolated strains are grouped according to their morphological characteristics and the presence of the molecular marker (100 bp) on the 23S rRNA gene.

| Group | Number of Strains | Morphological characteristics | | | Molecular marker (bp) |
| | | Macroscopic | | Microscopic | 23S rRNA |
		Pigmentation	Appearance	Ziehl-Neelsen	
1	29	Yellow	Creamy	−	250
2	10	White	Creamy	−	250
3	14	White	Dry	−	250
4	2	Salmon	Creamy	−	250
5	2	Salmon	Dry	−	250
6	2	White, dark	Creamy	−	250
7	2	White	Creamy	−	250
8	3	White, dark	Dry	−	250
9	4	White	Dry	−	250
10	10	White	Creamy, dry	−	250
11	10	White	Dry	+	350 and 250
12	7	Yellow	Creamy	+	350
13	13	White	Dry	−	250

−: absence of acid-fast bacilli; +: presence of acid-fast bacilli; Bp: base pairs.

TABLE 3: Comparison of 16S rRNA gene sequences of strains isolated from cattle with those documented in GenBank, using BLAST and EzTaxon.

Strain	Origin of the herd	Culture medium	Amplified fragment size (bp)	Similarity (Blast)	%	Similarity (EzTaxon)	%
1-AZ	2	Middlebrook	1428	M. neoaurum	98	M. neoaurum	98.3
2-AZ	2	Stonebrink	1408	M. neoaurum	99	M. neoaurum	99.1
3-AZ	2	Stonebrink	1428	M. neoaurum	98	M. neoaurum	98.2
5-AZ	3	Stonebrink	1416	M. neoaurum	99	M. neoaurum	99.2
8-AZ	4	Middlebrook	1415	M. neoaurum	99	M. neoaurum	99.0
12-AZ	2	Middlebrook	1415	M. neoaurum	99	M. neoaurum	99.4
4-AZ	4	Middlebrook-P	1420	M. parafortuitum	99	M. parafortuitum	98.2
9-AZ	3	Middlebrook	1415	M. parafortuitum	99	M. parafortuitum	98.9
10-AZ	4	Stonebrink	1411	M. parafortuitum	99	M. parafortuitum	98.4
11-AZ	3	Stonebrink	1414	M. parafortuitum	99	M. parafortuitum	98.2
6-AZ	2	Stonebrink	1455	M. moriokaense	99	M. moriokaense	98.2
13-AZ	4	Stonebrink	1417	M. moriokaense	98	M. moriokaense	98.2
7-AZ	2	Middlebrook-P	1420	M. confluentis	99	M. confluentis	99.1

2: Zacazonapan Holstein-F; 3: Zacazonapan Holstein-F; 4: Zacazonapan Holstein-F.

M. moriokaense, and, finally, 8% (1/13) had 99% similarity with *M. confluentis* (Table 3).

The phylogenetic tree was formed with the genus *Mycobacterium* and four of its species by which the phylogenetic relationships between the collection strains and the strains isolated in the present investigation were observed (Figure 1).

4. Discussion

The NTM species were isolated from samples of nasal exudate only, which eliminated the samples from one of the local farms of this study (Table 1). We found that the specific prevalence was 19.1% in herds of the south region of the State of Mexico. Similar studies in the United States, South Africa, Tanzania, and Brazil reported NTM prevalence values of

3.4%, 24.5%, 7%, and 7.8%, respectively; therefore, the prevalence value found in this study lies within the range reported previously [26–29]. In this study, 13 of the 39 analyzed strains were identified as the NTM species *M. neoaurum, M. moriokaense, M. confluentis*, and *M. parafortuitum*.

M. neoaurum, a member of the *Mycobacterium parafortuitum* complex, is responsible for a broad spectrum of illnesses, most of them device related infections such as Hickman catheters, BROVIAC catheters, PICC lines [30–33], arteriovenous fistula that included a polytetrafluoroethylene graft [34], pace makers [35], and prosthetic valve endocarditis [36]. Immunocompromised patients holding these devices are the principal hosts, for example, patients suffering from cancer [32] and diabetics with renal failure [31, 33, 34] and heart problems [35]. *M. neoaurum* has also been isolated from

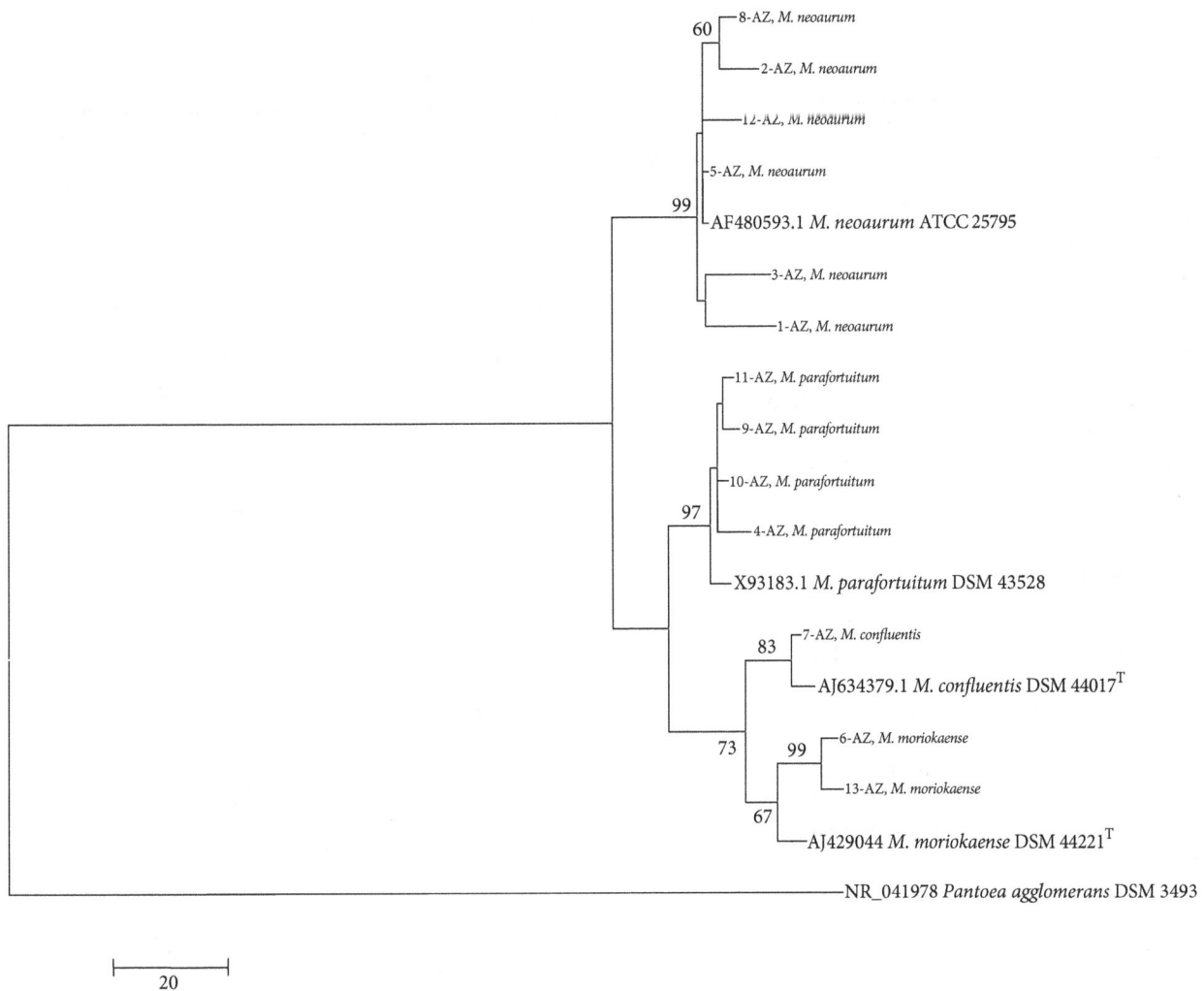

FIGURE 1: Phylogenetic tree constructed by comparing the 16S rRNA gene sequences from the isolated and reference strains.

patients with urinary infections [37], meningoencephalitis and alterations in the central nervous system [38], bacteremia and endocarditis [39], and pulmonary infection [40, 41]. Although it has been mainly isolated from clinical cases, there are also reports about its isolation from milk and cattle [28, 42, 43].

M. moriokaense was isolated from sputum sample [44]. Although it is considered nonpathogenic for humans, it has been associated with pulmonary diseases [45]. *M. confluentis* was isolated from sputum samples as well [46], and, along with *M. parafortuitum*, both are considered nonpathogenic species. *M. confluentis*, *M. moriokaense*, and *M. neoaurum* have been isolated from different bovine and wildlife tissues with tuberculous lesions, whereas *M. parafortuitum* has only been isolated from bovine milk [26, 28, 47–49]. However, in our work, *M. parafortuitum* was only isolated from nasal exudate samples.

The nutritional requirements of mycobacteria differ among various species, which was the reason for using different culture media. Notably, seven of the 13 strains identified in this study were isolated in Stonebrink medium, including

M. neoaurum, M. parafortuitum, and *M. moriokaense.* This result is consistent with that described by Sepúlveda et al. [50] who indicated that Stonebrink medium is suitable for the recovery of different species of the genus *Mycobacterium.* García-Martos and García-Agudo [51] reported that Middlebrook medium is optimal for the isolation of actinomycetes, which is in accord with the present investigation considering that two species, *M. neoaurum* and *M. parafortuitum*, were isolated in this medium. Notably, *M. confluentis* was isolated only in Middlebrook medium supplemented with sodium pyruvate; thus, the strategy of using different culture media was appropriate because it allowed the isolation of different species of the genus *Mycobacterium.*

The detection of the molecular marker present in the 23S rRNA gene of Gram-positive bacteria with HGC content allowed discrimination between strains of eubacteria and mycobacteria. The sequencing analysis of the 16S rRNA gene made the identification at the species level possible; therefore, the combination of these methodologies is appropriate for the identification of NTM species.

5. Conclusions

Using the methodology described in this study, four NTM species were isolated and identified: *M. confluentis, M. moriokaense, M. neoaurum,* and *M. parafortuitum.* These species were isolated for the first time from nasal exudates of bovines from the south region of the State of Mexico. Three of the identified species (*M. neoaurum, M. moriokaense,* and *M. confluentis*) are of public health and veterinary importance.

Disclosure

This work is derived from the thesis for the degree of Doctorate in Health Sciences (Universidad Autónoma del Estado de México), registered in the PNPC-CONACYT.

Acknowledgments

The authors would like to acknowledge the financial assistance from the Secretary of Research and Advanced Studies of Universidad Autónoma del Estado de México (UAEMex) through the following research grants: (i) "Implementation of Geographic Information Systems and Techniques of Molecular Biology, as tools in the detection and identification of *Mycobacterium* spp.," SIEA-UAEM 3486/2013CHT, and (ii) the network "Microbiología y química en las Ciencias de la Salud," 039/2014RIF.

References

[1] A. Aranaz, D. Cousins, A. Mateos, and L. Domínguez, "Elevation of *Mycobacterium tuberculosis* subsp. caprae Aranaz et al. 1999 to species rank as *Mycobacterium caprae* comb. nov., sp. nov," *International Journal of Systematic and Evolutionary Microbiology*, vol. 53, no. 6, pp. 1785–1789, 2003.

[2] M. H. Ho, C. K. Ho, and L. Y. Chong, "Atypical mycobacterial cutaneous infections in Hong Kong: 10-Year retrospective study," *Hong Kong Medical Journal*, vol. 12, no. 1, pp. 21–26, 2006.

[3] SAGARPA, "Norma Oficial Méxicana NOM-ZOO-031-1995 Campaña Nacional contra la Tuberculosis bovina *(M. bovis),*" *Diario Oficial de la Federación*, vol. 1996, pp. 12–32, 1995.

[4] O. R. G. Llamazares, C. B. G. Martín, D. A. Nistal, V. A. D. L. P. Redondo, L. D. Rodríguez, and E. F. R. Ferri, "Field evaluation of the single intradermal cervical tuberculin test and the interferon-γ assay for detection and eradication of bovine tuberculosis in Spain," *Veterinary Microbiology*, vol. 70, no. 1-2, pp. 55–66, 1999.

[5] SENASICA, "Informes de la Situación Zoosanitaria Nacional de 2016," 2016, http://www.gob.mx/cms/uploads/attachment/file/169575/SITUACION_ZOOSANITARIA_2016-11-8.pdf.

[6] M. D. Cave, K. D. Eisenach, P. F. McDermott, J. H. Bates, and J. T. Crawford, "IS6110: Conservation of sequence in the Mycobacterium tuberculosis complex and its utilization in DNA fingerprinting," *Molecular and Cellular Probes*, vol. 5, no. 1, pp. 73–80, 1991.

[7] S. R. Acosta, C. C. Estrada, and S. F. Milián, "Tipificación de cepas de *Mycobacterium bovis,*" *Técnica Pecuaria en México*, vol. 47, pp. 389–412, 2009.

[8] C. Roller, W. Ludwig, and K. H. Schleifer, "Gram-positive bacteria with a high DNA G+C content are characterized by a common insertion within their 23S rRNA genes," *Journal of General Microbiology*, vol. 138, no. 6, pp. 1167–1175, 1992.

[9] B. A. Zaragoza, C. M. Á. Karam, M. L. P. Bustamante, T. Á. H. Sandoval, and D. N. Ramírez, "Marcador molecular de actinomicetos utilizado para detectar micobacterias en muestras de esputo," *Revista Mexicana de Ciencias Farmacéuticas*, vol. 45, pp. 35–40, 2014.

[10] J. E. Clarridge, "Impact of 16S rRNA gene sequence analysis for identification of bacteria on clinical microbiology and infectious diseases," *Clinical Microbiology Reviews*, vol. 17, no. 4, pp. 840–862, 2004.

[11] D. O. Sanjay, M. D. Avani, and D. O. James, "Atypical *Mycobacterial cutaneous* infections," *Dermatologic Clinics*, vol. 27, no. 1, pp. 63–73, 2009.

[12] S. Weitzul, P. J. Eichhorn, and A. G. Pandya, "Nontuberculous mycobacterial infections of the skin," *Dermatologic Clinics*, vol. 18, no. 2, pp. 359–377, 2000.

[13] H. M. Al-Abdely, S. G. Revankar, and J. R. Graybill, "Disseminated *Mycobacterium simiae* infection in patients with AIDS," *Journal of Infection*, vol. 41, no. 2, pp. 143–147, 2000.

[14] H.-S. Jang, J.-H. Jo, C.-K. Oh et al., "Successful treatment of localized cutaneous infection caused by *Mycobacterium scrofulaceum* with clarithromycin," *Pediatric Dermatology*, vol. 22, no. 5, pp. 476–479, 2005.

[15] J. J. Meyer and S. S. Gelman, "Multifocal osteomyelitis due to *Mycobacterium szulgai* in a patient with chronic lymphocytic leukemia," *Journal of Infection*, vol. 56, no. 2, pp. 151–154, 2008.

[16] D. Wagner and L. S. Young, "Nontuberculous mycobacterial infections: a clinical review," *Journal of Infection*, vol. 32, no. 5, pp. 257–270, 2004.

[17] K. P. Redbord, D. A. Shearer, H. Gloster et al., "Atypical *Mycobacterium furunculosis* occurring after pedicures," *Journal of the American Academy of Dermatology*, vol. 54, no. 3, pp. 520–524, 2006.

[18] P. Tang, S. Walsh, C. Murray et al., "Outbreak of acupuncture-associated cutaneous *Mycobacterium abscessus* infections," *Journal of Cutaneous Medicine and Surgery*, vol. 10, no. 4, pp. 166–169, 2006.

[19] INEGI, "Censo Agrícola, Ganadero y Forestal 2007," 2007, http://www.inegi.org.mx/est/contenidos/proyectos/Agro/ca2007/Resultados_Agricola/default.aspx.

[20] B. A. Zaragoza, M. L. P. Bustamante, T. Á. H. Sandoval, and D. N. Ramírez, "Spatial analysis of bovine tuberculosis in the State of Mexico, Mexico," *Veterinaria Italiana*, vol. 53, no. 1, pp. 29–37, 2017.

[21] OPS, "Organización Panamericana de la Salud para el diagnóstico bacteriológico de la tuberculosis, Normas y guía técnica," Parte I Basiloscopia, 2008.

[22] T. A. Hall, "BioEdit: a user. friendly biologycal sequence alignment editor ana analysis program for Windows 95/98/NT," *Nucleic Acids Symposium Series*, vol. 41, no. 41, pp. 95–98, 1999.

[23] S. F. Altschul, T. L. Madden, J. Zhang, Z. Zhang, W. Miller, and D. J. Lipman, "Gapped BLAST and PSI-BLAST: a new generation of protein database search programs," *Nucleic Acids Research*, vol. 25, no. 17, pp. 389–402, 1997.

[24] J. Chun, J.-H. Lee, Y. Jung et al., "EzTaxon: a web-based tool for the identification of prokaryotes based on 16S ribosomal RNA gene sequences," *International Journal of Systematic and Evolutionary Microbiology*, vol. 57, no. 10, pp. 2259–2261, 2007.

[25] K. Tamura, J. Dudley, M. Nei, and S. Kumar, "MEGA4: molecular evolutionary genetics analysis (MEGA) software version 4.0," *Molecular Biology and Evolution*, vol. 24, no. 8, pp. 1596–1599, 2007.

[26] T. C. Thacker, S. Robbe-Austerman, B. Harris, M. V. Palmer, and W. R. Waters, "Isolation of mycobacteria from clinical samples collected in the United States from 2004 to 2011," *BMC Veterinary Research*, vol. 9, pp. 100–110, 2013.

[27] N. Gcebe, V. Rutten, N. C. Gey van Pittius, and A. Michel, "Prevalence and distribution of non-tuberculous mycobacteria (NTM) in cattle, African buffaloes (syncerus caffer) and their environments in South Africa," *Transboundary and Emerging Diseases*, vol. 60, supplement 1, pp. 74–84, 2013.

[28] B. Z. Katale, E. V. Mbugi, L. Botha et al., "Species diversity of non-tuberculous mycobacteria isolated from humans, livestock and wildlife in the Serengeti ecosystem, Tanzania," *BMC Infectious Diseases*, vol. 14, no. 1, pp. 1–8, 616, 2014.

[29] M. M. J. Franco, A. C. Paes, M. G. Ribeiro et al., "Occurrence of mycobacteria in bovine milk samples from both individual and collective bulk tanks at farms and informal markets in the southeast region of Sao Paulo, Brazil," *BMC Veterinary Research*, vol. 9, pp. 1–8, 2013.

[30] L. L. Washer, J. Riddell, J. Rider, and C. E. Chenoweth, "*Mycobacterium neoaurum* bloodstream infection: report of 4 cases and review of the literature," *Clinical Infectious Diseases*, vol. 45, no. 2, pp. e10–e13, 2007.

[31] H. Awadh, M. Mansour, and M. Shorman, "Bacteremia with an unusual pathogen: *Mycobacterium neoaurum*," *Case Reports in Infectious Diseases*, vol. 2016, Article ID 5167874, 3 pages, 2016.

[32] M. B. Davison, J. G. McCormack, Z. M. Blacklock, D. J. Dawson, M. H. Tilse, and F. B. Crimmins, "Bacteremia caused by *Mycobacterium neoaurum*," *Journal of Clinical Microbiology*, vol. 26, pp. 762–764, 1988.

[33] C.-C. Lai, C.-K. Tan, C.-C. Chen, and P.-R. Hsueh, "*Mycobacterium neoaurum* infection in a patient with renal failure," *International Journal of Infectious Diseases*, vol. 13, no. 5, pp. e276–e278, 2009.

[34] M. L. Becker, A. A. Suchak, J. N. Wolfe, R. Zarychanski, A. Kabani, and L. E. Nicolle, "*Mycobacterium neoaurum* bacteremia in a hemodialysis patient," *Canadian Journal of Infectious Diseases*, vol. 14, no. 1, pp. 45–48, 2003.

[35] E. J. Hayton, O. Koch, M. Scarborough, N. Sabharwal, F. Drobniewski, and I. C. Bowler, "Rapidly growing mycobacteria as emerging pathogens in bloodstream and device-related infection: a case of pacemaker infection with *Mycobacterium neoaurum*," *JMM Case Reports*, vol. 2, no. 1–3, 2015.

[36] A. Kumar, G. S. Pazhayattil, A. Das, and H. A. Conte, "*Mycobacterium neoaurum* causing prosthetic valve endocarditis: a case report and review of the literature," *Brazilian Journal of Infectious Diseases*, vol. 18, no. 2, pp. 235–237, 2014.

[37] S. Zanetti, R. Faedda, G. Fadda et al., "Isolation and identification of *Mycobacterium neoaurum* from a patient with urinary infection," *New Microbiologica*, vol. 24, no. 2, pp. 189–192, 2001.

[38] G. A. Heckman, C. Hawkins, A. Morris, L. L. Burrows, and C. Bergeron, "Rapidly progressive dementia due to *Mycobacterium neoaurum* meningoencephalitis," *Emerging Infectious Diseases*, vol. 10, no. 5, pp. 924–927, 2004.

[39] B. A. Brown-Elliott, R. J. Wallace Jr., C. A. Petti et al., "*Mycobacterium neoaurum* and *Mycobacterium bacteremicum* sp. nov. as causes of mycobacteremia," *Journal of Clinical Microbiology*, vol. 48, no. 12, pp. 4377–4385, 2010.

[40] Y. Morimoto, E. D. Chan, L. Heifets, and J. M. Routes, "Pulmonary infection with *Mycobacterium neoaurum* identified by 16S ribosomal DNA sequence," *Journal of Infection*, vol. 54, no. 4, pp. e227–e231, 2007.

[41] C.-K. Kim, S. I. Choi, B. R. Jeon, Y.-W. Lee, Y. K. Lee, and H. B. Shin, "Pulmonary infection caused by mycobacterium neoaurum: the first case in Korea," *Annals of Laboratory Medicine*, vol. 34, no. 3, pp. 243–246, 2014.

[42] S. A. Sgarioni, R. D. C. Hirata, M. Hiroyuki Hirata et al., "Occurrence of *Mycobacterium bovis* and non-tuberculous mycobacteria (NTM) in raw and pasteurized milk in the northwestern region of Paraná, Brazil," *Brazilian Journal of Microbiology*, vol. 45, no. 2, pp. 707–711, 2014.

[43] L. Padya, N. Chin'Ombe, M. Magwenzi, J. Mbanga, V. Ruhanya, and P. Nziramasanga, "Molecular identification of *mycobacterium* species of public health importance in cattle in zimbabwe by 16S rRNA gene sequencing," *Open Microbiology Journal*, vol. 9, pp. 38–42, 2015.

[44] M. Tsukamura, I. Yano, and T. Imaeda, "*Mycobacterium moriokaense* sp. nov., a rapidly growing, nonphotochromogenic Mycobacterium," *International Journal of Systematic Bacteriology*, vol. 36, no. 2, pp. 333–338, 1986.

[45] A. Somoskovi and M. Salfinger, "Nontuberculous mycobacteria in respiratory infections: advances in diagnosis and identification," *Clinics in Laboratory Medicine*, vol. 34, no. 2, pp. 271–295, 2014.

[46] P. Kirschner, A. Teske, K.-H. Schroder, R. M. Kroppenstedt, J. Wolters, and E. C. Bottger, "*Mycobacterium confluentis* sp. nov," *International Journal of Systematic Bacteriology*, vol. 42, no. 2, pp. 257–262, 1992.

[47] M. Pate, U. Zajc, D. Kušar et al., "*Mycobacterium* spp. in wild game in Slovenia," *Veterinary Journal*, vol. 208, pp. 93–95, 2016.

[48] L. Botha, N. C. Gey van Pittius, and P. D. van Helden, "Mycobacteria and disease in Southern Africa," *Transboundary and Emerging Diseases*, vol. 60, no. 26, pp. 147–156, 2013.

[49] J. J. Camarena Miñana and R. González Pellicer, "Micobacterias atípicas y su implicación en patología infecciosa pulmonar," *Enfermedades Infecciosas y Microbiología Clínica*, vol. 29, no. 5, pp. 66–75, 2011.

[50] A. Sepúlveda, P. M. García, M. J. Rodríguez, A. Márquez, and J. L. Puerto, "Evaluación del medio de Stonebrink para la recuperación de micobacterias," *Revista de Diagnóstico Biológico*, vol. 50, pp. 189–192, 2001.

[51] P. García-Martos and L. García-Agudo, "Infecciones por micobacterias de crecimiento rápido," *Enfermedades Infecciosas y Microbiología Clínica*, vol. 30, no. 4, pp. 192–200, 2012.

5

Multidrug-Resistant Bacteria Associated with Cell Phones of Healthcare Professionals in Selected Hospitals in Saudi Arabia

Saeed Banawas [iD],[1] Ahmed Abdel-Hadi [iD],[1,2] Mohammed Alaidarous [iD],[1] Bader Alshehri,[1] Abdul Aziz Bin Dukhyil,[1] Mohammed Alsaweed,[1] and Mohamed Aboamer[3]

[1]*Department of Medical Laboratory Sciences, College of Applied Medical Sciences, Majmaah University, Majmaah 11952, Saudi Arabia*
[2]*Department of Botany and Microbiology, Faculty of Science, Al-Azhar University, Assuit Branch, Cairo, Egypt*
[3]*Department of Medical Equipment Technology, College of Applied Medical Sciences, Majmaah University, Majmaah 11952, Saudi Arabia*

Correspondence should be addressed to Saeed Banawas; s.banawas@mu.edu.sa

Academic Editor: José A. Oteo

Cell phones may be an ideal habitat for colonization by bacterial pathogens, especially in hot climates, and may be a reservoir or vehicle in transmitting nosocomial infections. We investigated bacterial contamination on cell phones of healthcare workers in three hospitals in Saudi Arabia and determined antibacterial resistance of selected bacteria. A questionnaire was submitted to 285 healthcare workers in three hospitals, and information was collected on cell phone usage at the work area and in the toilet, cell phone cleaning and sharing, and awareness of cell phones being a source of infection. Screening on the Vitek 2 Compact system (bioMérieux Inc., USA) was done to characterize bacterial isolates. Of the 60 samples collected from three hospitals, 38 (63.3%) were positive with 38 bacterial isolates (4 Gram-negative and 34 Gram-positive bacteria). We found 38.3% of cell phones were contaminated with coagulase-negative staphylococci, particularly *Staphylococcus epidermidis* (10 isolates). Other bacterial agents identified were *S. aureus*, *S. hominis*, *Alloiococcus otitis*, *Vibrio fluvialis*, and *Pseudomonas stutzeri*. Antimicrobial susceptibility testing showed that most coagulase-negative staphylococci were resistant to benzylpenicillin, erythromycin, and rifampicin. Eight isolates were resistant to oxacillin, specifically *S. epidermidis* (3), *S. hominis* (2), and *S. warneri* (2). *A. otitis*, a cause of acute otitis media showed multidrug resistance. One isolate, a confirmed hetero-vancomycin intermediate-resistant *S. aureus*, was resistant to antibiotics, commonly used to treat skin infection. There was a significant correlation between the level of contamination and usage of cell phone at toilet and sharing. Our findings emphasize the importance of hygiene practices in cell phone usage among healthcare workers in preventing the transmission of multidrug-resistant microbes.

1. Introduction

The popularity of cell phones with healthcare professionals and lack of antiseptic practices make them potential routes of transmission of bacterial pathogens [1]. It has been reported that inanimate objects used by healthcare workers including cell phones act as important origins of nosocomial infections [2]. The cell phones of healthcare workers may act as reservoirs of nosocomial pathogens, which can be easily transmitted from the cell phone by the hands of a healthcare worker, thereby spreading bacterial isolates from one patient to another in various hospital wards [3]. Nosocomial infections are associated with significant morbidity and mortality. Studies have shown that the most common bacteria are coagulase-negative staphylococci, *Escherichia coli*, and *Pseudomonas* [4] Coagulase-negative staphylococci can invade the human body and cause serious infections, including hospital-acquired blood stream and skin infections [5]. The increasing significance of multidrug-resistant strains including staphylococci, among other etiologic agents of nosocomial infections, imposes on researchers the need to seek possible ways in the spread of these pathogens and ensure their robust and effective prevention. Therefore, the aim of the study was isolation and identification of bacteria from mobile phones. Moreover, we determined antibiotic resistance of the isolates.

2. Materials and Methods

2.1. Study Setting. This study was performed in three selected hospitals in Riyadh Province, Saudi Arabia. Sixty swab samples were collected from the cell phones of those volunteers who consented for two months between September and November 2017. Swab samples were collected by swabbing the top portion of the cell phones using the BD BBL™ culture swab™ collection and transport systems [6]. Aseptic practices were followed during the sampling process. Of the 60 samples collected, 23 samples were obtained from hospital A, 20 samples were from hospital B, and 17 samples were from hospital C. In addition, written informed consent was signed by all healthcare workers prior to sample collection. Deanship of Scientific Research at Majmaah University approved the study with approval ethical number (MUREC-Sept.25/COM-2017/120).

2.2. Bacterial Isolation and Characterization. Collected swab samples were inoculated on 5% sheep blood agar and MacConkey agar (Oxoid, UK) and incubated at 37°C for 48 hours. Different colonies were subcultured on nutrient agar and 5% sheep blood agar to get pure colonies of the isolates. The preliminary identification of all isolates was done using Gram stain and different biochemical tests including catalase, oxidase and coagulase tests [6].

2.3. Bacterial Identification. Identification of isolated bacteria at the species level was performed with the Vitek 2 Compact system (bioMérieux Inc., USA) according to the manufacturer's instruction. A bacterial suspension of each isolate was prepared by mixing the bacterial colony growing on blood agar with 0.45% saline sodium chloride solution to obtain a concentration of 0.5–0.63 McFarland units using the VITEK DensiCHEK™ colorimeter (bioMérieux). The suspensions (2 mL) were automatically loaded into the VITEK 2 ID system (bioMérieux), using GP ID REF21342 and GN ID REF21341 cards for the identification of Gram-positive and Gram-negative bacteria, respectively and the version 07.01 release software. The cards were read by kinetic fluorescence measurement, and the results reported within 3 h [7]. Quality control for Vitek was done using Gram-positive bacteria (*Enterococcus casseliflavus* ATCC 700327 and *Staphylococcus saprophyticus* BAA-750) and Gram-negative bacteria (*Enterobacter hormaechei* ATCC 700323 and *Stenotrophomonas maltophilia* ATCC 17666). Skim milk growth medium (20%) was used to store the identified isolates and frozen at −20°C [8].

2.4. Antimicrobial Susceptibility Testing. To determine antimicrobial susceptibility testing for the isolates, 145 μL of the bacterial suspension was drawn into 3 mL of 0.45% saline solution to further adjust the bacterial cell density. Vitek cards were inoculated with the suspension vials and loaded into the Vitek 2 automated reader-incubator using AST-P580 (*S.* spp., *Enterococcus* spp., and *S. agalactiae*) and AST-N291 (Gram-negative bacilli) cards. Results were interpreted using Vitek 2 Compact software version 07.01 [7].

2.5. Questionnaire. We asked 285 healthcare workers in selected hospitals to complete a questionnaire, which included usage of cell phones at the work area and toilet, cleaning cell phones by disinfectants, and awareness that cell phones can serve as a source of infection.

2.6. Statistical Analysis. The correlation matrix by using Pearson's linear correlation coefficient [9] to discover the correlation between the contamination level and questionnaire variables (the usage of cell phones at the work area and toilet, cleaning cell phones by disinfectants, sharing, restriction of using cell phone at work, and awareness that cell phones can serve as a source of infection). The value of the correlation equal −1 indicates perfect negative correlation, and the value equal +1 indicates perfect positive correlation; p value < 0.05 was considered statistically significant.

3. Results and Discussion

3.1. Level of Contamination. The results showed that 38 (63.3%) of the 60 cell phone sample swabs collected from three hospitals were infected (Figure 1). Generally, the frequency of contaminated cell phones varied between the three selected hospitals, with the greatest contamination found in hospital A, where 18 (78.23%) of 23 samples were contaminated. Similarly, we found 70% (14/20) contamination in hospital B, while 35.39% (6/17) of cell phone sample swabs from hospital C were contaminated. Contamination of the healthcare environment coupled with nosocomial infections can lead to contamination of the cell phones of healthcare workers [10]. The hands of healthcare workers can be contaminated with different bacterial pathogens, and healthcare workers utilize cell phones in laboratories, hospital halls, operating rooms, and intensive care units [11]. Through every phone call, SMS, or other use, there is a risk that the cell phone comes into contact with contaminated areas of the human body by hand-to-hand contact or by hand to other areas, such as the mouth and ears [3]. Furthermore, cell phones may act as a favorable habitat for bacteria to colonize, especially under high temperature and humid conditions [12].

3.2. Bacterial Identification. Thirty-eight bacterial isolates belonging to coagulase-negative staphylococci (CNS) (60.5%), *Staphylococcus aureus* (2.6%), others Gram-positive (26.4%) including *Alloiococcus otitis*, *Micrococcus luteus*, *Globicatella sulfidifaciens*, *Kocuria rosea*, *Dermacoccus nishinomiyaensis* and *Facklamia hominis*), and Gram-negative bacteria (10.53%) including *Vibrio fluvialis*, *Alcaligenes faecalis*, *Acinetobacter lwoffii*, and *Pseudomonas stutzeri* were identified as cell phone contaminants. Eighteen isolates were isolated from hospital A and 14 isolates from hospital B, while only 6

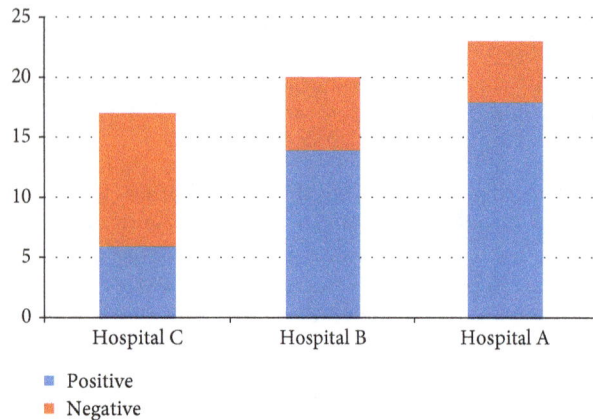

FIGURE 1: Bacterial frequency in collected samples from cell phones in selected hospitals.

isolates from hospital C. Samples from hospitals A and B had higher contamination rates than those from hospital C. In hospital A, 18 Gram-positive bacteria consisting of *S. hominis* subsp. *hominis* (18.4 %), *S. epidermidis* (18.4%), *S. capitis* (2.6%), *Micrococcus luteus* (2.6%), *Globicatella sulfidifaciens* (2.6%), and *Facklamia hominis* (2.6%) were identified. In hospital B, 11 Gram-positive bacteria, specifically *S. epidermidis* (5.3 %), *S. lentus* (2.6%), *M. luteus* (5.3%), *Alloiococcus otitis* (5.3%), *Dermacoccus nishinomiyaensis* (5.3%), and *Kocuria rosea* (2.6%), and 4 Gram-negative bacteria, specifically *Vibrio fluvialis* (2.6%), *Alcaligenes faecalis* subsp. *faecalis* (2.6%), *Acinetobacter lwoffii* (2.6%), and *Pseudomonas stutzeri* (2.6%), were identified. In hospital C, the 6 Gram-positive bacteria were identified as *S. aureus* (2.6%), *S. hominis* subsp. *hominis* (5.6%), *S. epidermidis* (2.6%), and *S. warneri* (5.3%) (Table 1).

Our study showed that coagulase-negative staphylococci were the most frequently isolated bacteria among healthcare workers (60.5%), particularly *S. epidermidis* and *S. hominis*. Our findings are similar to those of Zakai et al. [13] who reported coagulase-negative staphylococci were the most abundant isolates (68%) from contaminated cell phones of medical students in Saudi Arabia. It has been documented that handling contaminated inanimate objects during casual activities may cause hand-to-mouth transfer of pathogens. Furthermore, it has been predicted that cell phones can be an active origin of nosocomial infection as hand use to hold the phone comes in close contact with strongly contaminated body areas, such as the mouth, and ears [3]. In fact, nearly 30% of bacteria on cell phones are found on the hands of the owner [14]. Coagulase-negative staphylococci have the ability to create a biofilm on both animate and inanimate objects, which poses a particular threat for individuals receiving valve prostheses, implants, or catheters [15]. It was reported that coagulase-negative staphylococci are responsible for blood infections, of which *S. epidermidis* causes 67% of infections and other coagulase-negative staphylococci cause 33% [16].

3.3. Antimicrobial Susceptibility. Next, twenty-six Gram-positive bacteria were selected for antimicrobial

TABLE 1: Types of bacteria isolated from cell phones of healthcare workers in selected hospitals.

Total	Hospital C	Hospital B	Hospital A	Bacterium
1	1	—	—	*Staphylococcus aureus*
9	2	—	7	*Staphylococcus hominis* subsp. *hominis*
10	1	2	7	*Staphylococcus epidermidis*
1	—	1	—	*Staphylococcus lentus*
1	—	—	1	*Staphylococcus capitis*
2	2	—	—	*Staphylococcus warneri*
3	—	2	1	*Micrococcus luteus*
1	—	—	1	*Globicatella sulfidifaciens*
1	—	—	1	*Facklamia hominis*
2	—	2	—	*Alloiococcus otitis*
2	—	2	—	*Dermacoccus nishinomiyaensis*
1	—	1	—	*Kocuria rosea*
1	—	1	—	*Alcaligenes faecalis* subsp. *faecalis*
1	—	1	—	*Vibrio fluvialis*
1	—	1	—	*Acinetobacter lwoffii*
1	—	1	—	*Pseudomonas stutzeri*
38	6	14	18	**Total**

susceptibility testing including 15 isolates from hospital A (*S. hominis* subsp. *hominis* (7), *S. epidermidis* (7), and *S. capitis* (1)), 5 isolates from hospital B (*S. epidermidis* (2), *S. lentus* (1), and *A. otitis* (2)), and 6 isolates from hospital C (*S. aureus* (1), *S. hominis* subsp. *hominis* (2), *S. epidermidis* (1), and *S. warneri* (2)).

As shown in Table 2, our antimicrobial susceptibility results indicate that most of the coagulase-negative isolates from the three hospitals were resistant to benzylpenicillin (MIC ≥ 0.5), erythromycin (MIC ≥ 8), and fusidic acid (MIC ≥ 32), with intermediate resistance to rifampicin (MIC ≤ 0.5). Resistance to oxacillin (MIC ≥ 4) was observed in *S. epidermidis* (30 %), *S. hominis* (22.2%), *S. warneri* (100%), and *S. lentus* (100%). Similarly, Asaad et al. [17] reported that coagulase-negative staphylococci isolates from nosocomial bloodstream infections in Najran (Saudi Arabia) were highly resistant to penicillin, oxacillin, and erythromycin, exhibiting sensitivity to vancomycin and teicoplanin. It has been believed that coagulase-negative staphylococci are important reservoirs of antimicrobial resistance genes and resistance-associated mobile genetic elements, which can be transferred between staphylococcal species. *S. hominis*, *S. epidermidis*, and *S. haemolyticus* are reported to be multiple drug resistant coagulase-negative staphylococci [18, 19]. It was demonstrated that mecA gene is transferred from coagulase-negative staphylococcal species to *S. aureus* in vivo and has a role in emergence of more successful *S. aureus* clones, cell adherence, and invasion [20, 21].

Interestingly, one isolate was confirmed as hetero-vancomycin intermediate-resistant *S. aureus* (hVISA) by standard Etest methods [22]. It was resistant to antibiotics commonly used to treat skin infection including benzyl-penicillin (MIC ≥ 0.5), oxacillin (MIC ≥ 4), clindamycin (MIC $= 4$), and vancomycin (MIC $= 2$). A previous study

TABLE 2: Antibiotic susceptibility against selected Gram-positive bacteria.

Antibiotic	Staphylococcus aureus (1)			Staphylococcus hominis (9)			Staphylococcus epidermidis (10)			Staphylococcus lentus (1)			Staphylococcus warneri (2)			Alloiococcus otitis (2)		
	S	I	R	S	I	R	S	I	R	S	I	R	S	I	R	S	I	R
Benzylpenicillin	0	0	**1**	1	0	**8**	0	0	**10**	1	0	0	0	0	**2**	NA	NA	NA
Oxacillin	0	0	**1**	7	0	**2**	7	0	**3**	0	0	**1**	0	0	**2**	NA	NA	NA
Gentamicin	1	0	0	9	0	0	10	0	0	0	0	**1**	2	0	0	NA	NA	NA
Tobramycin	0	0	**1**	8	0	**1**	7	1	**2**	1	0	0	2	0	0	NA	NA	NA
Erythromycin	0	0	**1**	3	0	**6**	5	0	**5**	0	1	0	1	0	**1**	0	0	**2**
Clindamycin	1	0	0	6	0	**3**	7	0	**3**	0	0	**1**	2	0	0	0	0	**2**
Linezolid	1	0	0	9	0	0	10	0	0	1	0	0	2	0	0	2	0	0
Teicoplanin	1	0	0	7	2	0	8	2	0	1	0	0	2	0	0	0	0	**2**
Vancomycin	0	1	0	9	0	0	10	0	0	1	0	0	2	0	0	0	0	**2**
Tetracycline	1	0	0	5	0	**4**	8	0	**2**	1	0	0	2	0	0	2	0	0
Fosfomycin	0	0	**1**	0	0	**9**	8	0	**2**	0	0	**1**	0	0	**2**	NA	NA	NA
Fusidic acid	0	1	0	1	1	**7**	0	5	**5**	0	1	0	1	0	**1**	NA	NA	NA
Rifampicin	0	1	0	0	9	0	0	10	0	0	1	0	0	2	0	NA	NA	NA
Trimethoprim/sulfamethoxazole	1	0	0	9	0	0	10	0	0	1	0	0	2	0	0	0	2	0

Note. I, intermediate; NA, not applicable; R, resistant; S, susceptible. Values in brackets indicate number of isolates. Number of resistant isolates indicated in bold.

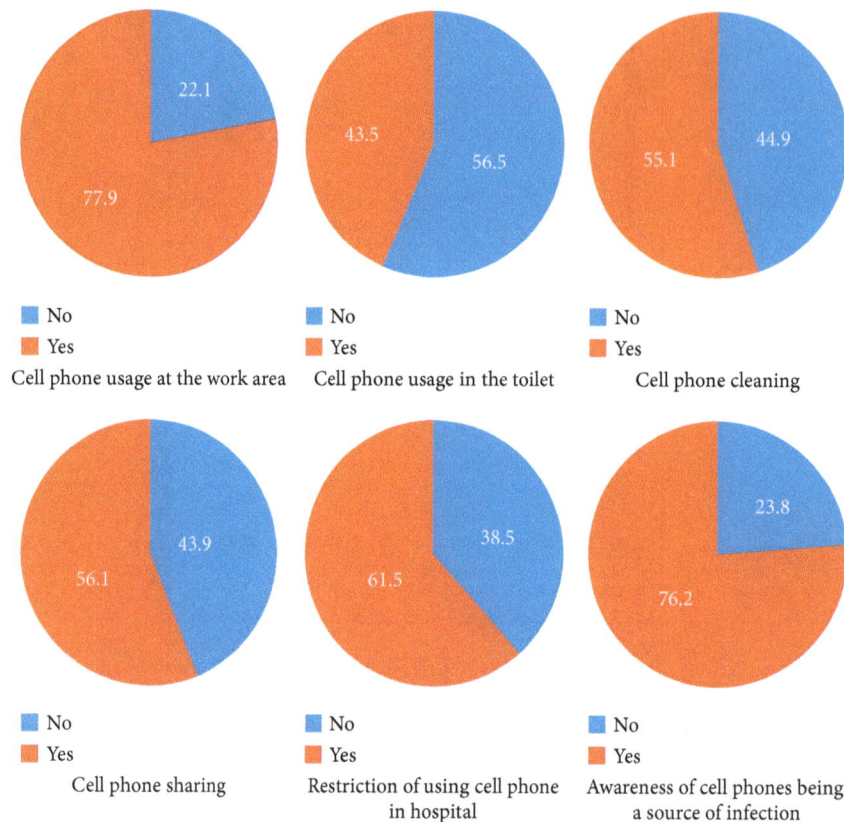

FIGURE 2: Survey results of cell phone use among healthcare workers ($n = 285$) at selected hospitals.

reported that hVISA may not only be associated with persistent bacteremia and treatment failure but may also be a precursor of the vancomycin intermediate *S. aureus* phenotype [23]. In Saudi Arabia, the occurrence of community- and hospital-acquired methicillin-resistant *S. aureus* infections is recorded; however, there are no available reports regarding hVISA [24].

We found that *A. otitis*, a cause of acute otitis media, was resistant to clindamycin (MIC = 4), erythromycin (MIC ≥ 8), vancomycin (MIC = 1), nitrofurantoin (MIC = 128), and teicoplanin (MIC = 4). *A. otitidis* has been frequently documented as one of the most prevalent bacteria in middle ear aspirates of patients with otitis media with effusion [25]. Recently, it was reported that *A. otitidis* plays a role in the pathogenesis of otitis media with effusion, in which it forms both single- and multi-species biofilms with other bacteria, thus promoting multidrug resistance [26].

3.4. Questionnaires. Based on completed questionnaires, we found that 222 (77.9%) participants used their cell phones at work, 160 (56.1%) shared their phone with colleagues, and 128 (44.9%) never cleaned their phones. In addition, 23.8% of participants (68/285) believed that cell phones could serve as a source of bacterial transmission, and over half of the participants (61.5%) reported that they agreed with restriction rules for using cell phones in the college. However, according to the opinions of participants, 110 (38.5%) did not agree with these rules (Figure 2).

Data on the correlation between contamination level and questionnaire variables are shown in Table 3. There was a significant correlation between the contamination level and usage of cell phone in toilet and sharing ($P < 0.05$). By contrast, no significant correlation was found between contamination level and the usage of cell phones at the work area, cleaning cell phones by disinfectants, restriction of using cell phone at work, and awareness that cell phones can serve as a source of infection. There was, however, a positive correlation between the contamination level and the usage of cell phones at the work area and cleaning cell phones by disinfectants. Mkrtchyan et al. [27] reported that *Staphylococcus* species are common toilets isolates, and 37.8% of the isolates were drug resistant which can be freely transferred to the environment. Bhoonderowa et al. [28] reported that sharing mobile phone within females was associated with high bacterial load. It was recommended by previous studies that the level of bacterial contamination on the cell phones of healthcare workers can be reduced by reduce sharing [29].

4. Conclusion

Our study demonstrably highlights that the cell phones of healthcare workers can be contaminated by a wide range of bacteria including multidrug resistance bacteria. Bacteria may be readily able to adhere to the surface of cell phones, and the heat emitted by the cell phone enhances bacterial growth. These bacteria can then be transferred to the owner

TABLE 3: Correlation between contamination of cell phone and questionnaire variables.

Contamination	Correlation	P value
Cell phone usage at work area	0.897	0.290
Cell phone usage in toilet	0.992	0.038*
Cell phone cleaning	0.830	0.375
Cell phone sharing	0.993	0.042*
Restriction of using cell phone at work	−0.961	0.176
Awareness of being a source of infection	−0.847	0.356

*Statistical analysis is significant, $P < 0.05$.

of the cell phone, patients, and the community. Based on our presented data, there is a lack of awareness of using cell phones in toilets and sharing among healthcare workers that may contribute to a significant risk of transmitting multidrug-resistant bacteria through unguarded cell phone use. The development of active preventive strategies is needed to reduce the risk of cross infection.

Authors' Contributions

Saeed Banawas and Ahmed Abdel-Hadi designed the study and drafted the manuscript. Bader Alshehri, Abdul Aziz Bin Dukhyil, and Mohammed Alsaweed contributed to the data collection. Ahmed Abdel-Hadi and Mohammed Alaidarous carried out sample collection, isolation, and identification of bacterial isolates. Saeed Banawas and Bader Alshehri were involved in sample collection, preparation of media, isolation, purification, and biochemical characterization of bacterial isolates. Abdul Aziz Bin Dukhyil, and Mohammed Alsaweed contributed to the identification of bacterial isolates, antimicrobial susceptibility testing, and data interpretation. Mohamed Aboamer carried out statistical analysis of the study. All authors approved the final version.

Acknowledgments

The authors thank the Deanship of Scientific Research and the Deanship of Community Service at Majmaah University, Kingdom of Saudi Arabia, for supporting this work. The authors thank Adil AL-Maqati, Abdullah Al-Rasheed, Abdulaziz Al-Anazi, Mohammad Almoharb, and Ahmad Alabdulwahab for participating in this work.

References

[1] O. Famurewa and O. David, "Cell phone: a medium of transmission of bacterial pathogens," World Rural Observations, vol. 1, pp. 69–72, 2009.

[2] A. A. Mahfouz, T. A. Al Azraqi, F. I. Abbag, M. N. Al Gamal, S. Seef, and C. S. Bello, "Nosocomial infections in a neonatal intensive care unit in south-western Saudi Arabia," Eastern Mediterranean Health Journal, vol. 16, no. 1, pp. 40–44, 2010.

[3] D. Mark, C. Leonard, H. Breen, R. Graydon, C. O'Gorman, and S. Kirk, "Mobile phones in clinical practice: reducing the risk of bacterial contamination," International Journal of Clinical Practice, vol. 68, no. 9, pp. 1060–1064, 2014.

[4] G. Ducel, J. Fabry, and L. Nicolle, Prevention of Hospital Acquired Infections: A Practical Guide, 2nd edition, 2002.

[5] A. Shittu, O. Oyedara, F. Abegunrin et al., "Characterization of methicillin-susceptible and –resistant staphylococci in the clinical setting: a multicentre study in Nigeria," BMC Infectious Diseases, vol. 12, no. 1, p. 286, 2012.

[6] K. O. Akinyemi, A. D. Atapu, O. O. Adetona, and A. O. Coker, "The potential role of mobile phones in the spread of bacterial infections," Journal of Infection in Developing Countries, vol. 3, no. 8, pp. 628–632, 2009.

[7] Y. Tian, B. Zheng, B. Wang, Y. Lin, and M. Li, "Rapid identification and multiple susceptibility testing of pathogens from positive-culture sterile body fluids by a combined MALDI-TOF mass spectrometry and vitek susceptibility system," Frontiers in Microbiology, vol. 7, p. 523, 2016.

[8] W. L. Cody, J. W. Wilson, D. R. Hendrixson et al., "Skim milk enhances the preservation of thawed −80°C bacterial stocks," Journal of Microbiological Methods, vol. 75, no. 1, pp. 135–138, 2008.

[9] C.-C. Lai, C.-C. Chu, A. Cheng, Y.-T. Huang, and P.-R. Hsueh, "Correlation between antimicrobial consumption and incidence of health-care-associated infections due to methicillin-resistant Staphylococcus aureus and vancomycin-resistant enterococci at a university hospital in Taiwan from 2000 to 2010," Journal of Microbiology, Immunology and Infection, vol. 48, no. 4, pp. 431–436, 2015.

[10] K. Fleming and J. Randle, "Toys-friend or foe? A study of infection risk in a paediatric intensive care," Pediatric Nursing, vol. 18, pp. 14–18, 2006.

[11] O. Karabay, E. Koçoglu, and M. Tahtaci, "The role of mobile phones in the spread of bacteria associated with nosocomial infections," Journal of Infection in Developing Countries, vol. 1, pp. 72–73, 2007.

[12] P. Srikanth, R. Ezhil, S. Suchitra, I. Anandhi, U. Maheswari, and J. Kalyani, "The mobile phone in a tropical setting emerging threat for infection control," in Proceedings of 13th International Congress on Infectious Diseases, Kuala Lumpur, Malaysia, June 2008.

[13] S. Zakai, A. Mashat, A. Abumohssin et al., "Bacterial contamination of cell phones of medical students at King Abdulaziz University, Jeddah, Saudi Arabia," Journal of Microscopy and Ultrastructure, vol. 4, no. 3, pp. 143–146, 2016.

[14] H. S. Selim and A. F. Abaza, "Microbial contamination of mobile phones in a healthcare setting in Alexandria, Egypt," GMS Hygiene and Infection Control, vol. 10, p. Doc03, 2015.

[15] M. Otto, "Staphylococcus epidermidis—the 'accidental' pathogen," Nature Reviews Microbiology, vol. 7, no. 8, pp. 555–567, 2009.

[16] S. G. Gatermann, T. Koschinski, and S. Friedrich, "Distribution and expression of macrolide resistance genes in coagulase-negative staphylococci," Clinical Microbiology and Infection, vol. 13, no. 8, pp. 777–781, 2007.

[17] A. M. Asaad, Q. M. Ansar, and H. S. Mujeeb, "Clinical significance of coagulase-negative staphylococci isolates from nosocomial bloodstream infections," Infectious Diseases, vol. 48, no. 5, pp. 356–360, 2016.

[18] O. Bouchami, W. Achour, M. A. Mekni, J. Rolo, and A. B. Hassen, "Antibiotic resistance and molecular characterization of clinical isolates of methicillin-resistant coagulase-negative staphylococci isolated from bacteremic patients in oncohematology," *Folia Microbiologica*, vol. 56, no. 2, pp. 122–130, 2011.

[19] K. Becker, C. Heilmann, and G. Peters, "Coagulase-negative staphylococci," *Clinical Microbiology Reviews*, vol. 27, no. 4, pp. 870–926, 2014.

[20] E. M. Harrison, G. K. Paterson, M. T. G. Holden et al., "A novel hybrid SCCmec-mecC region in *Staphylococcus sciuri*," *Journal of Antimicrobial Chemotherapy*, vol. 69, no. 4, pp. 911–918, 2013.

[21] E. Szczuka, S. Krzymińska, N. Bogucka, and A. Kaznowski, "Multifactorial mechanisms of the pathogenesis of methicillin-resistant *Staphylococcus hominis* isolated from bloodstream infections," *Antonie van Leeuwenhoek*, vol. 111, no. 7, pp. 1259–1265, 2017.

[22] S. W. Satola, M. M. Farley, K. F. Anderson, and J. B. Patel, "Comparison of detection methods for heteroresistant vancomycin-intermediate *Staphylococcus aureus*, with the population analysis profile method as the reference method," *Journal of Clinical Microbiology*, vol. 49, no. 1, pp. 177–183, 2010.

[23] A. M. Casapao, S. N. Leonard, S. L. Davis et al., "Clinical outcomes in patients with heterogeneous vancomycin-intermediate *Staphylococcus aureus* bloodstream infection," *Antimicrobial Agents and Chemotherapy*, vol. 57, no. 9, pp. 4252–4259, 2013.

[24] H. H. Abulreesh, S. R. Organji, G. E. H. Osman, K. Elbanna, M. H. K. Almalki, and I. Ahmad, "Prevalence of antibiotic resistance and virulence factors encoding genes in clinical *Staphylococcus aureus* isolates in Saudi Arabia," *Clinical Epidemiology and Global Health*, vol. 5, no. 4, pp. 196–202, 2017.

[25] C. L. Chan, D. Wabnitz, A. Bassiouni, P.-J. Wormald, S. Vreugde, and A. J. Psaltis, "Identification of the bacterial reservoirs for the middle ear using phylogenic analysis," *JAMA Otolaryngology–Head & Neck Surgery*, vol. 143, no. 2, pp. 155–161, 2017.

[26] C. Chan, K. Richter, P. Wormald, A. Psaltis, and S. Vreugde, "*Alloiococcus otitidis* forms multispecies biofilm with *Haemophilus influenzae*: effects on antibiotic susceptibility and growth in adverse conditions," *Front Cell Infect Microbiol*, vol. 7, p. 344, 2017.

[27] H. V. Mkrtchyan, C. A. Russell, N. Wang, and R. R. Cutler, "Could public restrooms Be an environment for bacterial resistomes?," *PLOS One*, vol. 8, no. 1, Article ID e54223, 2013.

[28] A. Bhoonderowa, S. Gookool, and S. D. Biranjia-Hurdoyal, "The importance of mobile phones in the possible transmission of bacterial infections in the community," *Journal of Community Health*, vol. 39, no. 5, pp. 965–967, 2014.

[29] M. Dogan, B. Feyzioglu, M. Ozdemir, and B. Baysal, "Investigation of microbial colonization of computer keyboards used inside and outside hospital environments," *Mikrobiyoloji Bülteni*, vol. 42, no. 2, pp. 331–336, 2008.

6

The Structure of *ampG* Gene in *Pseudomonas aeruginosa* and Its Effect on Drug Resistance

Qingli Chang,[1,3,4] Chongyang Wu,[1,3] Chaoqing Lin,[1,3] Peizhen Li,[3] Kaibo Zhang,[2] Lei Xu,[3] Yabo Liu,[3] Junwan Lu,[2] Cong Cheng,[2] Qiyu Bao,[1,3] Yunliang Hu,[1,3] Shunfei Lu ⓘ,[2] and Jinsong Li ⓘ[3]

[1]*The Second Affiliated Hospital and Yuying Children's Hospital, Wenzhou Medical University, Wenzhou 325027, China*
[2]*School of Medicine and Health, Lishui University, Lishui 323000, China*
[3]*School of Laboratory Medicine and Life Science, Institute of Biomedical Informatics, Wenzhou Medical University, Wenzhou 325035, China*
[4]*Department of Clinical Laboratory, The First Affiliated Hospital of Xinxiang Medical University, Xinxiang 453100, China*

Correspondence should be addressed to Shunfei Lu; lslsf@163.com and Jinsong Li; strongli72@sina.com

Academic Editor: Bruno Pozzetto

In order to study the relationship between the structure and function of AmpG, structure, site-specific mutation, and gene complementary experiments have been performed against the clinical isolates of *Pseudomonas aeruginosa*. We found that there are 51 nucleotide variations at 34 loci over the *ampG* genes from 24 of 35 *P. aeruginosa* strains detected, of which 7 nucleotide variations resulted in amino acid change. The *ampG* variants with the changed nucleotides (amino acids) could complement the function of *ampG* deleted PA01 (PA01ΔG). The ampicillin minimum inhibitory concentration (MIC) of PA01ΔG complemented with 32 *ampG* variants was up to 512 μg/ml, similar to the original PA01 (*P. aeruginosa* PA01). Furthermore, site-directed mutation of two conservative amino acids (I53 and W90) showed that when I53 was mutated to 53S or 53T (I53S or I53T), the ampicillin MIC level dropped drastically, and the activity of AmpC β-lactamase decreased as well. By contrast, the ampicillin MIC and the activity of AmpC β-lactamase remained unchanged for W90R and W90S mutants. Our studies demonstrated that although nucleotide variations occurred in most of the *ampG* genes, the structure of AmpG protein in clinical isolates is stable, and conservative amino acid is necessary to maintain normal function of AmpG.

1. Introduction

Pseudomonas aeruginosa is a common opportunistic pathogen and often infects people with low immunity. *P. aeruginosa* infection leads to a high fatality rate in burn patients or those needing mechanically assisted ventilation. *P. aeruginosa* also plays an important role in chronic respiratory infection, especially for those with cystic fibrosis (CF) and some other chronic respiratory system infections [1]. With the abused use of antibiotics in clinics and agriculture, some strains of *P. aeruginosa* become resistant to most if not all antibiotics, causing serious consequences especially for patients in the intensive care unit (ICU) or with chronic respiratory diseases. The main mechanism of resistance is selective mutations of the chromosome leading to a high yield of the cephalosporin lytic enzyme AmpC. *ampC* is located on the chromosome, its expression inducible by β-lactams, and is found in most *Enterobacteria*, *P. aeruginosa*, and other nonfermentative Gram-negative bacilli [2]. β-lactamases are normally expressed in low levels, but can be induced by β-lactam antibiotics especially cefoxitin and imipenem. The only exception is *Escherichia coli* and *Shigella* due to the lack of *ampR* [3]. Therefore, the prolonged and wide use of β-lactam antibiotics can result in multiple β-lactam-resistant bacteria that produce high levels of β-lactamases, causing therapeutic failures [4, 5].

The induction of AmpC production is intimately linked to peptidoglycan recycling [6]. A number of genes including *ampG*, *ampR*, *ampD*, and *ampE* are involved in the process [7]. *ampG* encodes a transmembrane protein functioning as a specific permease to transport 1,6-GldNAc-anhydro-MurNAc and 1,6-GldNAc-anhydro-MurNAc peptide, which are the signal molecules involved in *ampC* expression [8]. *ampR* encodes a DNA-binding protein belonging to the LysR superfamily [9]. There are two regulatory characteristics of *ampR*: in the absence of a β-lactam inducer, it binds to the UDP-MurNAc pentapeptide to promote the formation of an AmpR-DNA complex that represses *ampC* transcription, while in the presence of a β-lactam antibiotic, peptidoglycan fragments accumulate in the cytoplasm [10], and the 1,6-anhydro-MurNAc tripeptide (or pentapeptide) competitively displaces the UDP-MurNAc pentapeptide and converts AmpR into an activator, triggering the *ampC* expression or production of β-lactamase [9]. *ampD* encodes a cytosolic N-acetyl-anhydromuramyl-L-alanine amidase and specifically hydrolyzes the 1,6-anhydro-MurNAc peptide, thus inhibiting the *ampC* expression [11, 12]. *ampE* encodes a cytoplasmic membrane protein acting as a sensory transducer molecule required for *ampC* induction [13], but the exact role of AmpE is not fully understood. It has been shown that there are two *ampG* homologues in *P. aeruginosa*, *ampG* (PA4393) and *ampGh1* (PA4218), and only the product of *ampG* is a functional protein; the inactivation of *ampG* by mutation or deletion confers noninducible and low-level β-lactamase expression [14, 15]. Herein, we studied the relationship between the structure and function of *ampG* in wild type *P. aeruginosa* with different resistance levels against ampicillin. Our findings may provide more theoretical basis for identifying molecular features of AmpG and help design methods to screen candidate agents to inhibit the function of AmpG, thus prolonging the use of commonly used β-lactams in clinics.

2. Materials and Methods

2.1. Bacterial Strain and Plasmid. Two hundred and eleven (211) nonduplicate wild strains of *P. aeruginosa* were isolated from the clinical samples at the First Affiliated Hospital of Wenzhou Medial University, China, between 2009 and 2011. The strains were identified by the Vitek-60 microorganism autoanalysis system (BioMerieux Corporate, Lyon, France). *P. aeruginosa* PA01 and plasmids pUCP24 [14]were obtained from the Laboratory of Microbial Genetics, University of Florida, Gainesville, USA. The strains and plasmids used or constructed in this work are listed in Table 1.

2.2. Antibiotic Susceptibility Test. Minimal inhibitory concentrations (MICs) to the antimicrobial agents were determined by the agar dilution method for the control and recombinant strains in accordance with the guidelines of the Clinical and Laboratory Standards Institute (CLSI). Antimicrobial agents were obtained from the National Institute for the Control of Pharmaceutical and Biological Products (NICPBP) and the pharmaceutical companies in China.

E. coli ATCC 25922 was used as a quality control for the MIC test.

2.3. Cloning and Comparative Analysis of the ampG Genes. Genomic DNA was extracted from the strains using an AxyPrep Bacterial Genomic DNA Miniprep kit (Axygen Scientific, Union City, CA, USA) and PCR- (polymerase chain reaction-) amplified to clone the *ampG* genes. The primers were designed by using Primer 5.0, and a pair of flanking restriction endonuclease adapters were added at the 5′ end of the primers (*Bam*HI for the forward primer PA*ampG*-F and *Hind*III for the reverse primer PA*ampG*-R, respectively, Table 2) and synthesized by Shanghai Sunny Biotechnology Co., Ltd (Shanghai, China). PCR amplification was carried out under the following conditions, i.e., an initial 5 min denaturation at 95°C, followed by 35 cycles of denaturation (94°C for 45 s), annealing (65°C for 45 s), and extension (72°C for 90 s), and a final extension step at 72°C for 10 min. The PCR products of *ampG*s were first cloned into a pMD18-T vector. The recombinant plasmid (pMD18-*ampG*) was identified initially by PCR and then verified by sequencing. Blast programs from NCBI (http://www.ncbi.nlm.nih.gov/BLAST) and MEGA5.05 (molecular evolutionary genetics analysis software, http://www.megasoftware.net) were used to analyze the similarities of the *ampG* nucleotide sequences and the AmpG amino acid sequences.

2.3. Genetic Complementation Assays to Determine the Function of the Cloned ampG Genes. The verified recombinant pMD18-*ampG* plasmid was digested with *Bam*HI and *Hind*III restriction enzymes. The *ampG* fragment was recovered and then ligated into a pUCP24 vector digested with the same restriction enzymes (*Bam*HI and *Hind*III). The recombinant plasmid pUCP24-*ampG* was transformed into *E. coli* JM109, and the recombinant *E. coli* JM109-pUCP24-*ampG* was further identified by PCR. pUCP24-*ampG* was extracted and introduced into PA01Δ*ampG* as described previously [16]. MIC to ampicillin was performed for the recombinant PA01Δ*ampG*-pUCP24-*ampG* to detect the function of the cloned *ampG*s. PA01Δ*ampG* carrying the vector pUCP24 was used as a negative control.

2.4. Site-Directed Mutation of the Conservative Amino Acids in the ampG Gene. We used the *ampG* gene sequence of PA01 as the template to design primers for amplification of the 5′ and 3′ end fragments of the *ampG* gene, respectively. The forward primer for amplification of the 5′ end fragment (PA*ampG*-F with a *Bam*HI recognition site at the 5′ end) and the reverse primer for amplification of the 3′ end fragment (PA*ampG*-R with a *Hind*III recognition site at the 5′ end) were the same as described above (Table 2). The corresponding nucleotide mutations were inserted into the downstream primers of 5′ end and the upstream primer of 3′ end fragments of the *ampG* gene, and then the mixture of the PCR products of the 5′ end and the 3′ end fragments (mole ratio of 1:1) was used as the

TABLE 1: Bacterial strains and plasmids.

Strains or plasmids	Relevant characteristic (s)
Strains	
E. coli JM109	endA1 hsdR17 supE44 thi-1 recA1 gyrA96 relA1 (argF-lacZYA) U169 80dlacZ
PA01	Reference strain; genome completely sequenced
PA01Δ*ampG*	*ampG* (PA4393) deleted PA01[14]
Plasmids	
pMD18-*ampG*$_{1-35}$	pMD18 vectors carrying *ampG*s of 35 wild type *P. aeruginosa* strains, respectively (this work)
pMD18-*ampG*$_{PA}$	pMD18 vector carrying *ampG* of PA01 (this work)
pUCP24	pUC18-derived broad-host-range vector; Gm^r
pUCP24-*ampG*$_{1-35}$	*ampG* genes from pMD18-*ampG1-35* cloned into pUCP24, respectively; Gmr (this work)
pUCP24-*ampG*$_{PA}$	*ampG* gene of pMD18-*ampGPA* cloned into pUCP24; Gmr (this work)
pUCP24-*ampG*$_{mut}$	pUCP24 vector carrying site-directedly mutated *ampG* of PA01 (this work)
pUCP24-*ampG*$_{PA}$-I53S	
pUCP24-*ampG*$_{PA}$-I53T	
pUCP24-*ampG*$_{PA}$-W90R	
pUCP24-*ampG*$_{PA}$-W90S	

TABLE 2: Primers used in this work.

Primer	Sequence*	Purpose
PA$_{ampG}$-F	5′GGGATCCCAACGCGCACGCTTGCGCGAGGA 3′(BamHI)	Cloning of *ampG* of PA01
PA$_{ampG}$-R	5′GAAGCTTTCAGTGCTGCTCGGCG TTCTGGT3′(HindIII)	
PA$_{ampG}$-I53S	5′CCCAGCCAACTGGCGAAACCgctGGTATCC CGCGCCACGC3′	Forward primer for I53S
PA$_{ampG}$-I53T	5′CCCAGCCAACTGGCGAAACCggtGGTATC CCGCGCCACGC3′	Forward primer for I53T
PA$_{ampG}$-53R	5′GGTTTCGCCAGTTGGCTGGGGCTGGTGT ACGCCTTCAAGT3′	
PA$_{ampG}$-W90R	5′AGCACCTGCGAGAACACCAGccgGGAAC GGCGCCGGCCGA3′	Forward primer for W90R
PA$_{ampG}$-W90S	5′AGCACCTGCGAGAACACCAGcgaGGAACG GCGCCGGCCGA3′	Forward primer for W90S
PA$_{ampG}$-90R	5′CTGGTGTTCTCGCAGGTGCTGATCGCCC TGGGACTGCTCG3′	

*Underlined are restriction endonuclease sites; nucleotide sequence corresponding to the mutated amino acids is shown in lowercase.

template, and the upstream primer of the 5′ end and the downstream primer of the 3′ end were used as the primers for amplification of *ampG* variants with the point mutations. Different mutations in the primers are shown in Table 2. PCRs were performed under the following conditions: an initial 5 min denaturation at 95°C followed by 35 amplification cycles, each consisting of a 40 sec denaturation step at 95°C, a 30 sec annealing step at 55°C, and a 40 sec extension step at 72°C followed by a 10 min final extension at 72°C (ExTaq from TaKaRa, Dalian, China). The PCR products (*ampG*$_{mut}$) were purified and inserted into pMD18-T vectors. The recombinant plasmid pMD18-*ampG*$_{mut}$ was initially identified by PCR and then verified by sequencing. The verified pMD18-*ampG*$_{mut}$ recombinant plasmids were digested with *Bam*HI and *Hind*III. The *ampG*$_{mut}$ fragments were recovered and ligated into the pUCP24 vectors digested with the same restriction enzymes

(*Bam*HI and *Hind*III). The recombinant pUCP24-*ampG*$_{mut}$ was then transformed into PA01Δ*ampG* to detect the complementary effect of ampicillin resistance in the host.

2.5. Detection of β-Lactamase Activity. The detection procedures were performed as described in [14]. *P. aeruginosa* cells were induced for 1 h with 4 μg/ml cefoxitin (Calbiochem, San Diego, USA) and for 2 h with 50 μg/ml cefoxitin, respectively. Crude cell extracts were prepared by sonication, and the protein content of crude extracts was determined using BCA protein assay reagent (Pierce, USA) [17]. The β-lactamase activity was quantified with an UV spectrophotometer using 100 μM of nitrocefin as the substrate. The activity of the β-lactamase was defined as nanomole of nitrocefin hydrolyzed at 30°C per min by 1 g protein. All the induction experiments were performed in triplicate, and the result represents an average of the three replicates.

3. Results

3.1. Ampicillin MIC Detection of the P. aeruginosa Strains. The MIC to ampicillin for 211 strains of *P. aeruginosa* showed that most of the strains had a high resistance level. Only 2.84 % (6/211) strain had a low MIC level (≤128 μg/ml), and more than a half of them (61.61 %, 130/211) showed a very high MIC level of ≥2048 μg/ml (Figure 1).

3.2. Sequence Variations of the ampG Genes among the Strains with Different MIC Levels. To compare the *ampG* gene structure of *P. aeruginosa* strains with different ampicillin MIC levels, we cloned and sequenced the *ampG* gene of 35 strains with high MIC levels (512 to −≥8192 μg/ml). Compared with the *ampG* gene of PA01, a total of 51 nucleotide variations over 34 loci in 24 *ampG* genes were identified. Among these nucleotide variations, seven led to amino acid changes (Table 3). Three amino acids were located in the transmembrane regions, but none of them corresponded to the 51 conserved amino acids described in a recent report [18].

3.3. Function Analysis of ampG Variants from Clinically Isolated P. aeruginosa Strains. In order to detect the function of *ampG*s, the *ampG* genes from 24 strains with sequence variation were further cloned into pUCP24 and transformed into the PA01Δ*ampG* to perform genetic complementation analysis. All the cloned *ampG* genes complemented the function of the deleted *ampG* gene in PA01Δ*ampG*. The MIC levels for ampicillin were between 256 and 1024 μg/ml, close to the level of PA01 or PA01Δ*ampG*-pUCP24-*ampG*$_{PA}$ (512 μg/ml). The AmpC β-lactamase activity of the genetically complemented recombinants also showed similar results (Table 3). These data indicate that the cloned *ampG*s have similar function despite their structural differences.

3.4. Effect of the Mutations of the Conservative Amino Acids on AmpG Function. In order to analyze the correlation of the conservative amino acids with the function of AmpG, 2 conservative amino acids I53 and W90 located in the transmembrane regions 2 and 3, respectively, were randomly chosen for site-directed mutagenesis. According to the chemical properties of the amino acids, 4 to 6 different amino acid substitutions were designed for each conserved amino acid. Finally, a total of 4 mutated genes were successfully cloned; these mutants were transformed into the recipient cell PA01Δ*ampG*; their MIC levels to ampicillin and activities of AmpC type β-lactamase were tested (Table 4). PA01 Δ *ampG*-pUCP24-*ampG*PA-W90R and PA01 Δ *ampG*-pUCP24-*ampG*PA-W90S had high resistance level to ampicillin, similar to that of the original *P. aeruginosa* PA01, but significantly different from that of the I53S and I53T mutants that had much lower resistance level to ampicillin

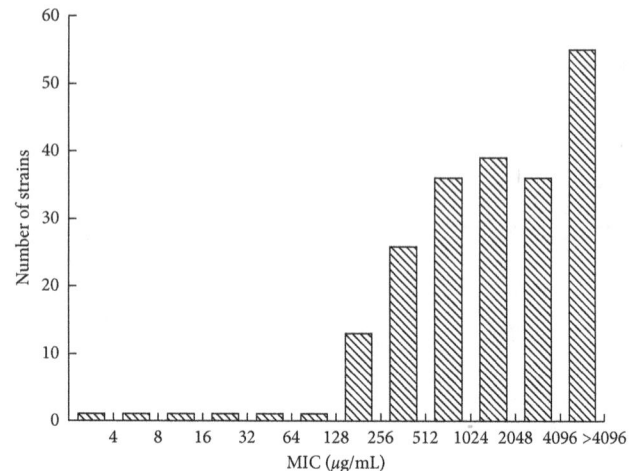

FIGURE 1: The MIC to ampicillin for 211 strains of *P. aeruginosa* had a high resistance level.

and showed significantly lower AmpC type β-lactamase activities (Table 4).

4. Discussion

The clinical isolates of *P. aeruginosa* often show resistance to most antibiotics [19, 20]. The mechanism of multiple resistance is mainly related to inactivated enzyme production, overexpression of efflux systems, antibiotic target alteration, biofilm formation, and acquisition of foreign drug-resistant genes by means of horizontal gene transfer [21–23]. The inactivating enzymes to β-lactam antibiotics produced by *P. aeruginosa* were AmpC, the extended spectrum β-lactamase (ESBLs), and the metalloenzyme (MBL), of which AmpC has attracted more attention because its production can be induced [24]. Besides being encoded in *P. aeruginosa*, *ampC* extensively exists in the chromosomes or plasmids of Gram-negative bacillus such as *Enterobacter*, *Citrobacter*, and *Acinetobacter* [25, 26]. The muropeptide derivatives are essential for the induction of AmpC type β-lactamase expression [27]. Schmidt et al. [28] used nitrosoguanidine (NTG) to induce mutations in *E. coli* SN0301 (carrying *ampC* and *ampR* of *E. cloacae*) and obtained three mutants with mutated *ampG* genes including *ampG1* (G151D), *ampG3* (G268D), and *ampG5* (G373D), respectively. They all belong to the conserved amino acids located on the transmembrane regions 5 (158G), 10 (419G), and 13 (544G), respectively, in AmpG of *P. aeruginosa* PA01 [18]. In this work, we also performed site-directed mutation for two conserved amino acids (I53 and W59). As a result, the AmpC activity of the mutated AmpGs (I53S or I53T) located in the transmembrane regions 2 was drastically lowered. Our findings suggest that the conserved amino acids play an important role in keeping the normal function of AmpG. A single amino acid might be enough to determine the substrate specificity and the transportation activity of AmpG. The length of the AmpG proteins from different species differs from each other and certainly the transmembrane regions of the AmpGs also vary [29, 30]. A previous work from our team showed that the longest AmpG protein was

TABLE 3: Sequence variation and function of *ampGs* in clinical *P. aeruginosa* strains.

	Nucleotide		Amino acid		MIC**
	Position	Variation	Position	Variation	(µg/ml)
PA01ΔampG-pUCP24-*ampG1*	618	C-A	206	/	512/512
PA01ΔampG-pUCP24-*ampG2*	715	C-T	239	/	512/1024
	1080	G-C	360	/	
	1317	C-T	439	/	
PA01ΔampG-pUCP24-*ampG3*	715	C-T	239	/	512/1024
	1080	G-C	360	/	
	1317	C-T	439	/	
PA01ΔampG-pUCP24-*ampG4*	715	C-T	239	/	512/1024
	1080	G-C	360	/	
	1317	C-T	439	/	
PA01ΔampG-pUCP24-*ampG7*	618	C-A	206	/	512/512
	916	G-C	306	D-H	
PA01ΔampG-pUCP24-*ampG8*	27	C-A	9	/	512/1024
PA01ΔampG-pUCP24-*ampG9*	27	C-A	9	/	512/512
PA01ΔampG-pUCP24-*ampG10*	1329	G-A	443	/	512/1024
PA01ΔampG-pUCP24-*ampG11*	666	C-T	222	/	256/512
	819	G-A	273	/	
	942	G-A	314	/	
	1062	A-G	354	/	
	1077	C-A	539	/	
	1113	C-T	371	/	
PA01ΔampG-pUCP24-*ampG12*	618	C-A	206	/	512/1024
PA01ΔampG-pUCP24-*ampG13*	1423	G-A	475	D-N	512/1024
PA01ΔampG-pUCP24-*ampG14*	1423	G-A	475	D-N	512/1024
PA01ΔampG-pUCP24-*ampG15*	336	C-T	112	/	512/4096
PA01ΔampG-pUCP24-*ampG16*	1747	G-A	583	/	512/1024
PA01ΔampG-pUCP24-*ampG17*	153	T-C	51	/	512/≥8192
PA01ΔampG-pUCP24-*ampG20*	213	G-A	71	/	256/4096
PA01ΔampG-pUCP24-*ampG24*	450	C-T	150	/	1024/4096
PA01ΔampG-pUCP24-*ampG25*	336	C-T	112	/	1024/≥8192
	1027	C-T	343	/	
PA01ΔampG-pUCP24-*ampG26*	1182	G-A	394	/	512/4096
PA01ΔampG-pUCP24-*ampG28*	657	C-T	219	/	512/≥8192
	729	C-T	243	/	
	837	C-T	279	/	
	990	C-T	330	/	
	1062	A-G	354	/	
	1239	T-C	443	/	
	1316	T-C	439	I-T(11)*	
PA01ΔampG-pUCP24-*ampG29*	1143	C-T	381	/	512/≥8192
PA01ΔampG-pUCP24-*ampG30*	27	C-A	9	/	512/≥8192
	1329	G-A	443	/	
PA01ΔampG-pUCP24-*ampG31*	27	C-T	9	/	256/4096
	558	G-A	186	/	
	1002	C-T	334	/	
	1062	A-G	354	/	
	1113	C-T	371	/	
PA01ΔampG-pUCP24-*ampG35*	617	C-T	206	T-I (6)*	512/≥8192
	708	T-A	236	/	
	1193	G-A	398	G-E (9)*	
	1364	T-C	455	L-P	
PA01ΔampG-pUCP24-*ampGPA*	/	/	/	/	512
PA01ΔampG	/	/	/	/	32
PA01	/	/	/	/	512
ATCC 25922	/	/	/	/	4

D: aspartic acid; H: histidine; N: asparagine; I: isoleucine; T: threonine; G: glycine; E: glutamate; L: leucine; P: proline; *transmembrane region; **MIC values of the cloned ORF/wild strain.

TABLE 4: MIC levels to ampicillin and AmpC β-lactamase activity of the site-directed mutants.

Strain	Amino acid variation	β-Lactamase activity	MIC (μg/ml)
PA01ΔampG-pUCP24-ampG$_{PA}$-I53S	Ile (atc)-Ser (agc)	69.8	32
PA01ΔampG-pUCP24-ampG$_{PA}$-I53T	Ile (atc)-Thr (acc)	56.7	16
PA01ΔampG-pUCP24-ampG$_{PA}$-W90R	Try (tgg)-Arg (cgg)	25296.4	512
PA01ΔampG-pUCP24-ampG$_{PA}$-WA90S	Try (tgg)-Ser (tcg)	12628.9	512
PA01	/	1981.6	512
PA01ΔampG	/	44.8	32
PA01ΔampG-pUCP24-ampG$_{PA}$	/	5019.3	1024
ATCC 25922	/	0	4

from *P. aeruginosa* (CDR92618), which consists of 598 amino acids and is predicted to have 14 transmembrane regions. The shortest was from *Microcoleus* with only 401 AA and 11 transmembrane regions. Most of the AmpG proteins contain 12 or 14 transmembrane regions. Analysis of the conservative amino acid against 134 AmpGs showed that there were 51 conserved amino acids identified in 12 transmembrane regions excluding the corresponding transmembrane regions 7 and 8 of PA01. In *P. aeruginosa* PA01, transmembrane regions 1, 2, and 4 contained more conserved amino acids (with 8, 7, and 9 conserved amino acids, respectively), and transmembrane regions 6, 11, 12, and 14 contained only 1 or 2 conserved amino acids. In this work, we sequenced 35 *ampG* genes from clinically isolated *P. aeruginosa* with different MIC levels to ampicillin (512 to $\geq$8192 μg/ml) and found 24 genes harboring 51 nucleotide variations over 34 loci. Among them, only 6 loci in 5 bacterial strains showed amino acid variations. Four strains had one amino acid difference, and one strain had 3 mutated amino acids. Amino acid change in PA01ΔampG-pUCP24-ampG28 (I439T) was located in transmembrane 11, and two of the three amino acid changes in PA01ΔampG-pUCP24-ampG35 (T206I and G398E) were located in transmembrane regions 6 and 9, respectively. They did not belong to the 51 conserved amino acids predicted in our previous work [18]. The MIC levels for ampicillin indicated that all of these 24 genes had normal functions, suggesting that these variations both in nucleotide and amino acid sequences did not affect the function of AmpGs.

In the recent years, the clinically isolated pathogens became more and more resistant to most antibiotics. Studies on the polymorphism and relationship between the structure and function of AmpGs will help to establish a theoretical basis for the development of inhibitors against AmpG. Effective inhibitors for AmpG will shed light on prolonging the clinical use of β-lactam antibiotics.

Abbreviations

ATCC: American Type Culture Collection
BLAST: Basic local alignment search tool
CF: Cystic fibrosis
CLSI: Clinical and Laboratory Standards Institute
ESBL: Extended spectrum β-lactamase
ICU: Intensive care unit
MIC: Minimum inhibitory concentration

NICPBP: National Institute for the Control of Pharmaceutical and Biological Products
ORF: Open reading frame
P. aeruginosa: *Pseudomonas aeruginosa*
PCR: Polymerase chain reaction.

Authors' Contributions

Qingli Chang and Chongyang Wu contributed equally to this work.

Acknowledgments

This study was supported by the Natural Science Foundation of Zhejiang Province, China (LY14C060005 and LQ17H190001), the Science and Technology Foundation of National Health and Family Planning Commission of China (WKJ2012-2-032), and the National Natural Science Foundation of China (81401702, 81501808, 80215049, and 31500109).

References

[1] R. Bodnar, A. Meszaros, M. Olah, T. Agh et al., "Inhaled antibiotics for the treatment of chronic *Pseudomonas aeruginosa* infection in cystic fibrosis patients: challenges to treatment adherence and strategies to improve outcomes," *Patient Preference and Adherence*, vol. 10, pp. 183–193, 2016.

[2] J. Xia, J. Gao, and W. Tang, "Nosocomial infection and its molecular mechanisms of antibiotic resistance," *BioScience Trends*, vol. 10, no. 1, pp. 14–21, 2016.

[3] S. Normark, "beta-Lactamase induction in gram-negative bacteria is intimately linked to peptidoglycan recycling," *Microbial Drug Resistance*, vol. 1, no. 2, pp. 111–114, 1995.

[4] G. Meletis, D. Chatzidimitriou, and N. Malisiovas, "Double- and multi-carbapenemase-producers: the excessively armored bacilli of the current decade," *European Journal of Clinical Microbiology and Infectious Diseases*, vol. 34, no. 8, pp. 1487–1493, 2015.

[5] S. S. Tang, A. Apisarnthanarak, and L. Y. Hsu, "Mechanisms of beta-lactam antimicrobial resistance and epidemiology of major community- and healthcare-associated multidrug-resistant bacteria," *Advanced Drug Delivery Reviews*, vol. 78, no. 3, pp. 3–13, 2014.

[6] K. F. Kong, A. Aguila, L. Schneper, K. Mathee et al., "*Pseudomonas aeruginosa* beta-lactamase induction requires two permeases, AmpG and AmpP," *BMC Microbiology*, vol. 10, no. 1, p. 328, 2010.

[7] Y. Luan, G.-L. Li, L.-B. Duo et al., "DHA-1 plasmid-mediated AmpC beta-lactamase expression and regulation of Klebsiella pnuemoniae isolates," *Molecular Medicine Reports*, vol. 11, no. 4, pp. 3069–3077, 2015.

[8] J. F. Fisher and S. Mobashery, "The sentinel role of peptidoglycan recycling in the beta-lactam resistance of the Gram-negative Enterobacteriaceae and *Pseudomonas aeruginosa*," *Bioorganic Chemistry*, vol. 56, pp. 41–48, 2014.

[9] O. Caille, D. Zincke, M. Merighi et al., "Structural and functional characterization of *Pseudomonas aeruginosa* global regulator AmpR," *Journal of Bacteriology*, vol. 196, no. 22, pp. 3890–3902, 2014.

[10] G. Vadlamani, M. D. Thomas, T. R. Patel et al., "The beta-lactamase gene regulator AmpR is a tetramer that recognizes and binds the D-Ala-D-Ala motif of its repressor UDP-N-acetylmuramic acid (MurNAc)-pentapeptide," *Journal of Biological Chemistry*, vol. 290, no. 5, pp. 2630–2643, 2015.

[11] J. Hwang and H. S. Kim, "Cell wall recycling-linked coregulation of AmpC and PenB beta-lactamases through *ampD* mutations in *Burkholderia cenocepacia*," *Antimicrobial Agents and Chemotherapy*, vol. 59, no. 12, pp. 7602–7610, 2015.

[12] Q. Cheng and J. T. Park, "Substrate specificity of the AmpG permease required for recycling of cell wall anhydro-muropeptides," *Journal of Bacteriology*, vol. 184, no. 23, pp. 6434–6436, 2002.

[13] S. Lindquist, M. Galleni, F. Lindberg, and S. Normark, "Signalling proteins in enterobacterial AmpC beta-lactamase regulation," *Molecular Microbiology*, vol. 3, no. 8, pp. 1091–1102, 1989.

[14] Y. Zhang, Q. Bao, L. A. Gagnon et al., "*ampG* gene of *Pseudomonas aeruginosa* and its role in beta-lactamase expression," *Antimicrobial Agents and Chemotherapy*, vol. 54, no. 11, pp. 4772–4779, 2010.

[15] L. Zamorano, T. M. Reeve, C. Juan et al., "AmpG inactivation restores susceptibility of pan-beta-lactam-resistant *Pseudomonas aeruginosa* clinical strains," *Antimicrobial Agents and Chemotherapy*, vol. 55, no. 5, pp. 1990–1996, 2011.

[16] G. Nigro, L. L. Fazio, M. C. Martino et al., "Muramylpeptide shedding modulates cell sensing of Shigella flexneri," *Cellular Microbiology*, vol. 10, no. 3, pp. 682–695, 2008.

[17] S. Trepanier, A. Prince, and A. Huletsky, "Characterization of the penA and penR genes of Burkholderia cepacia 249 which encode the chromosomal class A penicillinase and its LysR-type transcriptional regulator," *Antimicrobial Agents and Chemotherapy*, vol. 41, no. 11, pp. 2399–2405, 1997.

[18] D. J. Biedenbach, P. T. Giao, P. H. Van et al., "Antimicrobial-resistant *Pseudomonas aeruginosa* and *Acinetobacter baumannii* from patients with hospital-acquired or ventilator-associated pneumonia in Vietnam," *Clinical Therapeutics*, vol. 38, no. 9, pp. 2098–2105, 2016.

[19] C. Ding, Z. Yang, J. Wang et al., "Prevalence of *Pseudomonas aeruginosa* and antimicrobial-resistant *Pseudomonas aeruginosa* in patients with pneumonia in mainland China: a systematic review and meta-analysis," *International Journal of Infectious Diseases*, vol. 49, pp. 119–128, 2016.

[20] A. H. Holmes, L. S. P. Moore, A. Sundsfjord et al., "Understanding the mechanisms and drivers of antimicrobial resistance," *The Lancet*, vol. 387, no. 10014, pp. 176–187, 2016.

[21] V. K. Sharma, N. Johnson, L. Cizmas, T. J. McDonald, and H. Kim, "A review of the influence of treatment strategies on antibiotic resistant bacteria and antibiotic resistance genes," *Chemosphere*, vol. 150, pp. 702–714, 2016.

[22] J. Sun, Z. Deng, and A. Yan, "Bacterial multidrug efflux pumps: mechanisms, physiology and pharmacological exploitations," *Biochemical and Biophysical Research Communications*, vol. 453, no. 2, pp. 254–267, 2014.

[23] X. Zeng and J. Lin, "Beta-lactamase induction and cell wall metabolism in Gram-negative bacteria," *Frontiers in Microbiology*, vol. 4, p. 128, 2013.

[24] S. Luk, W.-K. Wong, A. Y.-M. Ho, K. C.-H. Yu, W.-K. To, and T.-K. Ng, "Clinical features and molecular epidemiology of plasmid-mediated DHA-type AmpC beta-lactamase-producing *Klebsiella pneumoniae* blood culture isolates, Hong Kong," *Journal of Global Antimicrobial Resistance*, vol. 7, pp. 37–42, 2016.

[25] M. H. Patel, G. R. Trivedi, S. M. Patel, and M. M. Vegad, "Antibiotic susceptibility pattern in urinary isolates of gram negative bacilli with special reference to AmpC beta-lactamase in a tertiary care hospital," *Urology Annals*, vol. 2, no. 1, pp. 7–11, 2010.

[26] N. D. Hanson and C. C. Sanders, "Regulation of inducible AmpC beta-lactamase expression among Enterobacteriaceae," *Current Pharmaceutical Design*, vol. 5, no. 11, pp. 881–894, 1999.

[27] H. Schmidt, G. Korfmann, H. Barth, and H. H. Martin, "The signal transducer encoded by ampG is essential for induction of chromosomal AmpC beta-lactamase in *Escherichia coli* by beta-lactam antibiotics and 'unspecific' inducers," *Microbiology*, vol. 141, no. 5, pp. 1085–1092, 1995.

[28] P. Li, J. Ying, G. Yang et al., "Structure-function analysis of the transmembrane protein AmpG from *Pseudomonas aeruginosa*," *PLoS One*, vol. 11, no. 12, article e0168060, 2016.

[29] A. Chahboune, M. Decaffmeyer, R. Brasseur, and B. Joris, "Membrane topology of the *Escherichia coli* AmpG permease required for recycling of cell wall anhydromuropeptides and AmpC beta-lactamase induction," *Antimicrobial Agents and Chemotherapy*, vol. 49, no. 3, pp. 1145–1149, 2005.

[30] R. S. Rosenthal, W. Nogami, B. T. Cookson, W. E. Goldman, and W. J. Folkening, "Major fragment of soluble peptidoglycan released from growing Bordetella pertussis is tracheal cytotoxin," *Infection and Immunity*, vol. 55, no. 9, pp. 2117–2120, 1987.

7

Molecular Characteristics of Methicillin-Resistant Staphylococci Clinical Isolates from a Tertiary Hospital in Northern Thailand

Thawatchai Kitti,[1] Rathanin Seng,[2] Natnaree Saiprom,[2] Rapee Thummeepak,[3] Narisara Chantratita,[2] Chalermchai Boonlao,[4] and Sutthirat Sitthisak ⓘ[3,5]

[1]*Faculty of Oriental Medicine, Chiang Rai College, Chiang Rai, Thailand*
[2]*Department of Microbiology and Immunology, Faculty of Tropical Medicine, Mahidol University, Bangkok, Thailand*
[3]*Department of Microbiology and Parasitology, Faculty of Medical Sciences, Naresuan University, Phitsanulok, Thailand*
[4]*Chiangrai Prachanukroh Hospital, Amphoe Meuang, Chiangrai, Thailand*
[5]*Centre of Excellence in Medical Biotechnology, Faculty of Medical Science, Naresuan University, Phitsanulok, Thailand*

Correspondence should be addressed to Sutthirat Sitthisak; sutthirats@nu.ac.th

Academic Editor: Louis DeTolla

Methicillin-resistant staphylococci are now recognized as a major cause of infectious diseases, particularly in hospitals. Molecular epidemiology is important for prevention and control of infection, but little information is available regarding staphylococcal infections in Northern Thailand. In the present study, we examined antimicrobial susceptibility patterns, detection of antimicrobial resistance genes, and SCC*mec* types of methicillin-resistant *S. aureus* (MRSA) and methicillin-resistant coagulase-negative staphylococci (MR-CoNS) isolated from patients in a hospital in Northern Thailand. The species of MRSA and MR-CoNS were identified using combination methods, including PCR, MALDI-TOF-MS, and *tuf* gene sequencing. The susceptibility pattern of all isolates was determined by the disk diffusion method. Antimicrobial resistance genes, SCC*mec* types, and ST239 were characterized using single and multiplex PCR. ST239 was predominant in MRSA isolates (10/23). All MR-CoNS (N = 31) were identified as *S. haemolyticus* (N = 18), *S. epidermidis* (N = 3), *S. cohnii* (N = 3), *S. capitis* (N = 6), and *S. hominis* (N = 1). More than 70% of MRSA and MR-CoNS were resistant to cefoxitin, penicillin, oxacillin, erythromycin, clindamycin, gentamicin, and ciprofloxacin. In MRSA isolates, the prevalence of *erm*A (78.3%) and *erm*B (73.9%) genes was high compared to that of the *erm*C gene (4.3%). In contrast, *erm*C (87.1%) and *qac*A/B genes (70.9%) were predominant in MR-CoNS isolates. SCC*mec* type III was the dominant type of MRSA (13/23), whereas SCC*mec* type II was more present in *S. haemolyticus* (10/18). Ten MRSA isolates with SCC*mec* type III were ST239, which is the common type of MRSA in Asia. This finding provides useful information for a preventive health strategy directed against methicillin-resistant staphylococcal infections.

1. Introduction

Staphylococcus is recognized as an important cause of nosocomial infection. The most prominent pathogen of the genus is the coagulase-positive *Staphylococcus aureus*, which causes osteomyelitis, endocarditis, septic arthritis, pneumonia, and skin infections [1]. However, coagulase-negative staphylococci (CoNS) such as *S. epidermidis*, *S. haemolyticus*, *S. lugdunensis*, *S. cohnii*, *S. capitis*, and *S. hominis* are also associated with various infections with possible fatal

outcomes in newborns or immunocompromised patients [2]. It is well established that staphylococcal infections in hospitals show an increasing prevalence of methicillin-resistant *S. aureus* (MRSA) and methicillin-resistant coagulase-negative staphylococci (MR-CoNS) isolates [3, 4]. Methicillin resistance in staphylococci results from the recombinase-mediated insertion of the staphylococcal chromosomal cassette *mec* (SCC*mec*), the mobile genetic element that carries *mec*A and various antibiotic resistance genes. The *mec*A gene encodes penicillin-binding protein

PBP2a that has a low affinity for β-lactam antibiotics [5]. To date, eleven SCC*mec* types (I–XI) have been identified. SCC*mec* types I, II, and III have been associated more frequently with hospital-acquired MRSA (HA-MRSA), while SCC*mec* types IV and V are the most dominant in MRSA infections acquired in the community (CA-MRSA) [6]. Previous studies reported the prevalence rate of these major clones varies markedly in different geographic regions; the predominant HA-MRSA clone in Asian countries is MRSA-ST239-III [7]. *S. epidermidis* has been found to harbor SCC*mec* types I, II, III, IV, and V. Likewise, SCC*mec* types II, III, and V have been discovered in *S. haemolyticus* [8]. It is generally accepted that the tolerance of chlorhexidine in *S. aureus* is associated with the family of the *qac* (*qac*A/B) gene, which encodes proton-motive force-dependent export pumps [9]. Recently, a study suggested that *qac*A/B carriage might contribute to an increasing global dominance of CC22 and ST239 clones [10]. Erythromycin resistance in staphylococci is predominantly caused by erythromycin resistance RNA methylase, whose action also affects resistance to other macrolides, lincosamides, and streptogramin B (MLS$_B$). This resistance is mediated by the *erm*-type genes, caused almost exclusively by *erm*A or *erm*C [11]. Little information is available on the molecular epidemiology of MRSA and MR-CoNS in Northern Thailand. This study was designed to characterize the antimicrobial resistance genes and SCC*mec* types of MRSA and MR-CoNS isolated from a hospital in Chiangrai Province located in Northern Thailand. These data will provide insights into the epidemiology of the MRSA and MR-CoNS in this region.

2. Materials and Methods

2.1. Bacterial Isolates. A total of 54 clinical isolates of staphylococci were collected from November 2015 to October 2016 from patients who were admitted to Chiangrai Prachanukroh Hospital, Chiangrai. The hospital is a (756-bed) teaching hospital that handles ~3,500 admissions per day, located in the north of Thailand. The isolates were collected from blood (39 isolates, 72.2%), pus (10 isolates, 18.5%), sputum (4 isolates, 7.4%), and other body fluids (1 isolate, 1.9%).

The bacteria were initially identified by colony morphology, mannitol fermentation, Gram characteristics, catalase test, coagulase test, and DNase activity. The phenotypic methicillin resistance was assessed using the cefoxitin disk diffusion method in accordance with the Clinical and Laboratory Standard Institute guidelines (CLSI M100-S24) at our clinical laboratory, which has been accredited by the College of American Pathologists [12]. *S. aureus* NCTC10442, *S. aureus* JCSC10442, and *S. aureus* WIS were used as reference strains for SCC*mec* typing. *S. aureus* COL was used as a positive control for *mec*A gene detection.

2.2. Species Identification of Methicillin-Resistant Staphylococci. All isolates were confirmed as staphylococci by a PCR method based on the 16S rRNA gene [13]. The *mec*A gene

was detected in all isolates to confirm the methicillin resistance [14]. MRSA was identified using PCR for detecting the *nuc* gene as previously described by Sasaki et al. [15]. The species level of MR-CoNS was identified by MALDI-TOF-MS [16] and *tuf* gene sequencing [17].

The direct colony of MALDI-TOF-MS analysis was analyzed as previously described [15]. The score identification criteria were used as follows: a score of 2.000 to 3.000 indicated species-level identification, a score of 1.700 to 1.999 indicated genus-level identification, and a score <1.700 indicated an unreliable identification [18].

2.3. Determination of Antibiotic Susceptibility. The antibiotic susceptibility patterns of bacteria to penicillin (P; 10 units), clindamycin (DA; 2 µg), chloramphenicol (C; 30 µg), gentamicin (CN; 10 µg), erythromycin (E; 15 µg), cefoxitin (FOX; 30 µg), sulfamethoxazole/trimethoprim (SXT; 1.25/23.75 µg), vancomycin (VA; 30 µg), rifampicin (RD; 5 µg), linezolid (LZD; 30 µg), mupirocin (MUP; 5 µg), ciprofloxacin (CIP; 5 µg), fusidic acid (FD; 10 µg), and novobiocin (NV; 5 µg) (Oxoid) were determined according to the antibiotic disk diffusion method (CLSI, 2014).

2.4. Determination of SCCmec Types. Multiplex PCR was carried out as described by Zhang et al. [19]. Amplification was performed in a total volume of 25 µl containing 3 µl of 10x buffer with 15 mM of Mg^{2+}, 2.5 µl of 2.5 mM dNTP, 0.2 µl of 5 U *Taq* polymerase, various concentrations of each primer, and 3 µl of the DNA template. The condition for thermal cycler was set as follows: denaturation at 94°C for 4 min followed by 30 cycles at 94°C for 20 sec, 55°C for 30 sec, and 72°C for 30 min and a final extension at 72°C for 5 min. All PCR products were visualized using gel electrophoresis with 1% agarose gel stained with ethidium bromide.

2.5. ST239 Identification. The ST239 was determined by the PCR method using two oligonucleotide primer sets as previously described by Feil et al. [20]. Amplification reaction was performed with the following condition: 1 cycle of predenaturation at 95°C for 15 min followed by 30 cycles at 95°C for 30 sec, 55°C for 30 sec, and 72°C for 30 sec and a final extension at 72°C for 7 min.

2.6. Detection of Antibiotic and Disinfectant Resistance Genes. The other antibiotic and disinfectant resistance genes including the *erm*A, *erm*B, *erm*C, and *qac*A/B genes (disinfectant) were detected by PCR as previously described [21–23]. The primer sets are shown in Supplementary Material 1. All PCR products were visualized using gel electrophoresis with 1% agarose gel stained with ethidium bromide. The absence of bias was ensured by the sequencing of each gene in the representative isolates.

3. Results

3.1. Species Distribution of Staphylococci. The species of all isolates were identified by combined methods, including biochemical tests, PCR, MALDI-TOF-MS, and DNA sequencing. All 23 MRSA isolates were confirmed by detection of the *nuc* gene, and all species of MR-CoNS isolates were confirmed by *tuf* gene sequencing. The species distribution of MR-CoNS is given in Figure 1. The species included methicillin-resistant *S. haemolyticus* ($n = 18$), methicillin-resistant *S. epidermidis* ($n = 3$), methicillin-resistant *S. cohnii* ($n = 3$), methicillin-resistant *S. capitis* ($n = 6$), and methicillin-resistant *S. hominis* ($n = 1$).

3.2. Antimicrobial Susceptibility Testing. All methicillin-resistant staphylococci were tested for their susceptibility against 15 commonly used antibiotics (Figure 2). All MRSA isolates were sensitive to linezolid, fusidic acid, novobiocin, and vancomycin. Prevalence of resistance among the isolates was as follows: cefoxitin (100%), penicillin (100%), oxacillin (95.7%), erythromycin (86.9%), clindamycin (86.9%), gentamicin (72.1%), ciprofloxacin (72.1%), sulfamethoxazole/trimethoprim (56.5%), mupirocin (13.1%), rifampicin (8.6%), and chloramphenicol (4.3%). Likewise, none of the MR-CoNS isolates were resistant to linezolid and vancomycin. However, prevalence of resistance among the isolates was as follows: oxacillin (100%), cefoxitin (100%), penicillin (100%), gentamicin (87.1%), erythromycin (86.9%), ciprofloxacin (77.4%), clindamycin (64.5%), sulfamethoxazole/trimethoprim (70.9%), mupirocin (41.9%), rifampicin (29.0%), fusidic acid (16.1%), chloramphenicol (9.7%), and novobiocin (6.5%).

3.3. Distribution of SCCmec Types and ST239 Type Detection. All 54 staphylococci were *mec*A-positive isolates. SCC*mec* types of all isolates were assigned by multiplex PCR according to the procedures and primer sets listed. As shown in Table 1, all MRSA isolates could be classified into six types of SCC*mec* elements: types I ($n = 6$), II ($n = 1$), III ($n = 13$), IVa ($n = 1$), IVb ($n = 1$), and V ($n = 1$). The distribution of SCC*mec* types in all MR-CoNS used in this study was ranked as types I ($n = 3$), II ($n = 10$), III ($n = 5$), IVa ($n = 3$), IVc ($n = 2$), and V ($n = 2$). SCC*mec* type II was the predominant clone (55.6%) in *S. haemolyticus*. The distribution of SCC*mec* types in each species is given in Table 1. Interestingly, using the multiplex PCR method, we could detect ST239 in 10 isolates of MRSA, and all of them were of SCC*mec* type III.

3.4. Disinfectant and Antibiotic Resistance Genes. Among the 54 methicillin-resistant staphylococci isolates as shown in Table 1, 28 isolates (51.9%) harbored *qac*A/B. These included 6 isolates (26.1%) of *S. aureus*, 13 isolates (72.2%) of *S. haemolyticus*, 3 isolates (100%) of *S. cohnii*, 5 isolates (83.3%) of *S. capitis*, and 1 isolate (100%) of *S. hominis*. The erythromycin resistance genes (*erm*A, *erm*B, and *erm*C) were also detected in MRSA and MR-CoNS. The prevalence of *erm*A, *erm*B, and *erm*C genes found in MRSA was 78.3% (18/23), 73.9% (17/23), and 4.3% (1/23), respectively, whereas 12.9% (4/31), 12.9% (4/31), and 87.1% (27/31) of *erm*A, *erm*B, and *erm*C, respectively, were present in MR-CoNS. The most prevalent *erm*C gene was detected in MR-CoNS, including 88.9% in *S. haemolyticus*, 100% in *S. cohnii*, 100% in *S. capitis*, and 100% in *S. hominis*. The *erm*A and *erm*B genes were found in *S. epidermidis* and *S. capitis* (Table 1).

4. Discussion

Methicillin-resistant staphylococci have dispersed worldwide and continue to be among the most common hospital pathogens. The prevalence and characterization of MRSA and MR-CoNS in hospitals have been reported from different parts of the world [24, 25]. However, the increase of antibiotic resistance in nosocomial isolates of MRSA and MR-CoNS aggravates this problem and poses a great challenge for the management of hospital-acquired infections. In the present study, we found that the 54 staphylococcal isolates belonged to 6 different species. The species distribution identification by MALDI-TOF-MS was consistent with the species identified by *tuf* gene sequencing, with the exception of one isolate (SP33) (Figure 1). Using MALDI-TOF-MS, this isolate was identified as *S. epidermidis*, but *tuf* gene sequencing identified it as *S. haemolyticus*. We assumed that the species assigned by *tuf* gene sequencing was more accurate because the score of MALDI-TOF-MS was only at the level of genus identification. Moreover, MALDI-TOF-MS could not identify 3 isolates of MR-CoNS. These 3 isolates were identified as *S. cohnii* by *tuf* gene sequencing. This result was consistent with a previous study reporting that MALDI-TOF-MS could not identify *S. cohnii* to the species level [26]. Additionally, a phylogenetic tree based on *tuf* gene sequencing was compared with the MALDI-TOF dendrogram for all 31 isolates of MR-CoNS (Figure 1). Interestingly, if the disagreement for one isolate (SP 33) was not considered, the structure of each species was broadly in alignment. Only *S. hominis* was located in different structures of both phylogenetic trees. To the best of our knowledge, this is the first comparison between phylogenetic tree based on *tuf* gene sequencing and MALDI-TOF dendrogram of MR-CoNS.

We found that MRSA and MR-CoNS isolates were resistant to multiple antibacterial agents (Figure 2). Among MR staphylococci isolates, 82.6% were resistant to 7–10 antibiotics (96.8% of MR-CoNS and 60.9% of MRSA). This result is similar to the findings in China and France with a high rate of antibiotic resistance within MRSA clinical isolates [27, 28]. In this study, all MRSA and MR-CoNS isolates were sensitive to vancomycin and linezolid. Thus, these drugs remain suitable options for the treatment of serious infections caused by MRSA and MR-CoNS.

The *mec*A gene, encoding a PBP variant which confers resistance to methicillin, was detected in 100% of staphylococci isolated in this study. *mec*A is carried by the mobile genetic element SCC*mec*. The distribution of different SCC*mec* types in methicillin-resistant staphylococci varied depending on the host species, bacterial clones, and possibly geographical locations [29]. SCC*mec* typing has become essential for the epidemiological characterization of MRSA and MR-CoNS clones. In this study, 54 methicillin-resistant staphylococci were investigated for their SCC*mec* types;

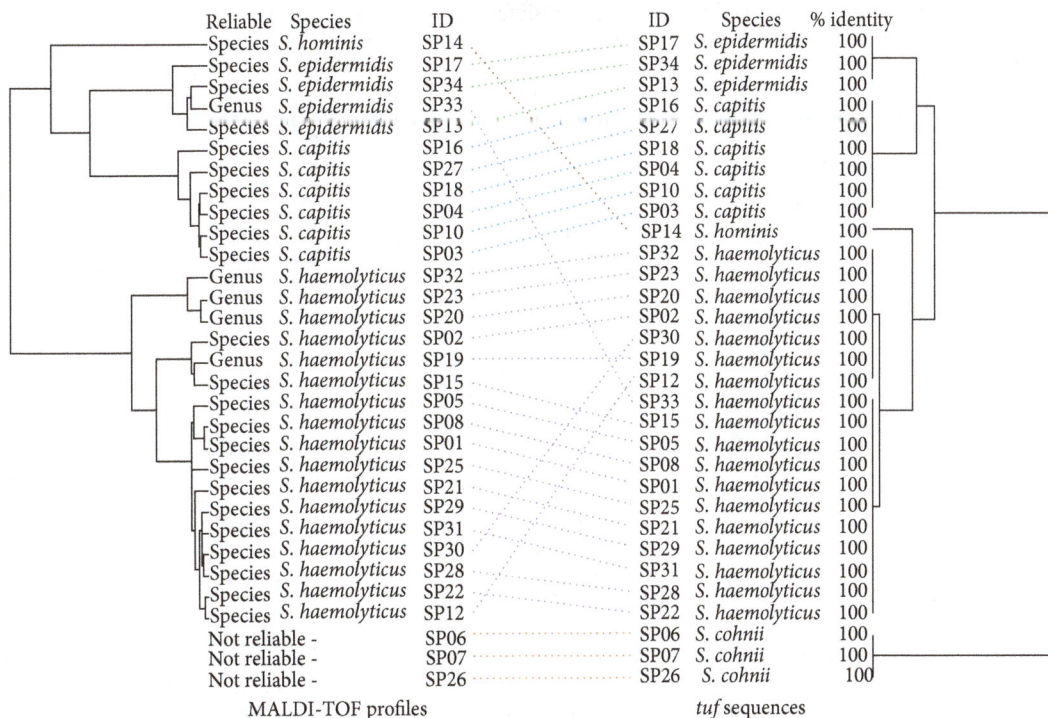

Figure 1: Species distribution of MR-CoNS isolates identified by MALDI-TOF and *tuf* gene sequencing.

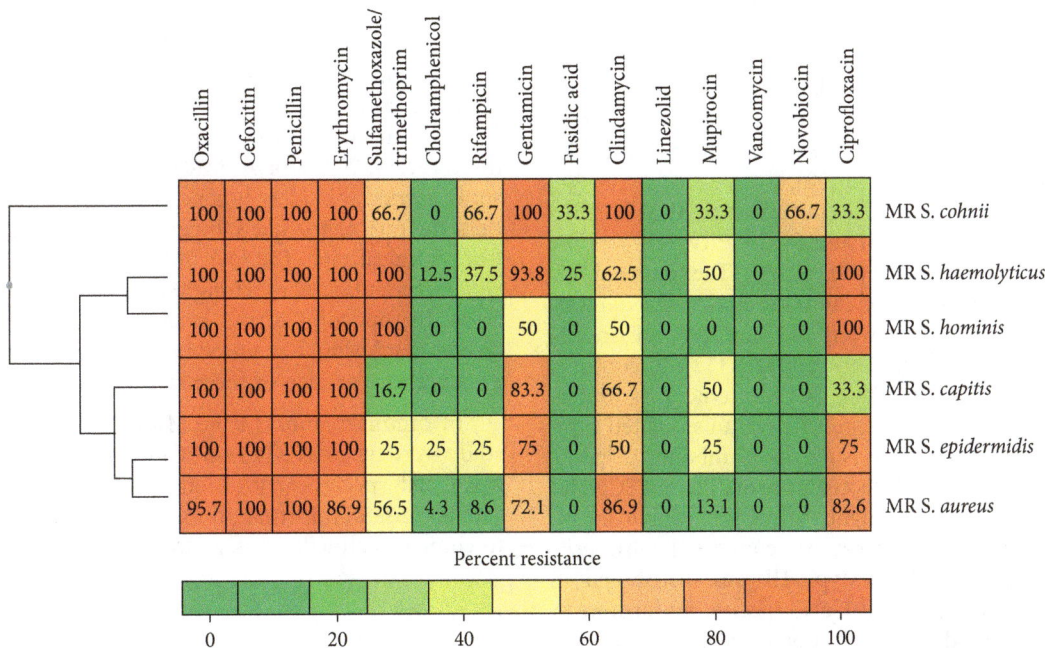

Figure 2: Antimicrobial resistance patterns of MRSA and MR-CoNS isolates to 15 antimicrobial agents.

SCC*mec* type III was found to be predominant, with a proportion of 56.5% (13/23) of MRSA isolates. Our results are in agreement with Chongtrakool et al., who reported SCC*mec* type III as the predominant type in many Asian countries such as Saudi Arabia, India, Sri Lanka, Singapore, Indonesia, Thailand, Vietnam, Philippines, and China, whereas SCC*mec* type I of MRSA isolates which shows high prevalence in Iran (56.9%) was found to be only 26.1% in our study [29, 30].

We found that ST239 was detected in 43.5% (10/23) MRSA isolates, and all positive clones carried SCC*mec* type III (ST239-SCC*mec* III). Previous studies have demonstrated that ST239-SCC*mec* III is the endemic HA-MRSA in many Asian countries, although a recent study showed that this clone is being steadily displaced by emerging CA-MRSA clones [24]. ST239-SCC*mec* III was also reported to be the dominant clone among MRSA clinical isolates in Singapore during 2006–2010. Similarly, because of its high prevalence

TABLE 1: Molecular characterization of SCCmec types, disinfectant resistance genes, and antibiotic resistance genes.

Gene	MRSA, n = 23 (%)	MR-CoNS					Total, n = 31 (%)
		S. haemolyticus, n = 18 (%)	S. epidermidis, n = 3 (%)	S. cohnii, n = 3 (%)	S. capitis, n = 6 (%)	S. hominis, n = 1 (%)	
SCCmec types							
I	6 (26.1)	0	0	0	3 (50.0)	0	3 (9.7)
II	1 (4.3)	10 (55.6)	0	0	0	0	10 (32.3)
III	13 (56.5)	0	0	3 (100)	1 (16.7)	1 (100)	5 (16.1)
IVa	1 (4.3)	3 (16.7)	0	0	0	0	3 (9.7)
IVb	1 (4.3)	0	0	0	0	0	0
IVc	0	0	2 (66.7)	0	0	0	2 (6.5)
IVd	0	0	0	0	0	0	0
V	1 (4.3)	0	0	0	2 (33.3)	0	2 (6.5)
Untypeable	0	5 (25.0)	1 (33.3)	0	0	0	6 (19.4)
ST239	10 (43.5)	–	–	–	–	–	–
qacA/B	6 (26.1)	13 (72.2)	0	3 (100)	5 (83.3)	1 (100)	22 (70.9)
Antimicrobial resistance							
ermA	18 (78.3)	0	1 (33.3)	0	3 (50.0)	0	4 (12.9)
ermB	17 (73.9)	0	1 (33.3)	0	3 (50.0)	0	4 (12.9)
ermC	1 (4.3)	16 (88.9)	1 (33.3)	3 (100)	6 (100)	1 (100)	27 (87.1)

(77.1%), ST239-SCCmec II was accounted for as the most dominant nosocomial MRSA clone in 18 hospitals in China [31]. It has been reported that ST239-SCCmec III was detected in at least 90% of HA-MRSA isolates in Sappasithiprasong Hospital, Northeast Thailand [20]. These dominant types were resistant to many antibiotics such as erythromycin, gentamicin, sulfamethoxazole/trimethoprim, and ciprofloxacin (Table 1). Similar to the finding of Shahsavan et al., 82% of clinical MRSA isolates in Iran were characterized as ST239, and all these strains were resistant to ciprofloxacin, erythromycin, gentamicin, sulfamethoxazole/trimethoprim, and tetracycline [32].

SCCmec types have been characterized in 31 MR-CoNS isolates, as shown in Table 1, and SCCmec type II was the dominant type of S. haemolyticus (62.5%). The results of this study are similar to those of Pinheiro et al., who demonstrated the association between SCCmec type II and S. haemolyticus isolated from blood cultures [33]. In contrast, Ruppe et al. demonstrated that SCCmec type V is preferentially associated with S. haemolyticus strains isolated from disparate geographical areas such as Cambodia, Algeria, Mali, and Moldova [34]. The occurrence of different SCCmec types in many countries might reflect the genetic background of S. haemolyticus strains, connected with geographical locations. SCCmec type III was distributed in various MRSA clones and MR-CoNS species, conforming to our results that found the distribution of SCCmec type III in various species such as S. cohnii, S. capitis, and S. hominis. Significantly, SCCmec type IV was associated with methicillin-resistant S. epidermidis (MRSE). This supported the finding of Wisplinghoff et al. that SCCmec type IV is distributed in many MRSE strains [35].

High prevalence of ermA (78.3%) and ermB (73.9%) genes was found in MRSA isolates, compared to the ermC (4.3%). The results of this study are similar to those of Lim et al. and Akpaka et al., which documented the high carriage of ermA and a lower prevalence of ermC in S. aureus isolates in Malaysian patients and Trinidad and Tobago patients, respectively [36, 37]. On the contrary, high prevalence of ermC (87.1%) was found in MR-CoNS isolates compared to the ermA (12.9%) and the ermB (12.9%) genes. Likewise, Bouchami et al. reported that the prevalence of ermC, ermA, and ermB of MR-CoNS isolated from bacteremic patients in oncohematology was 25.9%, 7.4%, and 7.4%, respectively [38].

We found that 26.1% of MRSA isolates carried the qacA/B gene. Its prevalence in the present study is higher than that in a previous report by Lu et al., who found 25 (7.8%) of the 321 MRSA isolates harboring qacA/B [39]. On the contrary, 70.9% of all MR-CoNS isolates in the present study carried the qacA/B gene. This prevalence was higher than the rate of the qacA/B gene carried by CoNS isolated from surgical sites (37.9%) [40], nurses (56.7%), and the general population in Hong Kong (13.5%) [23]. The increased proportion of the qacA/B gene in MR-CoNS indicates that hospital-acquired infections could exert selective pressure for carriage of these strains.

In summary, most of the MRSA isolates in the present study were typed as ST239-SCCmec type III, while different MR-CoNS species carry various SCCmec types. This finding provides useful information for a preventive health strategy to combat methicillin-resistant staphylococcal infections.

Acknowledgments

We would like to thank microbiology staff from Chiangrai Prachanukroh Hospital for specimen collection. We also acknowledge Dr. Keiichi Hiramatsu and Dr. Teruyo Ito for providing SCC*mec*-type strains. We thank Prof. Dr. Gavin Reynolds for editing the manuscript. This work was supported by a grant from the National Research Council of Thailand (R2560B064) to SS.

References

[1] S. Y. Tong, J. S. Davis, E. Eichenberger, T. L. Holland, and V. G. Fowler Jr., "*Staphylococcus aureus* infections: epidemiology, pathophysiology, clinical manifestations, and management," *Clinical Microbiology Reviews*, vol. 28, no. 3, pp. 603–661, 2015.

[2] C. von Eiff, G. Peters, and C. Heilmann, "Pathogenesis of infections due to coagulase-negative staphylococci," *Lancet Infectious Diseases*, vol. 2, no. 11, pp. 677–685, 2002.

[3] A. Japoni-Nejad, M. Rezazadeh, H. Kazemian et al., "Molecular characterization of the first community-acquired methicillin-resistant *Staphylococcus aureus* strains from Central Iran," *International Journal of Infectious Diseases*, vol. 17, no. 11, pp. e949–e954, 2013.

[4] R. Seng, T. Kitti, R. Thummeepak et al., "Biofilm formation of methicillin-resistant coagulase negative staphylococci (MR-CoNS) isolated from community and hospital environments," *PLoS One*, vol. 12, no. 8, Article ID e0184172, 2017.

[5] P. Tulinski, A. C. Fluit, J. A. Wagenaar et al., "Methicillin-resistant coagulase-negative staphylococci on pig farms as a reservoir of heterogeneous staphylococcal cassette chromosome *mec* elements," *Applied and Environmental Microbiology*, vol. 78, no. 2, pp. 299–304, 2012.

[6] E. Ghaznavi-Rad, M. Nor Shamsudin, Z. Sekawi, A. van Belkum, and V. A. Neela, "A simplified multiplex PCR assay for fast and easy discrimination of globally distributed staphylococcal cassette chromosome *mec* types in methicillin resistant *Staphylococcus aureus*," *Journal of Medical Microbiology*, vol. 59, no. 10, pp. 1135–1139, 2010.

[7] M. Xiao, H. Wang, Y. Zhao et al., "National surveillance of methicillin-resistant *Staphylococcus aureus* in China highlights a still-evolving epidemiology with 15 novel emerging multilocus sequence types," *Journal of Clinical Microbiology*, vol. 51, no. 11, pp. 3638–3644, 2013.

[8] Z. Zong, C. Peng, and X. Lü, "Diversity of SCC*mec* elements in methicillin-resistant coagulase-negative staphylococci clinical isolates," *PLoS One*, vol. 6, no. 5, Article ID e20191, 2011.

[9] S. Mayer, M. Boos, A. Beyer, A. C. Fluit, and F. J. Schmitz, "Distribution of the antiseptic resistance genes *qac*A, *qac*B and *qac*C in 497 methicillin-resistant and susceptible European isolates of *Staphylococcus aureus*," *Journal of Infection and Chemotherapy*, vol. 47, no. 6, pp. 896–907, 2001.

[10] J. A. Otter, A. Patel, P. R. Cliff et al., "Selection for *qac*A carriage in CC22, but not CC30, methicillin-resistant *Staphylococcus aureus* bloodstream infection isolates during a successful institutional infection control programme," *Journal of Antimicrobial Chemotherapy*, vol. 68, no. 5, pp. 992–999, 2013.

[11] A. C. Fluit, M. R. Visser, and F. J. Schmitz, "Molecular detection of antimicrobial resistance," *Clinical Microbiology Reviews*, vol. 14, no. 4, pp. 836–871, 2001.

[12] Clinical Laboratory Standards Institute, "Performance standards for antimicrobial susceptibility testing," in *Proceedings of Twenty-Fourth Informational Supplement: M100-S24*, Wayne, PA, USA, January 2014.

[13] P. Kohner, J. Uhl, C. Kolbert, D. Persing, and F. R. Cockerill, "Comparison of susceptibility testing methods with *mec*A gene analysis for determining oxacillin (methicillin) resistance in clinical isolates of *Staphylococcus aureus* and coagulase-negative *Staphylococcus* spp.," *Journal of Clinical Microbiology*, vol. 37, no. 9, pp. 2952–2961, 1999.

[14] C. Ryffel, W. Tesch, I. Birch-Machin et al., "Sequence comparison of *mec*A genes isolated from methicillin-resistant *Staphylococcus aureus* and *Staphylococcus epidermidis*," *Gene*.vol. 94, no. 1, pp. 137-138, 1990.

[15] T. Sasaki, S. Tsubakishita, Y. Tanaka et al., "Multiplex-PCR method for species identification of coagulase-positive staphylococci," *Journal of Clinical Microbiology*, vol. 48, no. 3, pp. 765–769, 2010.

[16] A. Bizzini and G. Greub, "Matrix assisted laser desorption ionization time of flight mass spectrometry, a revolution in clinical microbial identification," *Clinical Microbiology and Infection*, vol. 16, no. 11, pp. 1614–1619, 2010.

[17] A. J. Loonen, A. R. Jansz, J. N. Bergland et al., "Comparative study using phenotypic, genotypic, and proteomics methods for identification of coagulase-negative staphylococci," *Journal of Clinical Microbiology*, vol. 50, no. 4, pp. 1437–1439, 2012.

[18] V. Suttisunhakul, A. Pumpuang, P. Ekchariyawat et al., "Matrix-assisted laser desorption/ionization time-of-flight mass spectrometry for the identification of *Burkholderia pseudomallei* from Asia and Australia and differentiation between *Burkholderia* species," *PLoS One*, vol. 12, no. 4, e0175294 pages, 2017.

[19] K. Zhang, J. A. McClure, S. Elsayed, T. Louie, and J. M. Conly, "Novel multiplex PCR assay for characterization and concomitant subtyping of staphylococcal cassette chromosome *mec* types I to V in methicillin-resistant *Staphylococcus aureus*," *Journal of Clinical Microbiology*, vol. 43, no. 10, pp. 5026–5033, 2005.

[20] E. J. Feil, E. K. Nickerson, N. Chantratita et al., "Rapid detection of the pandemic methicillin-resistant *Staphylococcus aureus* clone ST 239, a dominant strain in Asian hospitals," *Journal of Clinical Microbiology*, vol. 48, no. 4, pp. 1520–1522, 2008.

[21] N. Ardic, M. Ozyurt, B. Sareyyupoglu, and T. Haznedaroglu, "Investigation of erythromycin and tetracycline resistance genes in methicillin-resistant staphylococci," *International Journal of Antimicrobial Agents*, vol. 26, no. 3, pp. 213–218, 2005.

[22] J. H. Youn, Y. H. Park, B. Hang'ombe, and C. Sugimoto, "Prevalence and characterization of *Staphylococcus aureus* and *Staphylococcus pseudintermedius* isolated from companion animals and environment in the veterinary teaching hospital in Zambia, Africa," *Comparative Immunology, Microbiology and Infectious Diseases*, vol. 37, no. 2, pp. 123–130, 2014.

[23] M. Zhang, M. M. O'Donoghue, T. Ito, K. Hiramatsu, and M. V. Boost, "Prevalence of antiseptic-resistance genes in *Staphylococcus aureus* and coagulase-negative staphylococci colonizing nurses and the general population in Hong Kong," *Journal of Hospital Infection*, vol. 78, no. 2, pp. 113–117, 2011.

[24] C. J. Chen and Y. C. Huang, "New epidemiology of *staphylococcus aureus* infection in Asia," *Clinical Microbiology and Infection*, vol. 20, no. 7, pp. 605–623, 2014.

[25] K. Becker, C. Heilmann, and G. Peters, "Coagulase-negative staphylococci," *Clinical Microbiology Reviews*, vol. 27, no. 4, pp. 870–926, 2014.

[26] T. F. Lee, H. Lee, C. M. Chen et al., ""Comparison of the accuracy of matrix-assisted laser desorption ionization–time of flight mass spectrometry with that of other commercial identification systems for identifying *Staphylococcus saprophyticus* in urine," *Journal of Clinical Microbiology*, vol. 51, no. 5, pp. 1563–1566, 2013.

[27] H. Kong, F. Yu, W. Zhang, X. Li, and H. Wang, "Molecular epidemiology and antibiotic resistance profiles of methicillin-resistant *Staphylococcus aureus* strains in a tertiary hospital in China," *Frontiers in Microbiology*, vol. 8, p. 838, 2017.

[28] F. Barbier, E. Ruppé, D. Hernandez et al., "Methicillin-resistant coagulase-negative staphylococci in the community: high homology of SCC*mec* IVa between *Staphylococcus epidermidis* and major clones of methicillin-resistant *Staphylococcus aureus*," *Journal of Infectious Diseases*, vol. 202, no. 2, pp. 270–281, 2010.

[29] P. Chongtrakool, T. Ito, X. X. Ma et al., "Staphylococcal cassette chromosome *mec* (SCC*mec*) typing of methicillin-resistant *Staphylococcus aureus* strains isolated in 11 Asian countries: a proposal for a new nomenclature for SCC*mec* elements," *Antimicrobial Agents and Chemotherapy*, vol. 50, no. 3, pp. 1001–1012, 2006.

[30] M. Moghadami, A. Japoni, A. Karimi, and M. Mardani, "Comparison of community and healthcare-associated MRSA in Iran," *Iranian Journal of Clinical Infectious Diseases*, vol. 5, no. 4, pp. 206–212, 2010.

[31] Y. Liu, H. Wang, N. Du et al., "Molecular evidence for spread of two major methicillin-resistant *Staphylococcus aureus* clones with a unique geographic distribution in Chinese hospitals," *Antimicrobial Agents and Chemotherapy*, vol. 53, no. 2, pp. 512–518, 2009.

[32] S. Shahsavan, L. Jabalameli, P. Maleknejad et al., "Molecular analysis and antimicrobial susceptibility of methicillin resistant *Staphylococcus aureus* in one of the hospitals of Tehran university of medical sciences: high prevalence of sequence type 239 (ST239) clone," *Acta Microbiologica et Immunologica Hungarica*, vol. 58, no. 1, pp. 31–39, 2011.

[33] L. Pinheiro, C. I. Brito, V. C. Pereira et al., "Susceptibility profile of *Staphylococcus epidermidis* and *Staphylococcus haemolyticus* isolated from blood cultures to vancomycin and novel antimicrobial drugs over a period of 12 years," *Microbial Drug Resistance*, vol. 22, no. 4, pp. 283–293, 2016.

[34] E. Ruppe, F. Barbier, Y. Mesli et al., "Diversity of staphylococcal cassette chromosome *mec* structures in methicillin-resistant *Staphylococcus epidermidis* and *Staphylococcus haemolyticus* strains among outpatients from four countries," *Antimicrobial Agents and Chemotherapy*, vol. 53, no. 2, pp. 442–449, 2009.

[35] H. Wisplinghoff, A. E. Rosato, M. C. Enright, M. Noto, W. Craig, and G. L. Archer, "Related clones containing SCC*mec* type IV predominate among clinically significant *Staphylococcus epidermidis* isolates," *Antimicrobial Agents and Chemotherapy*, vol. 47, no. 11, pp. 3574–3579, 2003.

[36] K. Lim, Y. Hanifah, M. Yusof, and K. Thong, "*erm*A, *erm*C, *tet*M and *tet*K are essential for erythromycin and tetracycline resistance among methicillin-resistant *Staphylococcus aureus* strains isolated from a tertiary hospital in Malaysia," *Indian Journal of Medical Microbiology*, vol. 30, no. 2, pp. 203–207, 2012.

[37] P. E. Akpaka, R. Roberts, and S. Monecke, "Molecular characterization of antimicrobial resistance genes against *Staphylococcus aureus* isolates from Trinidad and Tobago," *Journal of Infection and Public Health*, vol. 10, no. 3, pp. 316–323, 2017.

[38] O. Bouchami, W. Achour, M. A. Mekni, J. Rolo, and A. Ben Hassen, "Antibiotic resistance and molecular characterization of clinical isolates of methicillin-resistant coagulase-negative staphylococci isolated from bacteremic patients in oncohematology," *Folia Microbiologica (Praha)*, vol. 56, no. 2, pp. 122–130, 2011.

[39] Z. Lu, Y. Chen, W. Chen et al., "Characteristics of qacA/B-positive *Staphylococcus aureus* isolated from patients and a hospital environment in China," *Journal of Antimicrobial Chemotherapy*, vol. 70, no. 3, pp. 653–657, 2015.

[40] M. Temiz, N. Duran, G. G. Duran, N. Eryılmaz, and K. Jenedi, "Relationship between the resistance genes to quaternary ammonium compounds and antibiotic resistance in staphylococci isolated from surgical site infections," *Medical Science Monitor*, vol. 20, pp. 544–550, 2014.

8

Pathogenicity and Whole Genome Sequence Analysis of a Pseudorabies Virus Strain FJ-2012 Isolated from Fujian, Southern China

Xue-min Wu,[1] Qiu-yong Chen,[1] Ru-jing Chen,[1] Yong-liang Che,[1] Long-bai Wang,[1] Chen-yan Wang,[1] Shan Yan,[1] Yu-tao Liu,[1] Jin-sheng Xiu,[2] and Lun-jiang Zhou[1]

[1]*Institute of Animal Husbandry and Veterinary Medicine, Fujian Academy of Agriculture Sciences/Fujian Animal Disease Control Technology Development Center, Fuzhou 350013, China*
[2]*College of Animal Sciences, Fujian Agricultural and Forestry University, Fuzhou, Fujian 350002, China*

Correspondence should be addressed to Jin-sheng Xiu; xiujinsheng@163.com and Lun-jiang Zhou; lunjiang@163.com

Xue-min Wu and Qiu-yong Chen contributed equally to this work.

Academic Editor: Jialiang Yang

The outbreaks of pseudorabies have been frequently reported in Bartha-K61-vaccinated farms in China since 2011. To study the pathogenicity and evolution of the circulating pseudorabies viruses in Fujian Province, mainland China, we isolated and sequenced the whole genome of a wild-type pseudorabies virus strain named "FJ-2012." We then conducted a few downstream bioinformatics analyses including phylogenetic analysis and pathogenic analysis and used the virus to infect 6 pseudorabies virus-free piglets. FJ-2012-infected piglets developed symptoms like high body temperature and central nervous system disorders and had high mortality rate. In addition, we identified typical micropathological changes such as multiple gross lesions in infected piglets through pathological analysis and conclude that the FJ-2012 genome is significantly different from known pseudorabies viruses, in which insertions, deletions, and substitutions are observed in multiple immune and virulence genes. In summary, this study shed lights on the molecular basis of the prevalence and pathology of the pseudorabies virus strain FJ-2012. The genome of FJ-2012 could be used as a reference to study the evolution of pseudorabies viruses, which is critical to the vaccine development of new emerging pseudorabies viruses.

1. Introduction

Pseudorabies virus (PRV), also called Aujeszky's disease virus or *Suid herpesvirus* 1, is the causative agent of pseudorabies (PR), which infects a wide variety of animals from mollusks to mammals and damages world economy. PRV is a member of the subfamily Alphaherpesvirinae in the family Herpesviridae belonging to the genus *Varicellovirus* [1]. Though the virus was first described in cattle by Aujeszky in 1902, pigs are the natural reservoir for PRV [2, 3]. The clinical symptoms of PR in pigs are characterized by central nervous system (CNS) disorders in piglets, abortion in pregnant swine, and respiring signs in older pigs [4].

The PRV genome encompasses a unique long segment (UL) and a unique short region (US) flanked by the internal and terminal repeat sequences (IRS and TRS, resp.), encoding more than 70 proteins. The virulence of PRVs and the immunology mutual protection between them are determined by multiple genes, and thus the genome-wide analysis is necessary to define all the characteristics of the viruses [5, 6].

Pseudorabies had been well controlled in China due to the wide usage of gE-deleted vaccines and the serum distinguish test [7]. However, in late 2011, outbreaks of PR were reported in Bartha-K61-vaccinated farms, and the disease rapidly spread to 11 provinces from northern to eastern China including Heilongjiang, Jilin, Liaoning, Tianjin, Jiangsu, Zhejiang, and Fujian. A few studies showed that the current PR outbreaks on farms were caused by PRV variants, and the PR vaccine could not provide effective protection against the prevalence of PRV strains in China [8–10]. However, the complete genomes of the variants and their molecular characteristics are unclear, which is an obstacle in producing effective vaccines. As a result, the outbreaks have caused a great economic loss to swine-feeding industry in China.

In this study, we thoroughly assessed a pseudorabies virus named "PRV FJ-2012," which was isolated from a Bartha-K61-vaccinated pig farm in Fujian Province during a PR outbreak. The outbreak has the following characteristics: (1) the mortality of infections can be as high as 100% and (2) plenty of pregnant sows aborted. We have characterized the pathogenicity in pigs and analyzed the complete genome of the PRV FJ-2012 in order to characterize its molecular properties and virulence.

2. Materials and Methods

2.1. Virus, Cells, and Genomic Viral DNA Preparation. PRV FJ-2012 was isolated from pig brain samples collected from a Bartha-K61-vaccinated farm with a PR outbreak in Fujian Province, southern China, in 2012. The virus was determined to be a pseudorabies viral strain by the PCR analysis and the sequence analysis of its partial gE gene. Virus was propagated on PK-15 cells, cultured in Dulbecco's modified Eagle's medium (DMEM, Hyclone, USA) containing 1% fetal bovine serum (FBS, Gibco, USA), 100 IU/mL penicillin, and 100 μg/mL streptomycin at 37°C and 5% CO_2. Cells were harvested when the cytopathic effect (CPE) of PK-15 cells that were inoculated by PRV FJ-2012 strain reached 80%. After freeze-thaw for three times, the cell debris was removed by centrifugation at 5000 ×g for 30 min at 4°C. Then, the supernatant involving PRV was centrifuged by a Beckman ultracentrifuge (LE-80K) at 30,000 ×g for 2 h at 4°C; the supernatant was discarded, and the pellets were then resuspended in 2 mL PBS (0.01 mol/L, PH7.2). Discontinuous mass fraction sucrose gradients (30%, 35%, 40%, and 45%) that were formulated with PBS were further purified at 26,000 ×g for 2 h at 4°C. And then, the virus band (between 35% and 40%) was drawn to a centrifuge tube, and the sucrose was removed by centrifugation at 30,000 ×g for 1 h at 4°C. The purified virus particle was obtained and used to prepare genomic viral DNA using QIAamp DNA Mini Kit (QIAGEN, Germany) according to the manufacturer's instructions.

2.2. Experimental PRV Inoculation of Pigs. Ten healthy, 28-day-old Duroc × Landrace × Yorkshire (DLY) hybrid pigs were collected from PRV-free swine farm and confirmed to be serologically negative for PRV antibodies with a gB ELISA kit (IDEXX, USA). The pigs were randomly allocated to two groups, namely, the challenge and control group, and each group was housed in separate pens. Four pigs in Group 1 (the challenge group) were each inoculated intranasally (i.n.) with 1 mL 10^6 TCID50 FJ-2012 strain, and the other two pigs in Group 1 were i.n. with DMEM with the same dose as the cohabit infective test. The remaining four pigs were served as uninfected control. Clinical signs and rectal temperatures of pigs were recorded daily throughout the study. At 14 dpi, all surviving pigs were euthanized.

2.3. Tissue Sampling and Histological Analysis. After macroscopic examination, the tissue samples required for histological examination were obtained from the brains, kidneys, lungs, tonsils, livers, and lymph nodes (superficial inguinal). These samples were fixed in 10% formalin, processed routinely, and embedded in paraffin. Each paraffin sample was sectioned to 4-5 μm and stained with HE. The sections were viewed with a Motic BA210 microscope.

2.4. Genomic Sequencing, Assembly, Annotation, and Analysis. The genome of PRV FJ-2012 strain was sequenced with a Pacific Biosciences RS II sequencer (Pacific Biosciences, Menlo Park, CA, USA), using a single-molecule long-read sequencing technology with a 10K SMRTbell template library. We are fully aware that the long reads from the Pacific Biosciences RS II sequencer have some disadvantages like high error rate compared to short reads. However, we still prefer long reads since they are better at identifying gene isoforms and assembly, which are critical to this study. We then removed host reads by comparing the reads against the pigs (*Sus scrofa*) using BLAST. The remaining reads were de novo assembled; the obtained contigs were assembled with Celera software (https://sourceforge.net/projects/wgs-assembler/files/wgs-assembler/wgs-8.3/), and the scaffolds were constructed by comparing the contigs with reference PRV genomes (GenBank Accession # NC_006151) using the NCBI BLAST program. Finally, a Perl program was used to check gaps between the scaffolds, and the alignments were extremely high coverage with no gap.

The open reading frames (ORFs) of FJ-2012 genome were searched by ORF Finder (http://www.ncbi.nlm.nih.gov/gorf/), and genes were predicted and analyzed by GeneMarkS [11]. The ORF annotations of the FJ-2012 strain were created by BLAST homology-based transfer as previously described in [5, 12, 13]. The alignments were performed using the mVISTA genomic analysis tool with a LAGAN global alignment [14]. The phylogenetic trees were constructed using the neighbor-joining algorithm with 1000 bootstrap repetitions using the Kimura 2-parameter substitution model in MEGA 5.0 [15–17]. The distribution of polymorphic sites in eight PRV genomes was inferred using the software Base-By-Base [18].

3. Results

3.1. Pathogenicity of the PRV Strain FJ-2012 in Pigs. After intranasal infection of the 28-day-old PRV-free piglets, all pigs in the challenge group developed high fever beginning at 2 dpi with temperatures 41.9°C–42.5°C. The clinical signs were consistent with typical pseudorabies syndrome, from listlessness, anorexia, to high fever and then displayed respiratory symptoms such as cough, sneeze, and central nervous system (CNS) symptoms. Finally, all pigs in the challenge group exhibited opisthotonus and were dead in 8–14 dpi. The pigs in the cohabitation infection group also showed high fever with temperatures 41.9°C–42.5°C, but the time of onset was 4 days later and the clinical signs were milder than those in the challenge group. The pigs were also dead in the end (Table 1). In contrast, pigs in the control group remained healthy without any abnormal symptom.

TABLE 1: The outcome of the pigs inoculated intranasally (i.n.) with FJ-2012 strain or DMEM.

Groups	Dose (TCID50) 1 mL	Survival rate (day post infection)									Mortality (%)
		6	7	8	9	10	11	12	13	14	
PRV FJ-2012	10^6	4/4	4/4	3/4	3/4	2/4	2/4	1/4	1/4	0/4	100
Cohabitation	DMEM	2/2	2/2	2/2	2/2	2/2	2/2	1/2	1/2	1/2	50
Control	DMEM	4/4	4/4	4/4	4/4	4/4	4/4	4/4	4/4	4/4	0

3.2. Gross Lesions. The pigs in the FJ-2012-infected group showed multiple gross lesions. Macroscopic encephalic hemorrhages or encephalemia was observed in all pigs (4/4). Three of those pigs (3/4) showed pinpoint hemorrhages in the kidney. Small white foci were seen in the liver of four pigs (4/4). Diffuse reddened foci and edema of the lungs were observed in all pigs (4/4). The dark-red hemorrhage and congestion were noted in the lymph node of four pigs (4/4). Tonsil anabrosis was observed in three pigs (3/4). Two pigs in the cohabitation infection group showed milder lesions (such as slight hemorrhages in the brain and lung). No pig in the control group displayed gross lesions.

3.3. Histopathological Analysis. To further study the pathology of these organs, samples from brains, kidneys, livers, lungs, lymph nodes, and tonsils of pigs were stained with hematoxylin and eosin (H&E). On one hand, the histopathological examination showed multiple lesions in several organs of PRV-infected pigs. For example, nonsuppurative ganglioneuritis, characterized by gliosis, hemorrhage (Figure 1(a)), pronounced perivascular inflammatory infiltrates, and nerve cell necrosis were observed in the brain (Figure 1(b)). The lungs showed severe hemorrhage, congestion, and edema, and bronchiolar cavities were filled with cellular serous exudates that were red-stained (Figure 1(c)). Multiple small focal necrosis were discovered in the liver (Figure 1(d)) and the kidney with lymphocytic infiltration and congestion (Figure 1(e)). The striking changes in the lymph nodes include brownish-stained hemosiderosis and lymph follicle swelling (Figure 1(f)). The stratified squamous epithelium of tonsil appeared modified, necrosed and exfoliative (Figure 1(g)). On the other hand, the histopathological results of these organs from the control group had no significantly pathological changes (Figures 1(h)–1(n)).

3.4. Complete Genomic Characterization of the PRV FJ-2012 Strain. We performed the whole genome sequencing of FJ-2012 and performed a few downstream analyses on the sequencing data (Figure 2). The total length of its genome is 144,873 bp with a high G + C content of 73.5%. The overall genomic composition is the same as that of a few previously studied strains (Bartha, Kaplan, and Becker), consisting of a unique long (UL) region (position at 1–102,119), a unique short (US) region (118,893–128,096), internal repeat sequences (IRs, 102,120–118,892), and terminal repeat sequences (TRs, 128,097–144,873), which are located at the flank of the US region (Figure 1(a)). 70 open reading frames (ORFs) were identified, which relate to 70 genes that encode 68 different proteins (Figure 1(a)) since there are the two putative genes

(US1 and IE180). It is of note that US3 and US3.5 were treated as different genes due to their distinct functions [19].

The unique long regions containing 59 genes, most of which are involved in DNA replicative mechanisms and virus particle assembly and mature, are transcribed in both directions. Unique short regions containing 7 genes transcribed backward are likely affecting pathogenesis and host range functions. IRS and TRS containing US1 and IE180 genes, which function as an accessory regulatory protein and interact with the IE protein to enhance gene transactivation, are transcribed in reverse directions [20].

3.5. Comparison and Phylogenetic Analysis among PRV Strains. We compared the genomes of FJ-2012 with those of other 7 PRV strains including Kaplan, Becker, Bartha, JS-2012, HeN1, TJ, and ZJ01. The four strains JS-2012, HeN1, TJ, and ZJ01 were isolated from China (Table 2). As can be seen, FJ-2012 exhibited 94.2% to 98.32% nucleotide identity with other strains from China and 89.8% to 91.9% nucleotide identity with strains outside China. Specifically, FJ-2012 is highly homologous to TJ strains (98.32%) and shared only 89.8% identity with the strain Bartha, which is deemed as an excellent vaccine strain to control pseudorabies.

In addition, most genetic variations among the PRV strains are located in noncoding regions, internal repeat sequence regions, and terminal repeat sequence regions (Figure 3 and see Table S1 available online at https://doi.org/10.1155/2017/9073172). There are also variations in a few coding regions such as US1, UL36, gN, gB, and gC. There are overall 11,893, 12,621 and 14,956 genomic changes, including 3759, 3724, and 3789 single-nucleotide substitutions between FJ-2012 and three non-China-origin viruses Kaplan, Becker, and Bartha, respectively (Table 2). The genomic changes between FJ-2012 and non-China-origin viruses are higher than those between FJ-2012 and China-origin viruses. Specifically, there are 4649, 4628, 2445, and 8557 genomic changes, including 716, 560, 206, and 1025 single-nucleotide substitutions between FJ-2012 and four China-origin viruses JS-2012, HeN1, TJ, and ZJ01, respectively.

We then performed the phylogenetic analysis of the 8 viruses based on their full-length genome sequences, which indicates that the PRV strains can be separated into 2 major groups corresponding to their geographic locations, namely, group genotype I consisting of strains in China and group genotype II consisting of European and American strains (Figure 4). FJ-2012 is phylogenetically most close to TJ strain.

3.6. Distribution of Polymorphic Sites and Protein Coding Variations of PRVs. We used Base-by-Base software to infer

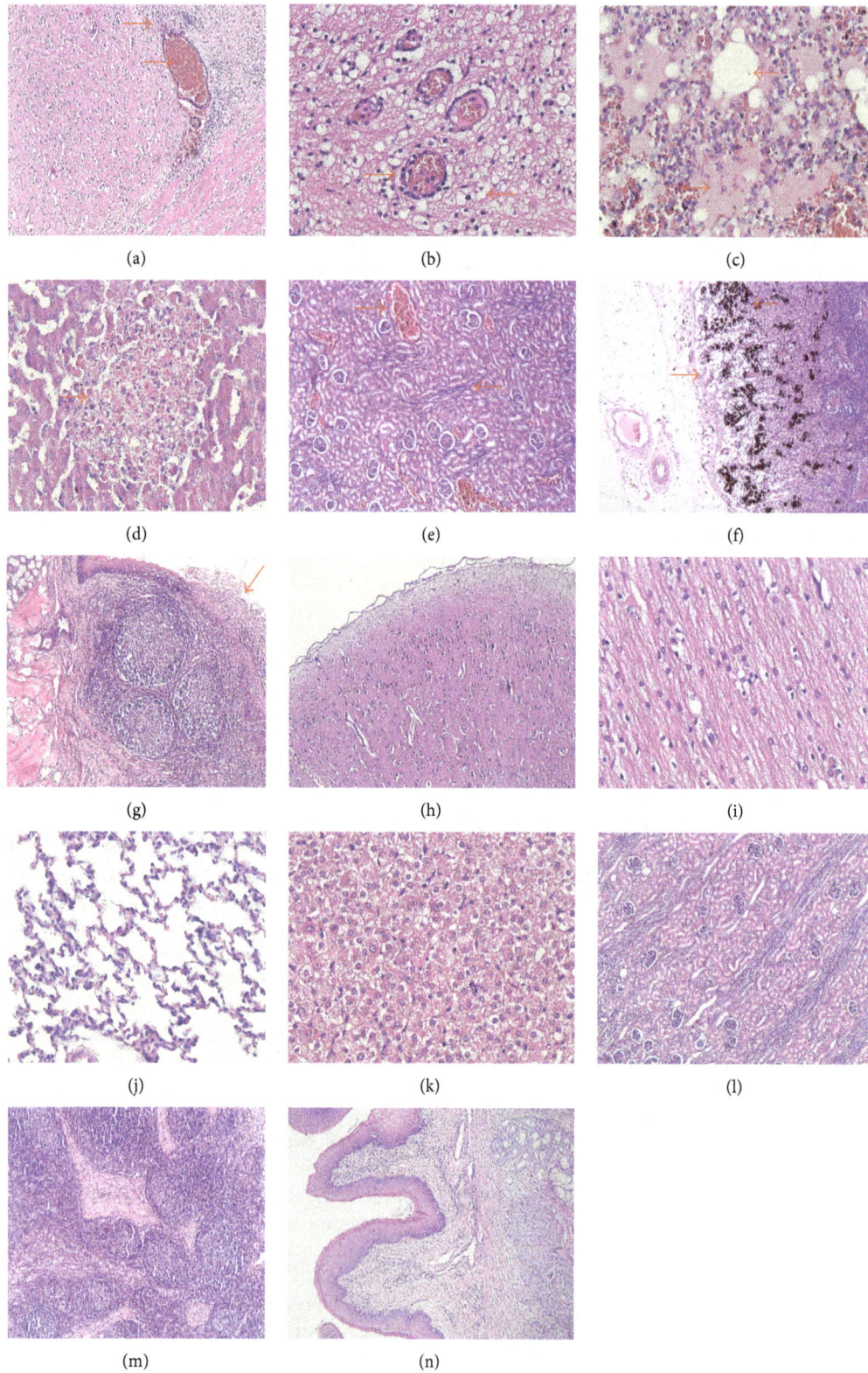

FIGURE 1: Histopathological findings of PRV-infected or control pigs. The pictures show representative tissue samples from the PRV-infected (a–g) and control (h–n) groups stained with H&E, 100x (a and h) and 400x (b–g, i–n). Brains (a, b, h, and i), lungs (c and j), livers (d and k), kidneys (e and l), lymph nodes (f and m), and tonsils (g and n).

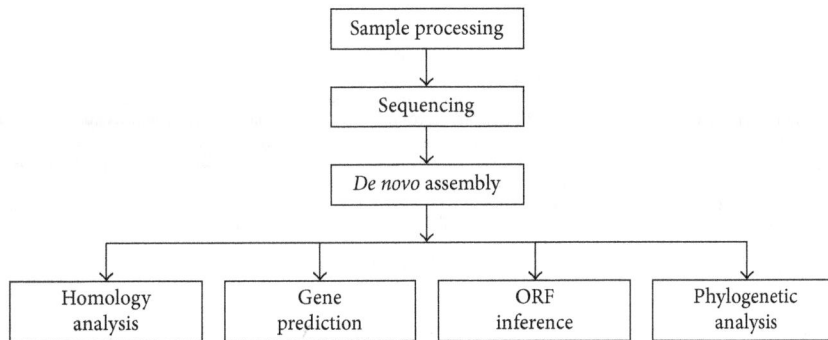

FIGURE 2: Data analysis flow for FJ-2012 sequence.

TABLE 2: Comparison of PRV FJ-2012 with other strains.

Genome	Kaplan	Becker	Bartha	JS-2012	HeN1	TJ	ZJ01
Identity (%)	91.89	91.44	89.82	96.84	96.82	98.32	94.17
Total changes	11,893	12,621	14,956	4649	4628	2445	8557
SNP	3759	3724	3789	716	560	206	1025

the distribution of polymorphic sites among the 8 PRVs. The changes between the genomic sequences of PRV FJ-2012 and those of non-China-origin PRV strains are predominantly substitutions, with a few insertions and deletions. However, the changes between FJ-2012 and China-origin strains JS-2012, HeN1, TJ, and ZJ01 are mainly insertions and substitutions (Figure 5). The sequence comparison revealed that PRV FJ-2012 genomes show great variations with other PRVs.

To further study the FJ-2012 genome, we compared its protein-coding regions with those of other viruses using local BLAST in BioEdit. The viruses in the group genotype I share 100% sequence identity with FJ-2012 for 16 ORFs and 94.7–99.9% identity for 53 ORFs. It is of note that HeN1 only shares 22.1% sequence identity with other strains on the protein IE180 due to a frame shift by upstream substitution. As for European and American strains (genotype II), FJ-2-12 shares 90.8–99.9% sequence identity in 69 ORFs (Table 2). The sequence alignment showed that FJ-2012 displayed extensive variations with previously isolated PRV strains including Kaplan, Becker, and the vaccine strain Bartha in most viral proteins, such as glycoproteins, for example, gN (UL49.5), gC (UL44), gL (UL1), gE (US8), and gB (UL27), tegument proteins, for example, UL36, UL46, UL16, and UL13, and nonstructural proteins, for example, IE180 and UL52 (Figure 5).

4. Discussion

Previous studies suggest that pseudorabies virus (PRV) can cause serious disease to piglets. The mortality rate is up to 100% for infected two-week old piglets with neurologic symptoms, while that for weaned piglets, the mortality rate is about 50% [19]. In this study, we tested the pathogenicity of FJ-2012 using six 28-day-old PRV-free piglets, four of

which were in the challenge group and the other two were in the cohabit group. The piglets in the challenge group received intranasal challenge with 1 mL $10^{6.0}$ 50% tissue culture infecting dose, and those in the cobabit group were inoculated intranasally with DMEM with the same dose. Unfortunately, all 4 piglets in the challenge group died on day 8, 10, 12, and 14 post infection (DPI), respectively, and one piglet in the cohabit group died on 12 DPI (Table 1). The clinical symptoms of the piglets in the challenge group were consistent with those of typical pseudorabies syndromes including listlessness, anorexia, and high fever and respiratory symptoms such as cough, sneeze, and central nervous system symptoms. In postmortem and histopathological examinations of dead piglets, multiple lesion sites were observed in several organs (Figure 1). The findings suggest that FJ-2012 strain can cause severe pathological changes, which are more serious than previously observed [19].

In general, the virulence of virus and the immune failure are potentially associated with gene mutations. Previous surveys have showed that gene variants of isolated viruses contributed to the epidemics of PRV [8–10, 21]. Therefore, it is important and necessary to further analyze the genetic variations of the current PR for disease control and surveillance. Here, we have sequenced the whole genome of the PRV strain FJ-2012 by a Pacific Biosciences RS II sequencer, and the resulting sequences were assembled, predicted, and annotated of genes. The resulting PRV FJ-2012 genome sequence is 144,873 bp in length with a high G + C content of 73.5% and contains 70 ORFs. The analysis of genome variations indicated that the isolate strain showed high variations with other abovementioned strains, including substitutions, insertions, and/or deletions that occurred in most proteins, revealing that the PRV strain in southern China is quite different from previous ones.

Additionally, the main antigen of gB, gC, and gD genes which induces the neutralization antibody is important for protecting PRV infection, and the genes of gE, gI, and TK are related to virus virulence [22, 23]. Our study showed that FJ-2012 has 96.9–97.4%, 93.1–93.3%, and 97.5–98.0% sequence identity with the 7 compared strains on gB, gC, and gD, respectively (see Table S1), while the sequence identities on gE, gI, and TK are 95.8–96%, 94.2–94.5%, and 99.4–99.7%, respectively. Moreover, the US1 protein, which functions as an accessory regulatory protein and

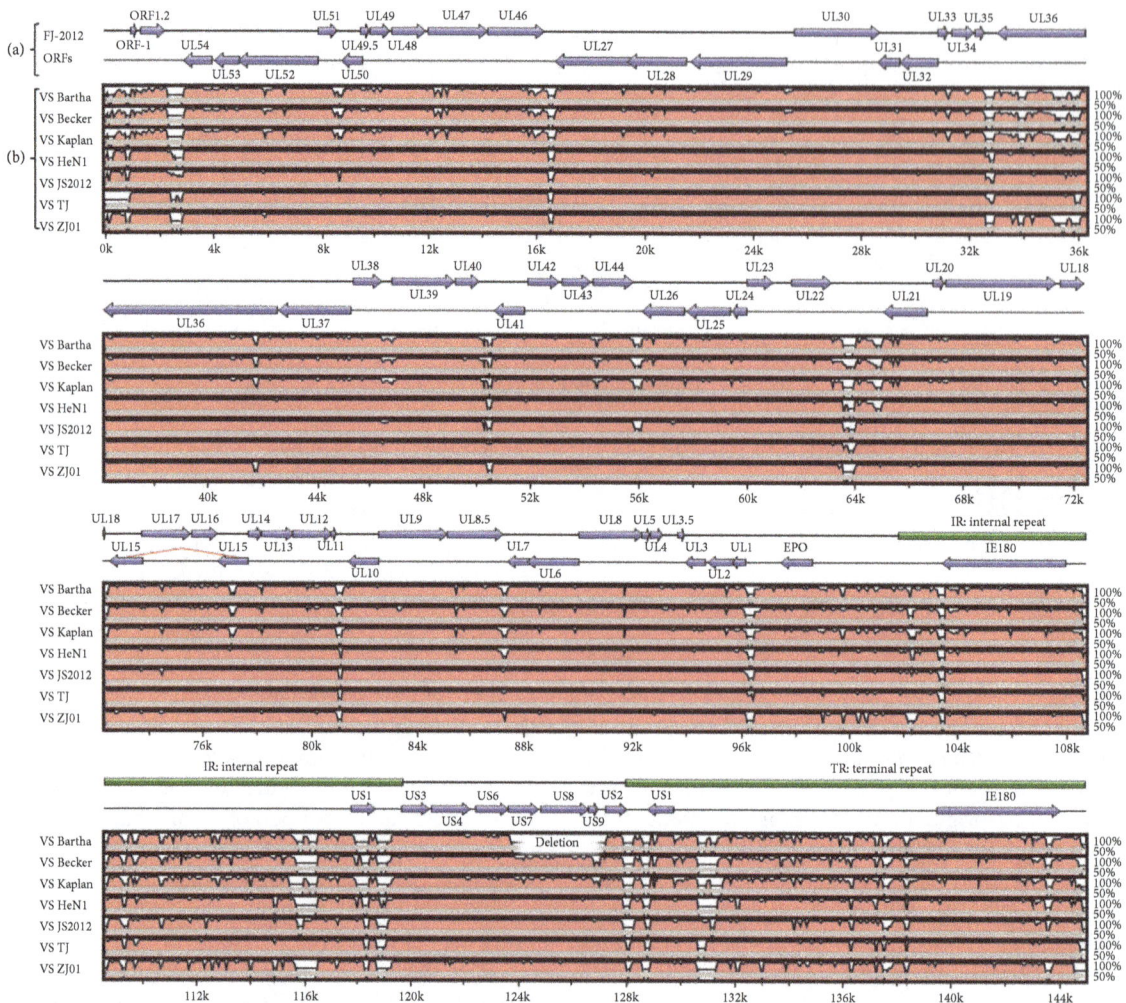

FIGURE 3: Genome organization of the PRV FJ-2012 and comparison of sequence conservation with other strains. (a) ORFs (horizontal bars in azure color) together with internal and terminal repeats (horizontal bars in green color) are depicted along with the genome. (b) Plots showing sequence conservation among PRV Bartha, Becker, Kaplan, HeN1, JS-2012, TJ, and ZJ01. Gene conservation was determined from a multiple sequence alignment, and the conservation score between any 2 genomes is plotted in a sliding 100 bp window.

interacts with the IE protein to enhance gene transactivation [20], and the UL36 protein, which is thought to function both in early infection and in later stages of viral maturation [24], showed the highest variability between genotype I and II PRV strains.

The envelope of PRV virion, glycoprotein N protein, is encoded by UL49.5 gene, a small O-glycosylated protein that forms a disulfide-linked complex with gM and functions in viral immune evasion [25, 26]. In veterinary varicelloviruses (PRV, EHV-1, and BHV-1), the UL49.5 gene product is an inhibitor of TAP, the transporter associated with processing antigens into peptides for presentation by major histocompatibility complex (MHC) class I molecules at the cell surface [26]. In this study, gN only shares 87.9% identity with the vaccine strain Bartha and shares high homology with other Chinese PRV strains (Table 2, Figure 3). The great variations between vaccine strains and novel Chinese strains might be a potential source of the novel isolate PRV strains to evade the immune response.

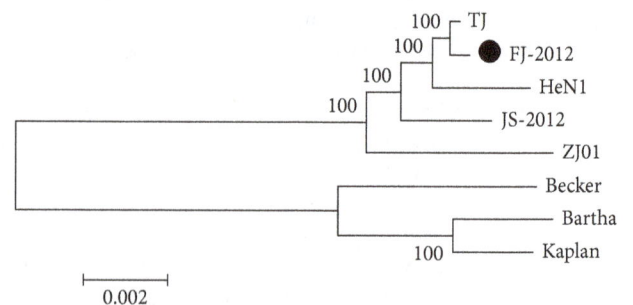

FIGURE 4: Phylogenetic comparison of PRVs. The sequences were aligned by Clustal, and the phylogenetic tree was constructed by MEGA 5.0 software using the neighbor-joining method with 1000 bootstraps. The nucleotide substitution model was chosen to be the Kimura 2-parameter substitution model.

Finally, the apparent genetic relationships among PRVs and the sufficient genomic variants in the field isolate strain FJ-2012 are identified to distinguish it from 2 major genotypes

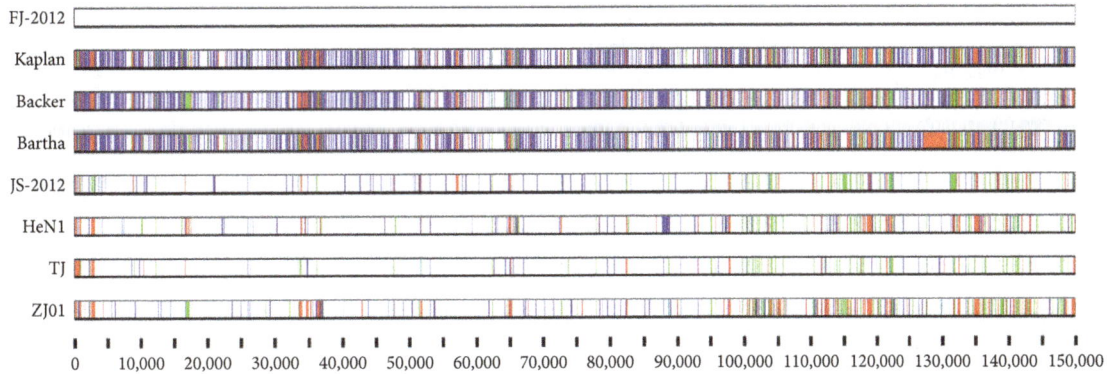

FIGURE 5: Distribution of polymorphic sites in eight PRV genomes. The genomes were aligned with CLC Genomics Workbench 8 and using Base-by-Base software. The sequence of the PRV strain FJ-2012 was used as the reference. Nucleotides in other 7 pseudorabies virus strains differing from the sequence of the PRV field isolate strain FJ-2012 are displayed: blue, nucleotide substitutions; green, insertions; and red, deletions.

based on phylogenetic analysis, which might be a factor contributing to the vaccination failure in a vaccinated farm.

5. Conclusions

Since late 2011, pseudorabies outbreaks have been reported and spread in many farms in China. However, all novel isolated PRV genome reports were isolated in northern China, and there is no systematic research in southern China. In this study, we observed that the PRV FJ-2012 isolated from Fujian Province, southern China, is highly pathogenic and has extensive variation in genomic sequence with the reference PRV. This study contributes to the study of epidemiology and genetic evolution on PRV and lays a scientific foundation for the development of new PR vaccine.

Authors' Contributions

Lun-jiang Zhou and Jin-sheng Xiu conceived the main idea of the research plan. Xue-min Wu and Qiu-yong Chen performed experiments. Ru-jing Chen and Yong-liang Che analyzed the data. Xue-min Wu and Qiu-yong Chen prepared the manuscript. Long-bai Wang, Shan Yan, Yu-tao Liu, and Chen-yan Wang contributed to the discussion. All authors have approved the final manuscript.

Acknowledgments

This study is partially supported by grants from the Natural Science Foundation project of Fujian Province, China (no. 2014J01107), and the Public Welfare projects of Fujian Province, China (no. 2015R1023-10), and the Innovative Research Team for Fujian Academy of Agriculture Science (no. STIT2017-3-10).

References

[1] L. E. Pomeranz, A. E. Reynolds, and C. J. Hengartner, "Molecular biology of pseudorabies virus: impact on neurovirology and veterinary medicine," *Microbiology and Molecular Biology Reviews*, vol. 69, no. 3, pp. 462–500, 2005.

[2] R. P. Hanson, "The history of pseudorabies in the United States," *Journal of the American Veterinary Medical Association*, vol. 124, no. 925, pp. 259–261, 1954.

[3] A. Marcaccini, M. López Peña, M. I. Quiroga, R. Bermúdez, J. M. Nieto, and N. Alemañ, "Pseudorabies virus infection in mink: a host-specific pathogenesis," *Veterinary Immunology and Immunopathology*, vol. 124, no. 3-4, pp. 264–273, 2008.

[4] J. Y. S. Lee and M. R. Wilson, "A review of pseudorabies (Aujeszky's disease) in pigs," *Canadian Veterinary Journal*, vol. 20, no. 3, pp. 65–69, 1979.

[5] B. G. Klupp, C. J. Hengartner, T. C. Mettenleiter, and L. W. Enquist, "Complete, annotated sequence of the pseudorabies virus genome," *Journal of Virology*, vol. 78, no. 1, pp. 424–440, 2004.

[6] T. Ben-Porat and A. S. Kaplan, "Molecular biology of pseudorabies virus," in *The Herpesviruses*, B. Roizman, Ed., pp. 105–173, Springer, New York, NY, USA, 1985.

[7] G. Z. Tong and H. C. Chen, "Pseudorabies epidemic status and control measures in China," *Chinese Journal of Veterinary Science*, vol. 19, pp. 1–2, 1999.

[8] R. Wu, C. Bai, J. Sun, S. Chang, and X. Zhang, "Emergence of virulent pseudorabies virus infection in Northern China," *Journal of Veterinary Science*, vol. 14, no. 3, pp. 363–365, 2013.

[9] X. Yu, Z. Zhou, D. Hu et al., "Pathogenic pseudorabies virus, China, 2012," *Emerging Infectious Diseases*, vol. 20, no. 1, pp. 102–104, 2014.

[10] T. Q. An, J. M. Peng, Z. J. Tian et al., "Pseudorabies virus variant in Bartha-K61-vaccinated pigs, China, 2012," *Emerging Infectious Diseases*, vol. 19, no. 11, pp. 1749–1755, 2013.

[11] J. Besemer, A. Lomsadze, and M. Borodovsky, "GeneMarkS: a self-training method for prediction of gene starts in microbial genomes. Implications for finding sequence motifs in regulatory regions," *Nucleic Acids Research*, vol. 29, no. 12, pp. 2607–2618, 2001.

[12] M. L. Szpara, Y. R. Tafuri, L. Parsons et al., "A wide extent of inter-strain diversity in virulent and vaccine strains of alpha-herpesviruses," *PLoS Pathogens*, vol. 7, no. 10, p. e1002282, 2011.

[13] J. Yang and L. Zhang, "Run probabilities of seed-like patterns and identifying good transition seeds," *Journal of Computational Biology*, vol. 15, no. 10, pp. 1295–1313, 2008.

[14] M. Brudno, C. B. Do, G. M. Cooper et al., "LAGAN and Multi-LAGAN: efficient tools for large-scale multiple alignment of genomic DNA," *Genome Research*, vol. 13, no. 4, pp. 721–731, 2003.

[15] K. Tamura, D. Peterson, N. Peterson, G. Stecher, M. Nei, and S. Kumar, "MEGA5: molecular evolutionary genetics analysis using maximum likelihood, evolutionary distance, and maximum parsimony methods," *Molecular Biology and Evolution*, vol. 28, no. 10, pp. 2731–2739, 2011.

[16] J. Yang, S. Grünewald, and X. F. Wan, "Quartet-net: a quartet-based method to reconstruct phylogenetic networks," *Molecular Biology and Evolution*, vol. 30, no. 5, pp. 1206–1217, 2013.

[17] J. Yang, S. Grünewald, Y. Xu, and X. F. Wan, "Quartet-based methods to reconstruct phylogenetic networks," *BMC Systems Biology*, vol. 8, p. 21, 2014.

[18] R. Brodie, A. J. Smith, R. L. Roper, V. Tcherepanov, and C. Upton, "Base-By-Base: single nucleotide-level analysis of whole viral genome alignments," *BMC Bioinformatics*, vol. 5, p. 96, 2004.

[19] G. Van Minnebruggen, H. W. Favoreel, L. Jacobs, and H. J. Nauwynck, "Pseudorabies virus US3 protein kinase mediates actin stress fiber breakdown," *Journal of Virology*, vol. 77, no. 16, pp. 9074–9080, 2003.

[20] W. A. Derbigny, S. K. Kim, H. K. Jang, and D. J. O'Callaghan, "EHV-1 EICP22 protein sequences that mediate its physical interaction with the immediate-early protein are not sufficient to enhance the trans-activation activity of the IE protein," *Virus Research*, vol. 84, no. 1-2, pp. 1–15, 2002.

[21] C. H. Wang, J. Yuan, H. Y. Qin et al., "A novel gE-deleted pseudorabies virus (PRV) provides rapid and complete protection from lethal challenge with the PRV variant emerging in Bartha-K61-vaccinated swine population in China," *Vaccine*, vol. 32, no. 27, pp. 3379–3385, 2014.

[22] F. A. Zuckermann, S. Martin, and R. Husmann, "Mechanisms of protective immunity against Aujeszky's disease virus," *Veterinary Research*, vol. 31, no. 1, p. 132, 2000.

[23] M. Ferrari, A. Brack, M. G. Romanelli et al., "A study of the ability of a TK-negative and gI/gE-negative pseudorabies virus (PRV) mutant inoculated by different routes to protect pigs against PRV infection," *Journal of Veterinary Medicine B, Infectious Diseases and Veterinary Public Health*, vol. 47, no. 10, pp. 753–762, 2000.

[24] V. Jovasevic, L. Liang, and B. Roizman, "Proteolytic cleavage of VP1-2 is required for release of herpes simplex virus 1 DNA into the nucleus," *Journal of Virology*, vol. 82, no. 7, pp. 3311–3319, 2008.

[25] A. Jöns, J. M. Dijkstra, and T. C. Mettenleiter, "Glycoproteins M and N of pseudorabies virus form a disulfide-linked complex," *Journal of Virology*, vol. 72, no. 1, pp. 550–557, 1998.

[26] D. Koppers-Lalic, E. A. Reits, M. E. Ressing et al., "Varicelloviruses avoid T cell recognition by UL49.5-mediated inactivation of the transporter associated with antigen processing," *Proceedings of the National Academy of Sciences of the United States of America*, vol. 102, no. 14, pp. 5144–5149, 2005.

9

Detection and Molecular Characterization of Human Adenovirus Infections among Hospitalized Children with Acute Diarrhea in Shanghai, China, 2006–2011

Lijuan Lu, Huaqing Zhong, Liyun Su, Lingfeng Cao, Menghua Xu, Niuniu Dong, and Jin Xu

Department of Clinical Laboratory, Children's Hospital of Fudan University, Shanghai 201102, China

Correspondence should be addressed to Jin Xu; jinxu_125@163.com

Academic Editor: Paul-Louis Woerther

Background: Human adenovirus (HAdV) is considered a significant enteropathogen associated with sporadic diarrhea in children. However, limited data are available regarding the epidemiology of HAdV in hospitalized children with viral diarrhea in Shanghai. The aim of this study was to characterize the epidemiology of HAdVs and describe their association with acute diarrhea in hospitalized children. *Methods*: A total of 674 fecal samples were subjected to PCR or RT-PCR to detect RVA, HuCV, HAstV, and HAdV. *Results*: HAdV infections were detected in 4.7% (32/674) of specimens, with detection rates of 13.4% (11/82), 4.6% (8/174), 3.2% (4/124), 4.1% (3/74), 2.0% (2/100), and 3.3% (4/120) from 2006 to 2011, respectively. Comprehensive detection of the four viruses revealed the presence of a high percentage (90.6%) of coinfections among HAdV-positive samples, where HAdV+RVA was the most prevalent coinfection. Of the 32 HAdV-positive samples, 50.0% (16/32) were classified as HAdV-41, and 18.8% (6/32) were classified as HAdV-3. Almost 94.0% of children infected with HAdV were less than 24 months of age. *Conclusions*: These results clearly indicated diversity across the HAdV genotypes detected in inpatient children with acute diarrhea in Shanghai and suggested that HAdVs play a role in children with acute diarrhea.

1. Introduction

Acute diarrhea is a major disease caused by various pathogenic bacteria, viruses, and parasites in all humans, but especially in children aged under 5 years. This condition remains a leading cause of morbidity and mortality worldwide, especially in developing areas. More than 50% of all diarrhea episodes have been found to be induced by viral pathogens [1]. Among the different kinds of diarrheal viruses, group A rotavirus (RVA) and human calicivirus (HuCV) have been identified as the major causes of acute diarrhea worldwide. Human adenovirus (HAdV) and human astrovirus (HAstV) have also been recognized as two additional primary causes of infectious diarrhea in pediatric patients [2, 3].

HAdVs are members of the genus *Mastadenovirus* in the family *Adenoviridae* and cause a wide spectrum of acute and chronic diseases, including acute diarrhea, respiratory illnesses, pneumonias, and pharyngoconjunctival fever [4]. HAdV is a linear, double-stranded DNA virus with a genome size of 26–45 kb. Following the development of phylogenetic and bioinformatic technologies, sequence-based typing strategies have been shown to serve as more rapid or sensitive methods than immunospecific methods for visualization via electron microscopy for HAdV detection. Over 70 HAdV genotypes in seven species (HAdV A–G) have been characterized and classified phylogenetically according to their nucleic acid characteristics and homologies as well as their hexon and fiber protein characteristics since HAdV was first isolated in 1953 [4, 5]. Among these species, HAdV-F types HAdV-40 and -41 have been found to be frequent causes of pediatric diarrhea and, as such, are known as enteric adenoviruses. Other adenoviruses are regarded as "nonenteric" adenoviruses. HAdV is not only considered a significant pathogen that occurs in association with sporadic acute diarrhea but is also a major enteropathogen responsible for nosocomial diarrhea in hospitals. HAdV diarrhea can be persistent and severe in immunocompromised hosts [6]. Thus, it is important to monitor the epidemiology of HAdV in hospitalized children with acute diarrhea.

Prior to this study, limited data were available regarding the epidemiology of HAdV in hospitalized children with viral diarrhea in Shanghai, and most studies have focused on RVA and HuCV infections [7–9]. Therefore, we conducted this study to evaluate the epidemiology of HAdV in hospitalized children in Shanghai upon the onset of viral diarrhea.

2. Materials and Methods

From January 2006 to December 2011, 674 stool samples were obtained from children under the age of 5 years with acute diarrhea enrolled at the Children's Hospital of Fudan University in Shanghai. All patients came from either the gastroenterology department, the infectious disease department, or the neonatal department. Each stool sample was collected from the patients when acute diarrhea was clinically suspected and stored at −70°C. Acute diarrhea cases were defined as three soft or liquid stools or three bouts of vomiting per 24 hours in a patient. When pus or blood was present in a sample, it was excluded, regardless of the identified fever conditions. Among the enrolled patients, 367 were male children, and 307 were female children. For subsequent data analysis, five different age groups were established: 0–12 months (504 samples), 13–24 months (104 samples), 25–36 months (29 samples), 37–48 months (27 samples), and 49–60 months (10 samples).

The fecal specimens were diluted to 10% suspensions with 0.9% physiological saline and then clarified via centrifugation at 8000 g for 10 min. The total RNA/DNA was extracted using the TIANamp Virus DNA/RNA Kit (Tiangen Biotech, Beijing, China) according to the manufacturer's instructions. The extracted viral RNA/DNA was dissolved in 40 μL of nuclease-free water and stored at −70°C until analysis.

The extracted DNA was subjected to PCR amplification using primers specific to HAdV. A 482 bp fragment of a conserved region (C4) in the HAdV hexon gene (nt: 1834–2296) was amplified using the Ad-1 (5′-TTCCCC-ATGGCICAYAACAC-3′) and Ad-2 (5′-CCCTGGTAKC-CRATRTTGTA-3′) primers [10]. The PCR cycling program was as follows: 94°C for 4 min, followed by 35 cycles of 94°C for 30 sec, 55°C for 30 sec, and 72°C for 1 min and a final extension cycle at 72°C for 7 min.

cDNA used for detecting HuCV and HAstV was synthesized using the extracted RNA and the PrimeScript™ RT Reagent Kit (Takara Bio Co., Dalian, China) according to the manufacturer's instructions. The obtained cDNA was used for the detection of HuCV and HAstV via PCR using specific primers, as previously described [9, 11].

The extracted RNA was also used as a template for the amplification of RVA via one-step reverse transcription PCR (RT-PCR) and seminested PCR with typing-specific primers, as reported in another paper [8].

Finally, all PCR products were electrophoresed in a 2% agarose gel with ethidium bromide and a DNA ladder of 100 bp (Takara Bio Co., Dalian, China).

The samples that were positive for HAdV, HuCV, and HAstV were subjected to nucleotide sequencing by the Shanghai Sunny Biotechnology Co., Ltd., and Sanger sequencing was carried out using the BigDye Terminator v3.1 Cycle Sequencing Kit (Thermo Fisher Scientific Inc., U.S.) according to the manufacturer's instructions. Phylogenetic analyses of the detected HAdVs were conducted using the MEGA version 6.0 software package. The phylogenetic tree was constructed using the Kimura two-parameter method. The reference HAdV strains and accession numbers used in this study were as follows: HAdV-1: AC_000017, AF534906, KC632723; HAdV-2: J01917; HAdV-3: AY599836, AY854176, KM458623, KX384958; HAdV-5: AY339865; HAdV-7: KM458626, KU361344, KC857700; HAdV-8: AB448767; HAdV-11: AY163756; HAdV-12: X73487; HAdV-14: AY803294; HAdV-16: AY601636; HAdV-17: AF108105; HAdV-18: GU191019; HAdV-21: KJ364591; HAdV-31: AB330112, AM749299, DQ149611; HAdV-34: AY737797; HAdV-35: AY128640; HAdV-37: AB448777, AB475144; HAdV-40: L19443, KU904311, AB330121, KU162869; HAdV-41: HQ326161, DQ315364, KF303070, KY316162; HAdV-49: DQ393829; HAdV-61: JF964962; HAdV-A: NC_001460; HAdV-B: NC_011202; HAdV-C: NC_001405; HAdV-D: AC_000006; HAdV-E: NC_003266; and HAdV-F: NC_001454.

3. Results

Thirty-two of the 674 (4.7%) children with acute diarrhea were infected with HAdV between 2006 and 2011. The prevalence rates of HAdV were 13.4% (11/82), 4.6% (8/174), 3.2% (4/124), 4.1% (3/74), 2.0% (2/100), and 3.3% (4/120) in 2006, 2007, 2008, 2009, 2010, and 2011, respectively. Of the 32 HAdV-infected cases, 29 (90.6%) were coinfected with other viruses, while only 3 (9.4%) cases consisted of monoinfections. The most frequently identified mixed infection was HAdV + RVA (28.1% of the 32 cases). We also detected 14 cases of triple gastrointestinal tract infections, including the combinations HAdV + RVA + HAstV (25% of the 32 cases) and HAdV + RVA + HuCV (18.8% of the 32 cases). All four of the viruses (HAdV, RVA, HuCV, and HAstV) were detected simultaneously in 5 cases.

The seasonal distribution of HAdV infections between 2006 and 2011 is shown in Figure 1. The HAdV detection rate presented distinct seasonal variation, with a higher detection rate identified in autumn and winter months.

In this study, 93.8% of children infected with HAdV were aged less than 24 months, and the highest detection rate was found in children between 13 and 24 months of age (6 of 104). Overall, HAdV infections were only detected in children less than 48 months of age (Figure 2).

A total of 32 HAdV sequences were phylogenetically analyzed based on the hexon gene-based classification scheme using MEGA 5.0. The phylogenetic tree analysis showed clear predominance of HAdV-41 (16 of 32),

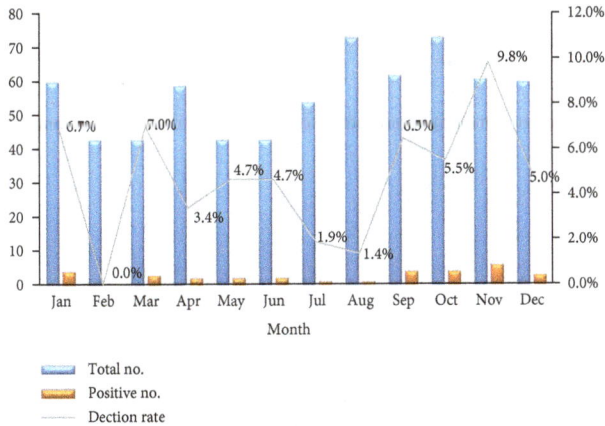

FIGURE 1: Monthly distribution of HAdV in hospitalized children with acute diarrhea in Shanghai between January 2006 and December 2011.

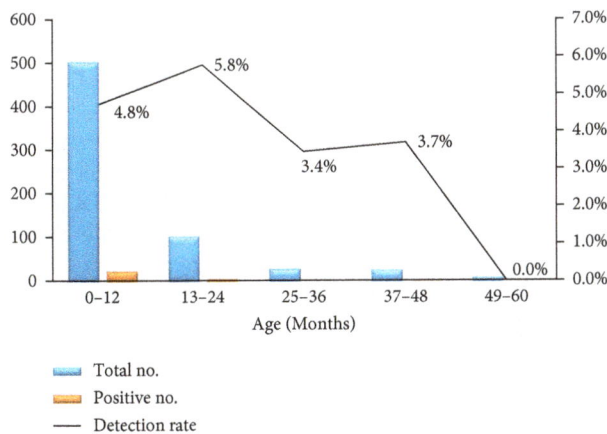

FIGURE 2: Age distribution of HAdV infection among hospitalized children with acute diarrhea in Shanghai between January 2006 and December 2011.

followed by HAdV-3 (6 of 32), whereas only one case of infection with HAdV-40 was detected from 2006 to 2011. Distinct differences in the prevalence of HAdV genotypes were observed by year. In 2006, 90.9% of HAdV-positive samples corresponded to HAdV-41, and only one HAdV-41 strain was detected. Various HAdV genotypes were detected in 2007, including HAdV-1, -3, -7, -31, -37, -41, and -61. The predominant HAdV genotype identified in 2008 and 2011 was HAdV-3. The HAdV-1, -31, and -41 genotypes of HAdV were detected in 2009. Finally, only two HAdV-41 strains were detected in 2010 (Figure 3 and Table 1).

4. Discussion

Prior to this study, no research aimed at determining the burden of HAdV-related diarrhea among children in Shanghai had been performed. We conducted this study to assess the infection status and HAdV distribution patterns of

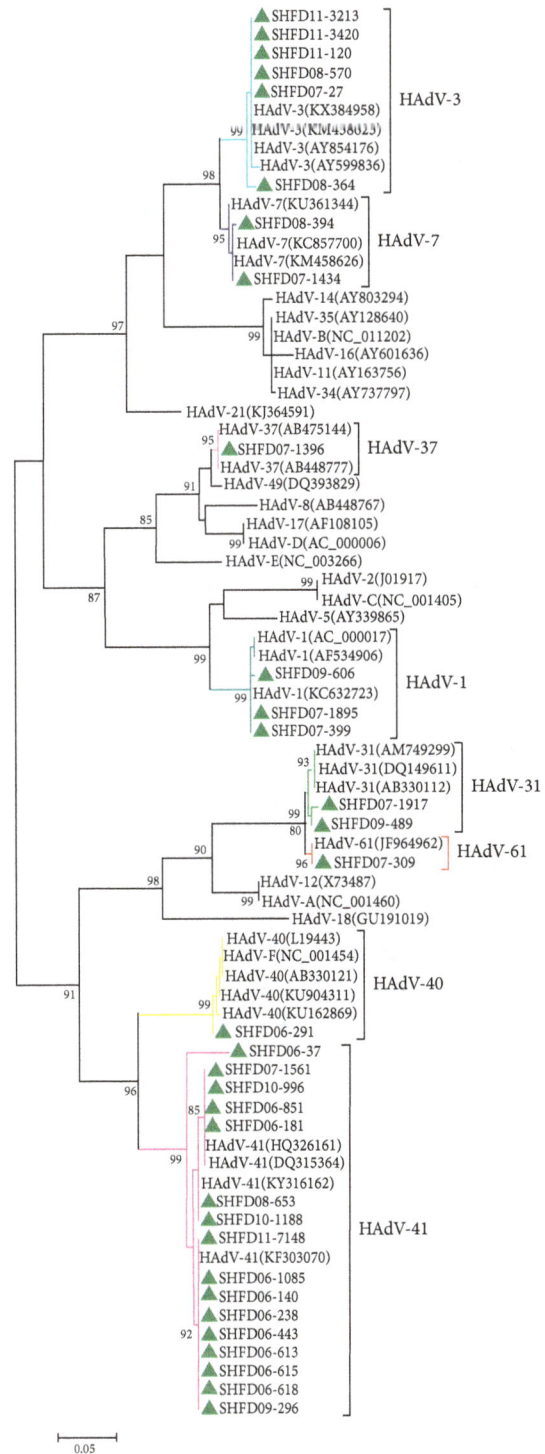

FIGURE 3: Phylogenetic tree based on partial nucleotide sequences (482 bp) of the hexon gene of HAdVs detected in hospitalized children with acute diarrhea in Shanghai, China, between January 2006 and December 2011. The delta symbol indicates the adenovirus strains detected in this study.

hospitalized children with acute diarrhea in Shanghai from January 2006 to December 2011. The proportion of participating children with acute diarrhea in whom HAdV was detected was 4.7%, which was similar to previously reported rates in most studies conducted in Bangladesh, South Korea,

TABLE 1: Distribution of HAdV genotypes in hospitalized children with acute diarrhea from 2006 to 2011.

Genotype	No. of HAdV-positive samples						
	2006 ($N = 82$)	2007 ($N = 174$)	2008 ($N = 124$)	2009 ($N = 74$)	2010 ($N = 100$)	2011 ($N = 120$)	Total ($N = 674$)
HAdV-1	0	2	0	1	0	0	3
HAdV-3	0	1	2	0	0	3	6
HAdV-7	0	1	1	0	0	0	2
HAdV-31	0	1	0	1	0	0	2
HAdV-37	0	1	0	0	0	0	1
HAdV-40	1	0	0	0	0	0	1
HAdV-41	10	1	1	1	2	1	16
HAdV-61	0	1	0	0	0	0	1
Total	11	8	4	3	2	4	32

N: total number tested each year.

Vietnam, and some other areas of China [12–19]. During the study period, the highest HAdV detection rate was observed in 2006, while the rate was lower than 5.0% in the remaining years. There was no evidence that HAdV led to an epidemic in 2006, as all of the HAdV-positive samples were distributed in 8 months (data not shown). The reasons for the decline observed from 2006 to 2011 may be improved environmental hygiene conditions and increased hygiene awareness. Similar to other studies [2, 3, 15, 20, 21], we found that most HAdV infections were detected in conjunction with RVA, HuCV, or HAstV, while monoinfection with HAdV alone was identified in only three samples. Additional research should be conducted in the future to determine whether coinfection with HAdV and other viruses serves as a characteristic feature of HAdV infection.

Our study also revealed that HAdV infections occurred throughout the year and peaked in the autumn and winter. This finding was in accordance with that of other studies conducted in Qingdao city and Hunan Province in China [22, 23]. However, in Tianjin, a northern city in China, HAdV infections are concentrated during the summer [16]. Although the reason for this difference remains unknown, more attention should be paid to the epidemiology of HAdV in Shanghai during different seasons to prevent HAdV outbreaks in hospitals.

In line with the findings of other studies [15–17], the majority of children with HAdV included in the present study were less than 2 years old. Similar trends have been detected in Tanzania and, in the case of the other three diarrhea viruses (RV, HuCV, and HAstV), in our previous studies [9, 24–26]. The reason that diarrhea-associated viral infections are much more likely to occur in younger children may be the immature immune function of infants and the fact that infections during infancy might result in protective immunity against reinfection at an older age [27, 28]. Furthermore, the high susceptibility of infants to pathogens may be influenced by differences in the intestinal microbiome, which changes over the first few of years of life [29–31].

According to the phylogenetic tree analysis conducted based on a partial genomic region of hexon, not only were species F (HAdV-40 and HAdV-41) strains detected, but

other "nonenteric" HAdVs, such as species B (HAdV-3), were also detected in our study. However, we failed to perform an analysis of the temporal relationship between HAdV cases, as the reference strains used in this study were prototype strains rather than epidemic strains from different areas and times. The molecular characterization of these HAdV strains showed a clear predominance of HAdV-41 (50.0%), which was in agreement with the results of studies including children from Bangladesh, other Asian countries, and Sweden [13, 16, 32, 33]. However, in Dhaka city, Bangladesh, HAdV-40 was found to dominate other genotypes, whereas only one patient was infected with HAdV-40 in our study [13]. The reason for this disparity may be regional divergence leading to a higher prevalence of HAdV-41 than HAdV-40. Fluctuations in the prevalence of HAdV-40 and HAdV-41 have also been observed in other studies [34, 35]. Although some studies have shown that the duration of diarrhea is longer in patients with HAdV-41 infection than in those with HAdV-40 infection [32], it was nearly impossible to compare the duration of diarrhea between patients infected with HAdV-41 and HAdV-40 strains in this study because of the limited number of HAdV-40-positive samples.

In this study, one HAdV-61 strain belonging to the species A adenoviruses was detected in 2007. HAdV-61, resulting from an intraspecies recombination event between HAdV-12 and HAdV-31, was first isolated from a patient with acute diarrhea in Japan [36, 37]. The present study provides the first report of the epidemiology of HAdV-61 in China. Although this genotype has not expanded to show widespread prevalence in humans since it was discovered in 2004, more extensive research must be conducted in the future to prevent outbreaks. In addition, further studies are essential for understanding the full mechanisms of recombination in HAdV. We also detected two strains of HAdV-31, which is another enteric adenovirus that was found in association with diarrhea in an earlier study [38].

Interestingly, HAdV-3, the second leading HAdV genotype detected in the children included in our study (18.8%), is usually regarded as a pathogen that causes acute febrile pharyngitis, pharyngoconjunctival fever, acute respiratory disease, and even gastrointestinal symptoms [39]. A similarly high incidence of HAdV-3 was detected in outpatients in Korea and in a previous study conducted by our group in patients diagnosed with community-acquired diarrhea [35, 40]. According to the medical history of the patients included in our study, two patients exhibited monoinfections and were diagnosed only with diarrhea. In addition to HAdV-3, other "nonenteric" HAdV strains (HAdV-1, -7, and -37) were also detected in these hospitalized children with diarrhea. Moreover, a similar situation regarding the prevalence of "nonenteric" HAdVs (e.g., HAdV-1, -2, -3, -5, -6, and -8) has been found to occur in children with diarrhea in many other regions [13, 16, 38, 40]. As it has been established that respiratory types of HAdVs, such as HAdV-1, -2, and -3, can be shed in the feces of an infected person for months after the initial infection when these HAdVs infect respiratory sites [41, 42], the role of these "nonenteric" HAdVs in the onset of children's diarrhea requires further research.

5. Conclusions

In conclusion, this is the first report of the burden of HAdV-related diarrhea in Shanghai among hospitalized children younger than 5 years of age during the period from 2006 to 2011. The results of the present study showed that an increasing number of HAdV genotypes were detected in children with acute diarrhea. The rate at which HAdV was detected in conjunction with other diarrhea-causing viruses was relatively high in our study. Together, these findings underscore the importance of monitoring the epidemiology of HAdV infection and protecting vulnerable patients as part of the suite of infection prevention strategies in hospitals.

Acknowledgments

This work was supported by the Program of the National Natural Science Foundation of China under Grant no. NSFC81273204.

References

[1] E. J. Anderson, "Prevention and treatment of viral diarrhea in pediatrics," *Expert Review of Anti-Infective Therapy*, vol. 8, no. 2, pp. 205–217, 2010.

[2] Z. Ren, Y. Kong, J. Wang, Q. Wang, A. Huang, and H. Xu, "Etiological study of enteric viruses and the genetic diversity of norovirus, sapovirus, adenovirus, and astrovirus in children with diarrhea in Chongqing, China," *BMC Infectious Diseases*, vol. 13, no. 1, p. 412, 2013.

[3] C. Gasparinho, M. M. Mirante, S. Centeno-Lima et al., "Etiology of diarrhea in children younger than 5 years attending the Bengo General Hospital in Angola," *Pediatric Infectious Disease Journal*, vol. 35, no. 2, pp. e28–e34, 2016.

[4] L. J. Ferreyra, M. O. Giordano, L. C. Martínez et al., "Tracking novel adenovirus in environmental and human clinical samples: no evidence of endemic human adenovirus type 58

[5] W. P. Rowe, R. J. Huebner, L. K. Gilmore, R. H. Parrott, and T. G. Ward, "Isolation of a cytopathogenic agent from human adenoids undergoing spontaneous degeneration in tissue culture," *Proceedings of the Society for Experimental Biology and Medicine*, vol. 84, no. 3, pp. 570–573, 1953.

[6] T. Lion, "Adenovirus infections in immunocompetent and immunocompromised patients," *Clinical Microbiology Reviews*, vol. 27, no. 3, pp. 441–462, 2014.

[7] J. Xu, Y. Yang, J. Sun, and Y. Ding, "Molecular epidemiology of norovirus infection among children with acute gastroenteritis in Shanghai, China, 2001–2005," *Journal of Medical Virology*, vol. 81, no. 10, pp. 1826–1630, 2009.

[8] J. Xu, Y. Yang, J. Sun et al., "Molecular epidemiology of rotavirus infections among children hospitalized for acute gastroenteritis in Shanghai, China, 2001 through 2005," *Journal of Clinical Virology*, vol. 44, no. 1, pp. 58–61, 2009.

[9] L. J. Lu, H. Q. Zhong, M. H. Xu et al., "Molecular epidemiology of human calicivirus infections in children with acute diarrhea in Shanghai: a retrospective comparison between inpatients and outpatients treated between 2006 and 2011," *Archives of Virology*, vol. 159, no. 7, pp. 1613–1621, 2014.

[10] K. Ebner, W. Pinsker, and T. Lion, "Comparative sequence analysis of the hexon gene in the entire spectrum of human adenovirus serotypes: phylogenetic, taxonomic, and clinical implications," *Journal of Virology*, vol. 79, no. 20, pp. 12635–12642, 2005.

[11] J. S. Noel, T. W. Lee, J. B. Kurtz, R. I. Glass, and S. S. Monroe, "Typing of human astroviruses from clinical isolates by enzyme immunoassay and nucleotide sequencing," *Journal of Clinical Microbiology*, vol. 33, no. 4, pp. 797–801, 1995.

[12] T. A. Nguyen, F. Yagyu, M. Okame et al., "Diversity of viruses associated with acute gastroenteritis in children hospitalized with diarrhea in Ho Chi Minh City, Vietnam," *Journal of Medical Virology*, vol. 79, no. 5, pp. 582–590, 2007.

[13] S. K. Dey, H. Shimizu, T. G. Phan et al., "Molecular epidemiology of adenovirus infection among infants and children with acute gastroenteritis in Dhaka City, Bangladesh," *Infection, Genetics and Evolution*, vol. 9, no. 4, pp. 518–522, 2009.

[14] J. W. Huh, W. H. Kim, S. G. Moon et al., "Viral etiology and incidence associated with acute gastroenteritis in a 5-year survey in Gyeonggi province, South Korea," *Journal of Clinical Virology*, vol. 44, no. 2, pp. 152–156, 2009.

[15] Y. Jin, W. X. Cheng, X. M. Yang et al., "Viral agents associated with acute gastroenteritis in children hospitalized with diarrhea in Lanzhou, China," *Journal of Clinical Virology*, vol. 44, no. 3, pp. 238–241, 2009.

[16] Y. Ouyang, H. Ma, M. Jin et al., "Etiology and epidemiology of viral diarrhea in children under the age of five hospitalized in Tianjin, China," *Archives of Virology*, vol. 157, no. 5, pp. 881–887, 2012.

[17] Q. Lin, Y. Jin, J. S. Zhou et al., "Molecular epidemiological study on viral diarrhea among pediatric patients under five years old in Nanjing, 2009-2010," *Chinese Journal of Evidence Based Pediatrics*, vol. 7, no. 1, pp. 31–36, 2012.

[18] A. Banerjee, P. De, B. Manna, and M. Chawla-Sarkar, "Molecular characterization of enteric adenovirus genotypes 40 and 41 identified in children with acute gastroenteritis in Kolkata, India during 2013-2014," *Journal of Medical Virology*, vol. 89, no. 4, pp. 606–14, 2017.

[19] A. Sanaei Dashti, P. Ghahremani, T. Hashempoor, and A. Karimi, "Molecular epidemiology of enteric adenovirus

gastroenteritis in under-five-year-old children in Iran," *Gastroenterology Research and Practice*, vol. 2016, Article ID 2045697, 5 pages, 2016.

[20] C. E. Ferreira, S. M. Raboni, L. A. Pereira, M. B. Nogueira, L. R. Vidal, and S. M. Almeida, "Viral acute gastroenteritis: clinical and epidemiological features of co-infected patients," *Brazilian Journal of Infectious Diseases*, vol. 16, no. 3, pp. 267–272, 2012.

[21] M. T. Mitui, G. Bozdayi, S. Ahmed, T. Matsumoto, A. Nishizono, and K. Ahmed, "Detection and molecular characterization of diarrhea causing viruses in single and mixed infections in children: a comparative study between Bangladesh and Turkey," *Journal of Medical Virology*, vol. 86, no. 7, pp. 1159–1168, 2014.

[22] D. Su, Y. L. Liu, F. H. Ai et al., "Epidemiology in children with diarrhea infection by EADV in Qingdao in winter and spring," *Acta Aacademiae Medicinae Qingdao Universitatis*, vol. 44, no. 2, pp. 175-176, 2008.

[23] J. Li, S. F. Zhou, Y. Z. Liu et al., "Etiological study on viral diarrhea among infants and young children in surveillance hospitals of Hunan Province from 2009 to 2010," *Practical Preventive Medicine*, vol. 19, no. 3, pp. 337–341, 2012.

[24] L. J. Lu, H. Q. Zhong, L. Y. Su et al., "Molecular characterization of group A Rotavirus genotypes in children hospitalized with diarrhea in Shanghai, during 2008–2011," *Chinese Journal of Evidence Based Pediatrics*, vol. 8, no. 2, pp. 135–141, 2013.

[25] L. J. Lu, J. Xu, H. Q. Zhong, L. Su, L. Cao, and M. Xu, "Characteristics of molecular epidemiology of human astrovirus in hospitalized and outpatient children with acute diarrhea," *Chinese Journal of Infectious Diseases*, vol. 34, no. 8, pp. 463–468, 2016.

[26] S. J. Moyo, K. Hanevik, B. Blomberg et al., "Prevalence and molecular characterisation of human adenovirus in diarrhoeic children in Tanzania; a case control study," *BMC Infectious Diseases*, vol. 14, no. 1, p. 666, 2014.

[27] L. Sai, J. Sun, L. Shao, S. Chen, H. Liu, and L. Ma, "Epidemiology and clinical features of rotavirus and norovirus infection among children in Ji'nan, China," *Virology Journal*, vol. 10, no. 1, p. 302, 2013.

[28] A. Thongprachum, S. Takanashi, A. F. Kalesaran et al., "Four-year study of viruses that cause diarrhea in Japanese pediatric outpatients," *Journal of Medical Virology*, vol. 87, no. 7, pp. 1141–1148, 2015.

[29] J. E. Koenig, A. Spor, N. Scalfone et al., "Succession of microbial consortia in the developing infant gut microbiome," *Proceedings of the National Academy of Sciences of the United States of America*, vol. 108, no. 1, pp. 4578–4585, 2011.

[30] T. Yatsunenko, F. E. Rey, M. J. Manary et al., "Human gut microbiome viewed across age and geography," *Nature*, vol. 486, no. 7402, pp. 222–227, 2012.

[31] G. Clarke, S. M. O'Mahony, T. G. Dinan, and J. F. Cryan, "Priming for health: gut microbiota acquired in early life regulates physiology, brain and behaviour," *Acta Paediatrica*, vol. 103, no. 8, pp. 812–819, 2014.

[32] I. Uhnoo, G. Wadell, L. Svensson, and M. E. Johansson, "Importance of enteric adenoviruses 40 and 41 in acute gastroenteritis in infants and young children," *Journal of Clinical Microbiology*, vol. 20, no. 3, pp. 365–372, 1984.

[33] L. Li, T. G. Phan, T. A. Nguyen et al., "Molecular epidemiology of adenovirus infection among pediatric population with diarrhea in Asia," *Microbiology and Immunology*, vol. 49, no. 2, pp. 121-128, 2005.

[34] L. Li, H. Shimizu, L. T. Doan et al., "Characterizations of adenovirus type 41 isolates from children with acute gastroenteritis in Japan, Vietnam, and Korea," *Journal of Clinical Microbiology*, vol. 42, no. 9, pp. 4032–4039, 2004.

[35] H. Shimizu, T. G. Phan, S. Nishimura, S. Okitsu, N. Maneekarn, and H. Ushijima, "An outbreak of adenovirus serotype 41 infection in infants and children with acute gastroenteritis in Maizuru City, Japan," *Infection, Genetics and Evolution*, vol. 7, no. 2, pp. 279–284, 2007.

[36] Y. Matsushima, H. Shimizu, T. G. Phan, and H. Ushijima, "Genomic characterization of a novel human adenovirus type 31 recombinant in the hexon gene," *Journal of General Virology*, vol. 92, no. 12, pp. 2770–2775, 2011.

[37] C. Zhou, H. Tian, X. Wang et al., "The genome sequence of a novel simian adenovirus in a chimpanzee reveals a close relationship to human adenoviruses," *Archives of Virology*, vol. 159, no. 7, pp. 1765–1770, 2014.

[38] J. D. Grydsuk, E. Fortsas, M. Petric, and M. Brown, "Common epitope on protein VI of enteric adenoviruses from subgenera A and F," *Journal of General Virology*, vol. 77, no. 8, pp. 1811–1819, 1996.

[39] H. Faden, M. Wilby, Z. D. Hainer et al., "Pediatric adenovirus infection: relationship of clinical spectrum, seasonal distribution, and serotype," *Clinical Pediatrics*, vol. 50, no. 6, pp. 483–487, 2011.

[40] L. J. Lu, R. Jia, H. Q. Zhong et al., "Molecular characterization and multiple infections of rotavirus, norovirus, sapovirus, astrovirus and adenovirus in outpatients with sporadic gastroenteritis in Shanghai, China, 2010-2011," *Archives of Virology*, vol. 160, no. 5, pp. 1229–1238, 2015.

[41] C. T. Garnett, D. Erdman, W. Xu, and L. R. Gooding, "Prevalence and quantitation of species C adenovirus DNA in human mucosal lymphocytes," *Journal of Virology*, vol. 76, no. 21, pp. 10608–10616, 2002.

[42] W. Wold and M. Horwitz, "Adenoviruses," in *Fields Virology*, D. M. Knipe and P. M. Howley Eds., Lippincott Williams & Wilkins Press, Philadelphia, PA, USA, 2007.

10

Bifidobacterium lactis Ameliorates the Risk of Food Allergy in Chinese Children by Affecting Relative Percentage of Treg and Th17 Cells

Qingbin Liu ⓘ, Wei Jing, and Wei Wang

Department of Pediatric, Affiliated Hospital of Changchun University of Traditional Chinese Medicine, Changchun 130021, China

Correspondence should be addressed to Qingbin Liu; liuqingbincc@163.com

Academic Editor: Lucia Lopalco

We aimed to explore the therapeutic effect of *Bifidobacterium lactis* on food allergy by investigating the percentage of Treg and Th17 cells in Chinese children and related molecular mechanisms. A total of 256 children with food allergy were evenly assigned into two groups: BG, the children received 10 ml *B. lactis* (1×10^6/ml) daily, and CG, the children received the solution without *B. lactis* daily for three months. Allergic symptoms, serum IgE, and food antigen-specific IgE were measured. A mouse allergy model was established by using shrimp tropomyosin and treated with *B. lactis*. Relative mRNA levels of Treg- and Th17-associated cytokines were measured by using quantitative PCR. The percentage of Treg and Th17 cells in spleen were measured by using flow cytometry. After 3-month therapy, the allergic symptoms of the BG were remarkably reduced when compared with the CG ($P < 0.05$). Serum levels of IgE and food antigen-specific IgE were decreased too ($P < 0.05$). Similar results were also found in a mouse allergy model. After *B. lactis* treatment, the relative mRNA level of FoxP3 was significantly enhanced in the *B. lactis* therapy group when compared to positive controls. In addition, relative mRNA levels of FoxP3 and TGF-β associated with Treg cells were increased, whereas relative mRNA levels of IL-17A and IL-23 associated with Th17 were reduced. *B. lactis* treatment significantly increased the ratio of Treg and Th17 cells in a mouse allergy model ($P < 0.05$). *B. lactis* effectively alleviates allergic symptoms by increasing the ratio of Treg and Th17 cells.

1. Introduction

The prevalence of food allergy (FA) has significantly increased in the pediatric population. However, the effective treatment is still lacking [1]. The etiology of food allergy is complex with individual differences in different patients [2]. The pathogenesis of food allergy involves many aspects, including immunity [3], genetics [4], *Helicobacter pylori* infection [5], and environment [6].

Food allergens are the main reason for causing allergic disorders. Among shellfish family, crustacean food can cause a large amount of allergic responses. For instance, shrimp has high-level tropomyosin, which is the factor for causing food allergies [7]. Shrimp [8] and crab [9] allergens are among the major types of food allergens reported by the Food and Agriculture Organization (FAO). Both crustaceans have

tropomyosin [10], arginine kinase [11, 12], myosin [13, 14], and sarcoplasmic calcium-binding protein allergens [15, 16]. The incidence of crustacean allergy is very common with 38% in food allergy [17]. In crustaceans, shrimp is favored by most consumers worldwide because it is delicious and rich in nutrients; however, shrimp causes the most allergic reaction with more than 50% of crustacean allergy. The prevalence of crustacean allergy is varied in different geographical locations [18]. Many studies have found that the allergic reaction is mainly Th2-induced inflammatory response [19]. Recently, it has been found that the imbalance between regulatory T cells (Treg) and Th17 in T-lymphocyte subsets also leads to immune disorders [20].

Th17 and Treg cells are the two main subsets of CD4$^+$ T cells and participate in allergy responses [21]. FoxP3 is an intracellular transcription factor of Treg cells [22]. TGF-β

plays a critical role in Treg cell development and can affect the number and function of Treg cells [23]. IL-17A is an important factor that accompanies pathogen infection and mainly produced by Th17 cells [24]. IL-23 is another important cytokine associated with Th17 cells [25]. Both IL-17 and IL-23 can affect the balance of Th17/Treg cells [26]. Thus, these cytokines were measured in mouse allergy models.

Treg cells can avoid excessive immune response by activating T cells expressing IL-2 receptor alpha-chains (CD25) and secreting cytokines such as IL-10 and TGF-β [27]. Th17 cells are a new type of CD4$^+$ T cells [28] and mainly exert inflammatory action by secreting orphan nuclear receptor yt (RORyt) and other effector cytokines such as IL-17A and IL-6, which can induce allergic asthma, systemic lupus erythematosus, rheumatoid arthritis, and other allergic diseases [29, 30]. A strong Th17-type immune response is induced, and a large number of inflammatory cytokines (IL-17, IL-6, IL-23, etc.) will be released [31, 32] when a food allergic reaction occurs.

Probiotics, as a kind of beneficial active microorganisms, have been fully affirmed in immune function by generating short-chain fatty acids [33], polysaccharides [34, 35], and cell wall components (peptidoglycan and lipoteichoic acid) [36]. Previous studies indicated that *Bifidobacterium* regulated the components of gut microbiota. The changes in *Dorea* and *Ralstonia* bacteria were closely associated with the Th2/Treg ratio and contributed to the reduction of tropomyosin-induced allergic responses. *Bifidobacterium* can alleviate food allergy and regulate gut immune homeostasis [37]. *Bifidobacterium lactis* is one of the main probiotics in yogurt, and it is safe and well tolerated [38]. *B. lactis* has been approved to be effective in the prevention of ovalbumin (OVA)-induced allergy in a mouse model [39]. However, its mechanism remains unclear. In the present study, we investigated the therapeutic effect of *B. lactis* on the allergic reaction in infants, the percentage of Treg and Th17 cells, and related cytokines to provide theoretical basis in the prevention of food allergy.

2. Materials and Methods

2.1. Participants. Before the present experiment, all procedures were approved by the Human Research Committee of Changchun University of Traditional Chinese Medicine (Changchun, China). The children's parents and caretakers were ready to help all children strictly adhere to all protocols and signed informed consent form. Intent-to-treat (ITT) population and the per-protocol (PP) population were the same.

2.2. Allergy Skin Test. Hypersensitivity response of each patient was assessed by using conventional skin prick tests against 16 common aeroallergens according to an earlier report [40]. Skin prick tests were performed according to the methods introduced by Gislason and Gislason [41]. The test would be regarded as clinically significant if allergens reactions were more than 10 among 16 common aeroallergens.

2.3. Measurement of Serum IgE. Serum IgE is an important indicator to determine food and aeroallergen sensitization in the children with food allergy [42]. Thus, serum IgE was measured in the children with food allergy. 3 ml venous blood was obtained from each patient, and serum was isolated via centrifugation. Serum IgE was measured by using ELISA kits from Thermo Fisher Scientific (Cat. no.: 88-50610-22, Carlsbad, CA, USA).

2.4. Measurement of Allergic Reactions on Food-Specific IgE of Food. Antigen-specific IgE that specifically binds to food allergens was measured by using the allergen diagnostic kit (MEDIWISS Analytic GmbH, Moers, Germany). This kit could be used to detect antigen-specific IgE of 9 kinds of food allergens in human serum, including egg, milk, shrimp, beef, shellfish, crab, mango, cashew nuts, and pineapple. Food-specific allergen was adsorbed on the surface of nitrocellulose membrane and placed on the reaction tank. The allergen-specific IgE antibody in the sample reacted with the allergen and bound to the nitrocellulose membrane. After excess antibody was eluted, biotin-labeled anti-human IgE antibody was added and incubated at room temperature. Alkaline phosphatase-labeled streptavidin was added and incubated at room temperature. After the addition of the BCIP/NBT substrate, a specific enzyme color reaction occurred and a precipitate appeared on the strip. The color intensity was proportional to specific antibody content of the serum sample and serum IgE. The color intensity was measured by using a densitometer (BioRad, Hercules, CA, USA). If the OD$_{490nm}$ values were more than two by the immunodot method, the food allergen-specific IgE reaction was regarded as positive.

2.5. Inclusion Criteria. The following patients were included: the patients who were clinically diagnosed with food allergy and a history of food allergy more than 1 year; the patients who were aged from 4 to 12 years; allergen-specific IgE responses that were more than 10 in food allergy test (20 allergen-specific IgEs could be tested each time). Total serum IgE levels were more than 4.5 μg/ml. The patients had normal food allergies, such as cutaneous manifestation (rash and eczema) and gastrointestinal symptoms (abdominal cramps, abdomen pain, and vomiting). The severity of atopic rash was measured by using the National Cancer Institute Common Terminology Criteria for Adverse Events version 3.0 (NCI CTCAE v3.0) (grades 1–5) [43]. Atopic eczema was measured by a dermatologist by using severity scoring of atopic dermatitis (SCORAD) (scores 0–103) [44]. Abdominal cramps and pain were measured by electrolyte disturbance (scores 0–45) [45]. Incidence of nausea and vomiting was measured using a 4-point scale (0 = asymptomatic, 1 = mild (subjective nausea was present and recovery was achieved without drug treatment), 2 = moderate (subjective nausea was present and recovery was achieved using antiemetics), and 3 = severe (subjective symptoms such as nausea and vomiting were present, and gastric contents were released)) by selecting the highest one at the time when the measurement was performed [46]. The patients had more than 6 events of food allergy (rash and eczema, abdominal cramps, abdomen pain, vomiting, and so on) within one month, and the symptoms duration was more than half an hour at each time.

2.6. Exclusion Criteria.

2.6. Exclusion Criteria. The following patients were excluded: the patients had pharmacological and medical therapy within three months, including vitamin, minerals, glucocorticoid drugs, and antibiotics; the patients were allergic to yogurt or dairy products; the patients had cardiac failure, renal failure, or other serious organ disorders; and the patients had irritable bowel syndrome (IBS) and inflammatory bowel diseases (IBD).

2.7. Study Intervention. B. lactis yogurt culture was purchased from Inner Mongolia Yili Industrial Group Company (Yili, China). The strain was isolated, identified by 16S rRNA, and inoculated in the MRS medium (Hangzhou Shuangtian Biological Co., Ltd.) for 24 h at 37°C in anaerobic environment. The bacterial suspension was centrifuged at 2000 ×g at 4°C for 10 min, pelleted with PBS (phosphate buffer saline) at the concentration of 10^9 CFU/ml, and stored at 4°C. A total of 256 children with food allergy were evenly assigned into two groups in a double-blind clinical study: B. lactis group (BG, those who received 10 ml B. lactis (1×10^6/ml) daily, $n = 128$) and control group (CG, those who received the solution without B. lactis, $n = 128$).

The study duration was three months. Allergic children meeting exclusion and inclusion criteria were recruited in the present experiment. The detailed history of patients was obtained from his or her guider and examined by two experts. All subjects were inquired to write down any unwanted adverse effects in the 3-month follow-up. All patients were visited before this study as the first visit, after one month as the second visit, and after 3-month follow-up as a final visit. Allergy symptoms were recorded at each time.

2.8. Establishment of Allergy Model. Before the present experiment, all procedures were approved by the animal research committee of Changchun University of Traditional Chinese Medicine (approval no. 20161206XYZ). Tropomyosin of Chinese shrimp (*Penaeus orientalis*) was purified according to a previous report [47]. BALB/c mice (4 weeks old, 18–22 g) were purchased from the animal center of the Changchun University of Traditional Chinese Medicine and raised in our animal facility. The mice were maintained at 20–22°C under a 12-h light and 12-h dark condition with free access to food and water. A total of 24 BALB/c mice were randomly divided into 3 groups ($n = 8$ in each group): negative control group (NG), positive control group (PG), and experiment group (EG). After one-week acclimatization, the mice from PG and EG were intracutaneously injected with 100-µg tropomyosin and 10-µg cholera toxin (Sigma) as an adjuvant in 0.1 ml of PBS buffer twice weekly for a month. The mice from NG were intracutaneously injected with 10-µg cholera toxin in PBS buffer twice weekly

for a month. Subsequently, the mice from EG were orally administrated with 0.5-ml (1×10^6/ml) B. lactis in 0.9% saline solution for 28 d. The mice from NG and PG received equal volume of saline solution. After 28 d, the mice were sacrificed by cervical dislocation. The spleen was isolated and exteriorized.

2.9. Evaluation of Systemic Anaphylaxis in Mouse Allergy Models. The symptoms of systemic anaphylaxis were measured before and after tropomyosin challenge and scored based on a scoring system [48]: 0, no symptoms; 1, scratch and rub nose and head; 2, swelling eyes and mouth, diarrhea, slow or no activity with an increased respiratory rate after prodding; 3, wheezing and cyanosis around the mouth and the tail; 4, no activity; and 5, death.

Considering serum tropomyosin-specific IgE variation, 100 µl venous blood was obtained from the tail of each mouse weekly after the establishment of an allergic model. Serum was isolated via brief centrifugation of the whole blood. Serum levels of tropomyosin-specific IgE were measured twice by using an ELISA kit. The ELISA plate was washed by using PBS buffer, 200 µl blocking solution was added and incubated for 2 h at 37°C. Horseradish peroxidase- (HRP-) conjugated rabbit anti-mouse secondary antibodies were added. After one-hour incubation at 37°C, TMB (3, 3′, 5, 5′-tetramethylbenzidine) was developed. The absorbance of IgE was measured at 490 nm.

2.10. Quantitative PCR Assay. A reverse transcription kit and SYBR Mix was purchased from Takara Company (Dalian, China). Total RNA was isolated by using the RNA isolation kit (Qiagen, Valencia, CA, USA). RNA purity was determined by using NanoDrop2000 (Thermo Scientific Company, Fremont, CA, USA). cDNA was synthesized from one-µg RNA by using a cDNA synthesis kit (Pharmacia Biotech, Piscataway, NJ, USA). Relative mRNA levels of IL-17A, IL-23, Treg-related transcription factor FoxP3, and cytokine TGF-β were measured by using quantitative PCR assay via the primers from Table 1. PCR reaction mixtures were set in 20-µl volumes: SYBR Mix 10 µL, primer (µm) 0.4 µL, cDNA 2 µL, and ddH$_2$O 7.2 µL. PCR amplification conditions were: 95°C 3 min; 95°C 20 s, 60°C 20 s, 72°C 20 s, and 40 cycles. The relative level of gene expression was calculated by using the 2-AACt method [49].

2.11. Measurement of T-Cell Subsets. Rabbit anti-human IgE antibodies were purchased from Southern Biotech (Birmingham, AL, USA); FITC-labeled CD4 (Cat#11-0047-42 for anti-human antibody and Cat# 11-0042-86 for anti-mouse antibody), FoxP3 PerCP-CY5.5 (Cat # 45-4776-42 for anti-human antibody and Cat # 45-5773-82 for anti-mouse antibody), PE-IL-17A (Cat # 12-7178-42 for anti-human antibody and Cat # 25-7177-82 for anti-mouse antibody), and PE CD25 (Cat # 12-0259-42 for anti-human antibody and Cat # 12-0251-82 for anti-mouse antibody) were purchased from American eBioscience Company (San Diego, CA, USA); mouse spleen was sterilely ground to

TABLE 1: The primers used for real-time PCR.

Genes	Forward primer sequence (5′-3′)	Reverse primer sequence (5′-3′)
The primers for human		
FoxP3	TTGAACCCCATGCCACCATC	CATCCACCGTTGAGAGCTGG
TGF-β	GGGCTTCTCCTACCCCTAC	CTTCCCCTTCTGGGATCTTG
IL-17A	CCCGGACTGTGATGGTCAAC	GGAGGCTCCCTGCGCAGGAC
IL-23	GATGAAGAGACTACAAATG	GAGGCATGAAGCTGGCCCAC
β-Actin	GGGCGTGATGGTGGGCATG	TCGGTCAGCAGCACGGGGTG
The primers for mouse		
FoxP3	TTTCCAAGAACGGGCATTA	TGTGGCTGACTGAGGGTGT
TGF-β	ACCGCAACAACGCCATCTAT	GCACTGCTTCCCGAATGTCT
IL-17A	AGGGAGAGCTTCATCTGTGG	AGATTCATGGACCCCAACAG
IL-23	TGCTGGATTGCAGAGCAGTAA	GCATGCAGAGATTCCGAGAGA
β-Actin	CGCAAAGACCTGTATGCCAAT	GGGCTGTGATCTCCTTCTGC

prepare cell suspension. After the cell lysis, the cell concentration was adjusted to 10^7 cells/ml and incubated with FITC-CD4, PE- CD25, FoxP3 PerCP-CY5.5, and PE-IL-17A. After washing with PBS buffer, the spleen cells were suspended in PBS buffer, and CD4$^+$ T-cell subsets of spleen cells were detected by flow cytometry (Beckman Coulter, USA).

2.12. Statistical Analysis. All data were presented as mean values ±SD. The chi-squared (χ^2) test was used to compare the number difference between two groups. Student's t-test was used to compare mean quantitative differences between two groups. All analyses were performed by using SPSS 20.0 statistical package (IBM Software, NY, USA). The statistical difference was significant if $P < 0.05$.

3. Results

3.1. Measurement of Food Allergy. Table 2 shows the allergens in the food and the incidence of food allergy varied from 4.3% to 79.3% among 9 kinds of food. All different-age groups were compared with each other, and the statistical difference was insignificant between the group of 4~7 years old and the group of 8~12 years old ($P < 0.05$, Table 3).

3.2. Clinical Characters. Table 4 shows that there was no significant difference between two groups in age and sex ($P > 0.05$). There was no significant difference in symptoms, allergy grades, and serum IgE ($P > 0.05$). The statistical differences for other parameters were insignificant between two groups, either ($P > 0.05$, Table 4). After one-month follow-up, 2 and 4 persons were withdrawn from BG and CG, respectively. After three-month follow-up, further 3 and 4 persons were withdrawn from BG and CG, respectively.

3.3. B. lactis Treatment Reduced Allergy Symptoms in the Children with Food Allergy. Allergic symptoms were alleviated in BG when compared with CG ($P < 0.05$, Table 5). After three-month therapy, the therapeutic results for allergic symptoms were still stable and statistical difference was significant between BG and CG ($P < 0.05$, Table 5). Rash grades, eczema scores, abdominal cramps/pain scores, and

vomiting grades were reduced significantly after long-term *B. lactis* consumption ($P < 0.05$, Table 5). The levels of serum IgE showed similar results and reduced significantly after long-term *B. lactis* consumption ($P < 0.05$, Table 5).

3.4. Serum Levels of IgE in the Children with Food Allergy. Before therapy, the statistical difference for serum levels of IgE was insignificant between control and *B. lactis* groups ($P > 0.05$, Figure 1(a)). After 3-month therapy, the levels of IgE were reduced in the *B. lactis* group and the statistical difference for serum levels of IgE was significant between control and *B. lactis* groups ($P < 0.05$, Figure 1). After 3-month therapy, the statistical difference for serum levels of IgE was significant between control and *B. lactis* groups ($P < 0.05$, Figure 1). All these results indicated that *B. lactis* effectively alleviated the allergic effect by regulating the levels of IgE in the children with food allergy.

3.5. B. lactis Consumption Increased the Percentage of Treg Cells and Reduced the Percentage of Th17 Cells. Before the probiotics consumption, the statistical difference for the percentage of Treg cells (Figure 2(a)) and Th17 cells (Figure 2(b)) and the ratio of Treg/Th17 cells (Figure 2(c)) was insignificant between two groups ($P > 0.05$) in the children with food allergy. After three-month probiotic consumption, *B. lactis* consumption increased the percentage of Treg cells (Figure 2(a)) and reduced the percentage of Th17 cells (Figure 2(b)) and the ratio of Treg/Th17 cells (Figure 2(c)) ($P < 0.05$).

3.6. B. lactis Consumption Reduced Anaphylaxis Scores in Mouse Allergy Models. Allergic symptoms were promoted within 30 min after tropomyosin challenge. The model mice scratched and rubbed around nose, with reduced activity or no activity after prodding. Diarrhea was found after 45-min challenge. After two-hour challenge, anaphylaxis scores were higher in a model group than those in the group treated with *B. lactis* or negative controls ($P < 0.05$, Figure 3).

3.7. Serum Levels of IgE in Mouse Allergy Models. To confirm the changes for the serum levels of IgE, an allergy animal model was established. Allergy symptoms were seen from

TABLE 2: Allergic reactions on food-specific IgE of food.

	Egg	Crab	Shrimp	Beef	Cashew	Milk	Mango	Pineapple	Shellfish
Positive number	203	123	134	56	29	21	14	11	79
Percent (%)	79.3	48.0	52.3	21.9	11.3	8.2	5.5	4.3	30.9

TABLE 3: IgE in different age groups.

Parameters	Egg	Crab	Shrimp
4~7 yr, n (%)	127 (62.6)	75 (61.0)	81 (60.4)
8~12 yr, n (%)	76 (37.4)	48 (39.0)	53 (39.6)
Total case, n	203	123	134
χ^2		0.174	
P values		0.917	

TABLE 4: Clinical characteristics.

Parameters	BG	CG	χ^2 and t value	P value
Gender, male/female	72/56	76/52	0.256	0.613
Age, yr	10.89 ± 3.26	10.23 ± 2.78	−1.313	0.109
Body mass index, weight (kg)/height^2 (m^2)	24.67 ± 4.18	24.13 ± 3.95	0.689	0.412
Allergy symptoms				
Rash, grades	2.51 ± 1.36	2.62 ± 1.43	−0.718	0.362
Eczema, scores	32.70 ± 11.26	30.54 ± 12.03	−0.964	0.358
Abdominal cramps/pain, scores	22.11 ± 9.34	24.26 ± 8.73	0.648	0.723
Vomiting, grades	1.22 ± 0.87	1.14 ± 0.79	0.452	0.612
IgE (μg/ml)	10.23 ± 5.18	10.36 ± 5.31	0.246	0.482

Note. BG, the patients received *B. lactis* treatment; CG, the patients received solution without *B. lactis* treatment. n=128 for each group. All data were presented as mean ± SD (standard derivation). The statistical difference was significant if $P < 0.05$ when compared with the control group.

TABLE 5: The effects of *B. lactis* on pediatric allergy.

Parameters	One-month follow-up		P value	Three-month follow-up		P value
	BG	CG		BG	CG	
Allergy symptoms						
Rash, grades	1.51 ± 1.13	2.56 ± 1.67	<0.001	1.46 ± 1.29	2.59 ± 1.85	<0.01
Eczema, scores	11.70 ± 9.36	32.41 ± 14.61	<0.001	11.59 ± 10.88	32.52 ± 15.99	<0.01
Abdominal cramps/pain, scores	8.11 ± 6.73	22.16 ± 8.41	<0.001	6.03 ± 5.26	22.09 ± 11.44	<0.01
Vomiting, grades	1.05 ± 0.97	2.23 ± 1.65	<0.001	1.16 ± 1.08	2.31 ± 1.89	<0.01
IgE (μg/ml)	2.27 ± 1.94	5.82 ± 3.90	<0.001	1.53 ± 1.38	5.96 ± 4.97	<0.01

Note. BG, the patients received *B. lactis* treatment; CG, the patients received the solution without *B. lactis* treatment; TSS, total allergy symptom score. n = 126 and 124 for BG and CG groups, respectively, after one-month follow-up. n = 123 and 120 for BG and CG, respectively, after three-month follow-up. All data were presented as mean ± SD (standard derivation). The statistical difference was significant if $P < 0.05$ when compared with the control group.

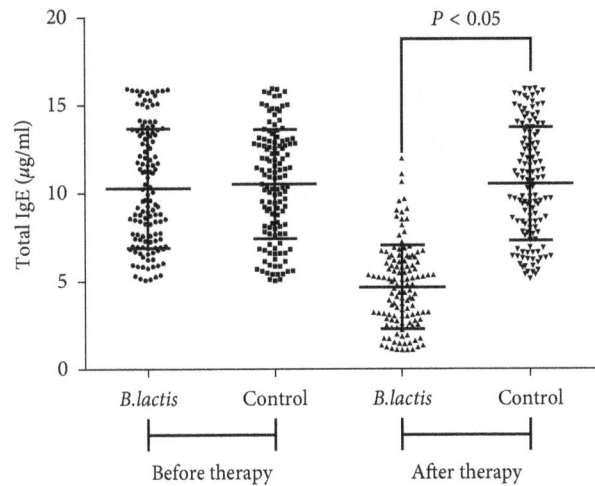

FIGURE 1: The effects of *B. lactis* on serum levels of IgE in the children with food allergy. *B. lactis* group: the patients received *B. lactis* treatment. Control group: the patients received the solution without *B. lactis* treatment. n = 128 for each group. The statistical difference was significant if $P < 0.05$.

animal models when compared with the negative control group, and both groups have varying degrees of diarrhea. *B. lactis* treatment alleviated allergic symptoms significantly ($P < 0.05$). In the NG, serum levels of IgE (Figure 4) were lowest when compared with other two groups ($P < 0.05$). In the PG, serum levels of IgE (Figure 4) were increased significantly when compared with the NG ($P < 0.05$). After *B. lactis* treatment, serum levels of IgE (Figure 4) were reduced significantly when compared with the PG ($P < 0.05$). *B. lactis* effectively alleviated the allergic responses caused by the original tropomyosin of shrimp in the mouse allergy models.

3.8. The Effects of B. lactis on Relative mRNA Levels of Treg- and Th17-Related Cytokine. In the PG, relative mRNA levels of FoxP3 (Figure 5(a)) and TGF-β (Figure 5(b)) were lowest when compared with other two groups ($P < 0.05$). In the NG, relative mRNA levels of FoxP3 (Figure 5(a)) and TGF-β (Figure 5(b)) were increased significantly ($P < 0.05$). After *B. lactis* treatment, relative mRNA levels of FoxP3 (Figure 5(a)) and TGF-β (Figure 5(b)) were increased significantly when compared with the PG ($P < 0.05$). In contrast, relative mRNA levels of IL-17A (Figure 5(c)) and IL-23 (Figure 5(d)) were highest in the PG when compared with other two groups ($P < 0.05$). In the NG, relative mRNA levels of IL-17A (Figure 5(c)) and IL-23 (Figure 5(d)) were decreased significantly ($P < 0.05$). After *B. lactis* treatment, relative mRNA levels of IL-17A (Figure 5(c)) and IL-23 (Figure 5(d)) were significantly reduced when compared

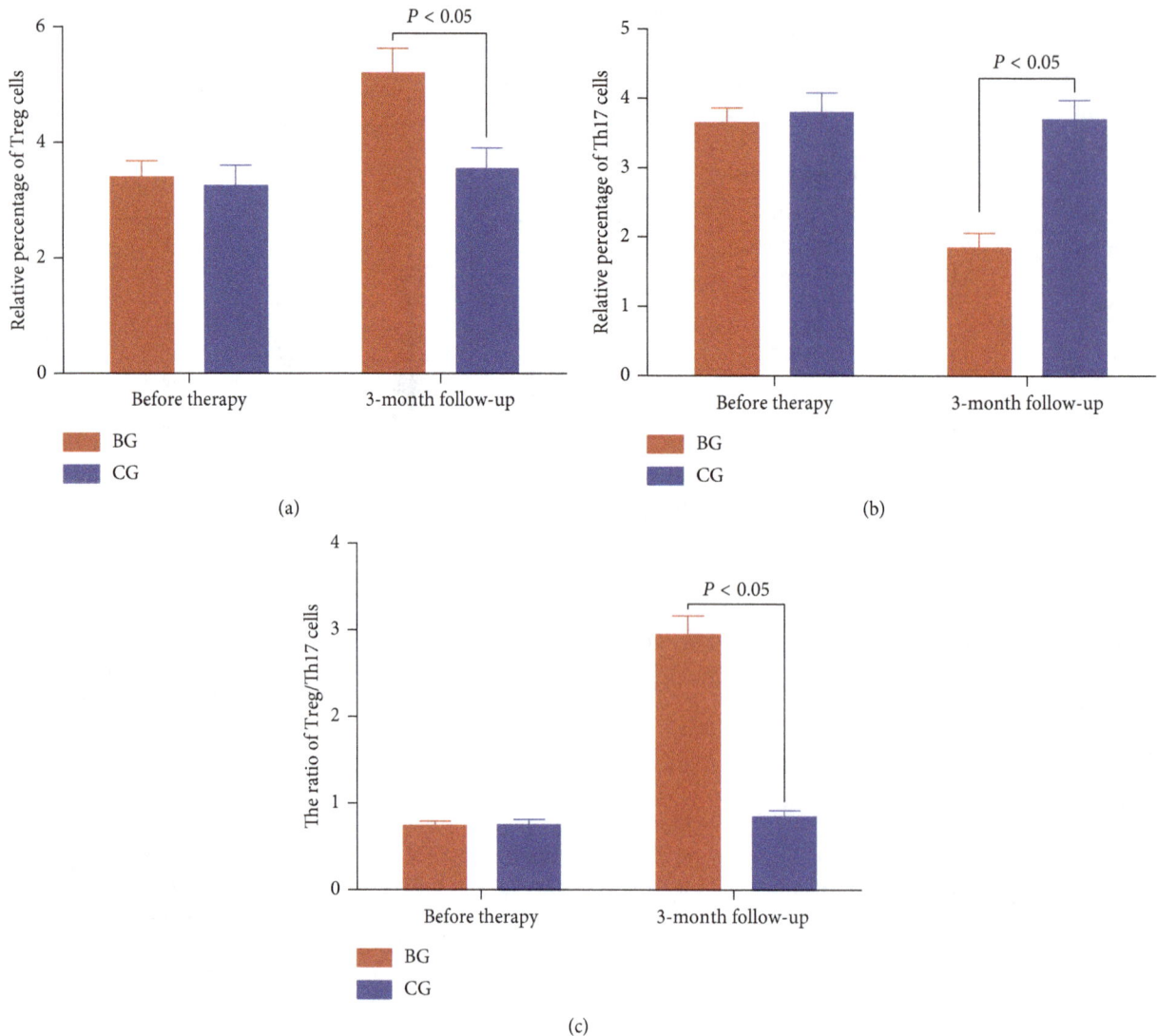

FIGURE 2: The effects of *B. lactis* on the percentage of Treg cells and Th17 cells in the children with food allergy. (a) The percentage of Treg cells. (b) The percentage of Th17 cells. (c) The ratio of Treg/Th17 cells. The statistical difference was significant if $P < 0.05$.

with the PG ($P < 0.05$). These results suggest *B. lactis* treatment may affect the balance of Th17/Treg cells since these cytokines are main indicators of the two subsets of T cells. The mouse allergy model may have imbalance of Treg/Th17 cells, and *B. lactis* may regulate the balance. Thus, the effects of *B. lactis* on the balance of Treg/Th17 cells were further explored.

3.9. The Effects of B. lactis on the Balance of Treg/Th17 Cells. To determine the effect of *B. lactis* on the number of Treg and Th17 cells in children with food allergy, Treg and Th17 cells were measured in three groups. Figure 6 shows that the percentage of Treg cells in the NG were significantly higher than that in the PG ($P < 0.05$, Figures 4(a), 4(b), and 4(d)), indicating that Treg cell differentiation was inhibited in allergy models. After *B. lactis* treatment, the contents were significantly increased when compared with the PG ($P < 0.05$, Figures 4(b) and 4(d)). The results indicated that

B. lactis treatment increased the levels of Treg cells. Figure 7 shows that the percentage of Th17 cells in the NG was significantly lower than that in the PG ($P < 0.05$, Figures 5(a), 5(b), and 5(d)), indicating that Th17 cell differentiation was promoted in allergy models. After *B. lactis* treatment, the percentage of Th17 significantly was reduced when compared with PG ($P < 0.05$, Figures 5(b) and 5(d)). The present findings demonstrated that allergic animal models had less T lymphocytes with Treg cells differentiation and more Th17 differentiation of T lymphocytes. *B. lactis* treatment induced a significant tolerance reaction for allergy symptoms by increasing Treg cells differentiation and suppressing Th17-type cells differentiation.

4. Discussion

As people's lifestyle changes [50] and environmental pollution aggravates [51], the therapy of allergic diseases is increasingly challenging and has become a serious disease

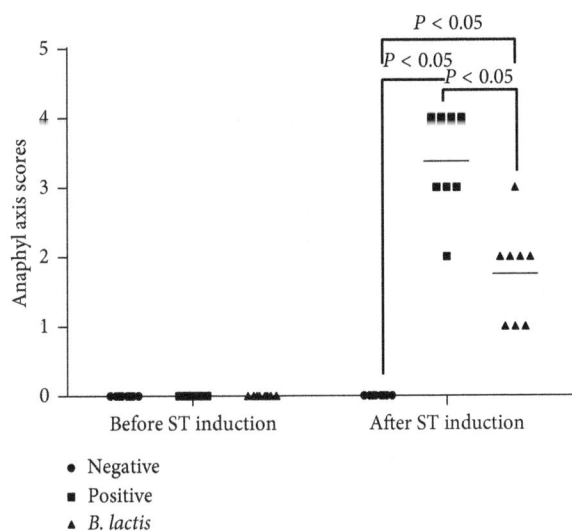

FIGURE 3: Shrimp tropomyosin-induced anaphylaxis in the mice among different groups. A total of 24 BALB/c mice were randomly divided into 3 groups ($n = 8$ in each group): negative control group (NG), positive control group (PG), and experiment group (EG). The statistical difference was significant if $P < 0.05$.

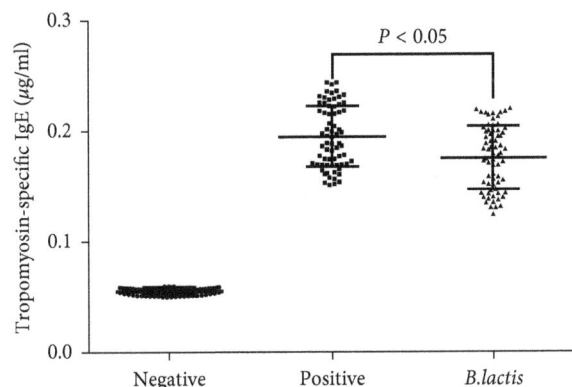

FIGURE 4: The effects of B. lactis on serum levels of IgE in mouse allergy models. BALB/c mice were randomly divided into 3 groups ($n = 8$ in each group): negative control group (NG), positive control group (PG), and experiment group (EG). The mice from PG and EG were individually immunized with tropomyosin and cholera toxin. The mice from NG received cholera toxin in PBS. Subsequently, the mice from EG received B. lactis. $n = 8$ for each group. The statistical difference was significant if $P < 0.05$.

threatening public health. Food allergies can occur in people of all ages, and high-risk groups are mainly infants and children. Food allergy can cause digestion, skin, nerves, respiratory disorders, and other symptoms [52]. Food allergy is closely related to genetic factors [53], the digestive system [54], environmental elements [55], and gut microbiota [56]. The nine kinds of food in this study are common food in daily life but are susceptible to allergies in children. Egg with high-level protein can cause severe allergy, followed by seafood, beef, milk, and fruit (Table 2). The results are different with previous reports: the allergic events caused by seafood are higher than those caused by eggs [57]. The consumption of eggs, shrimp, and crab is closely related to

the environment and life habits, which may be the reason causing the difference.

Different age groups are closely associated with the events of food allergy [58]. The statistical difference for the incidence of allergy symptoms was insignificant between different age groups from 4 to 7 years old and 8 to 12 years old ($P < 0.05$). The age differences for the two groups may not be better criteria for exploring the effects of age on food allergy. Furthermore, nine kinds of common food were selected as targets, but food allergy in children is much more complicated. Further work is highly demanded to address these issues. Food antibodies should be detected as soon as possible if some food allergies were suspected. The children should be prohibited from taking the same food and prevented from receiving further allergic damage and other allergic diseases.

Gut microbiota may also play an important role in egg allergy [59]. Probiotics is a potential way to improve the distribution of gut microbiota [60]. B. lactis is a main probiotics in dairy yogurt and has been proved to be effective to improve immune function by improving NK cell function and IFN-gamma levels [61]. The present findings demonstrated that B. lactis consumption reduced allergy symptoms of children with food allergy by reducing the serum levels of IgE (Table 5 and Figure 1). There was an improvement in all parameters in BG patients, which was consistent with previous reports. Dietary consumption of B. lactis can improve gut microecology and function of the digestive system and reduce the prevalence of rash [62]. Meanwhile, modulation of B. lactis for gut microecology may provide an alternative in the prevention of eczema [63]. On the other hand, the consumption of B. lactis can reduce abdominal pain (cramps), discomfort, and vomiting symptoms [64, 65]. Furthermore, Bifidobacterium species has been reported to inhibit IgE production [66].

Shrimp allergen tropomyosin is one of the main molecules for causing food allergy [10, 67]. According to early reports, shrimp tropomyosin was useful in exploring the mechanisms underlying food allergy in human subjects and assessing efficacy and safety of some therapeutic approaches. Some food allergy models were established by using shrimp tropomyosin [68, 69].

Further experiment showed that B. lactis reduced allergy symptoms of animal models with food allergy by reducing the serum levels of IgE (Figure 4). B. lactis increased relative mRNA levels of FoxP3 (Figure 5(a)) and TGF-β (Figure 5(b)) and reduced the relative mRNA levels of IL-17A (Figure 5(c)) and IL-23 (Figure 5(d)). All these cytokines are associated with the levels of Treg and Th17 cells. Th17 cells are associated with the pathogenesis of Th2-mediated allergic disorders [70]. Th17 cells regulate neutrophil recruitment and play an important role in allergy pathogenesis [71]. Th17 and Treg cells play a critical role in atopic disease [72]. Just as we supposed, B. lactis induced a significant tolerance reaction for allergy symptoms by increasing Treg cells differentiation (Figure 6) and suppressing Th17-type cells differentiation (Figure 7). The results were consistent with a previous report that B. lactis promoted potentially antiallergenic processes through

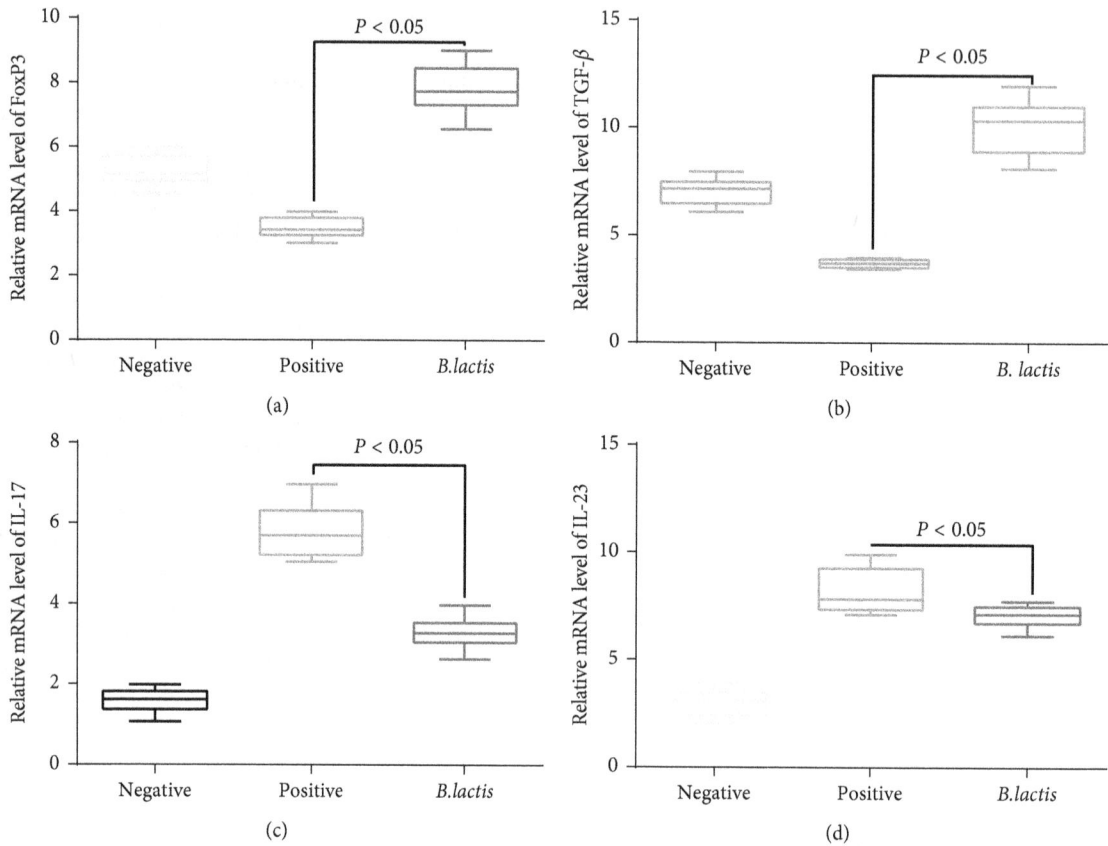

FIGURE 5: The effects of *B. lactis* on relative mRNA levels of Treg- and Th17-related cytokines in mouse allergy models. (a) The effects of *B. lactis* on mRNA levels of FoxP3 in mouse allergy models. (b) The effects of *B. lactis* on relative mRNA levels of TGF-β in mouse allergy models. (c) The effects of *B. lactis* on relative mRNA levels of IL-17A in mouse allergy models. (d) The effects of *B. lactis* on relative mRNA levels of IL-23 in mouse allergy models. The statistical difference was significant if $P < 0.05$.

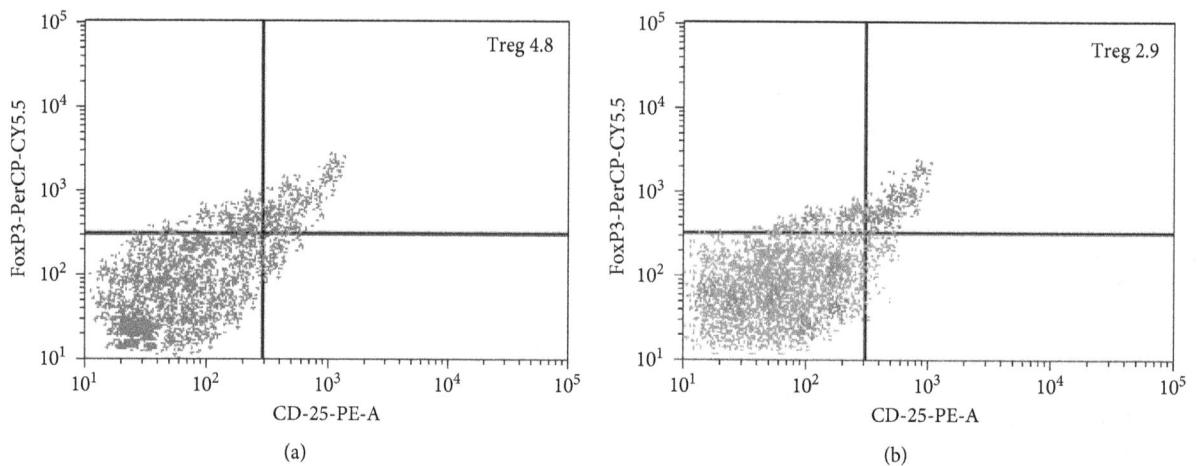

FIGURE 6: Continued.

(c)   (d)

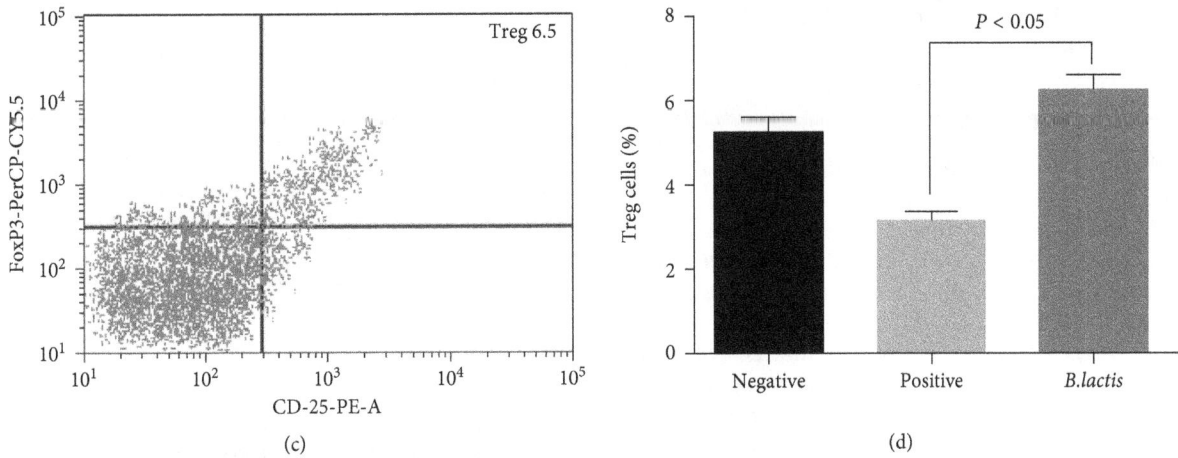

FIGURE 6: The effects of *B. lactis* on the percentage of Treg cells in mouse allergy models. (a) The percentage of Treg cells in the NG. (b) The percentage of Treg cells in the PG. (c) The percentage of Treg cells in the EG. (d) The effects of *B. lactis* on the percentage of Treg cells. BALB/c mice were randomly divided into 3 groups ($n = 8$ in each group): negative control group (NG), positive control group (PG), and experiment group (EG). The mice from PG and EG were individually immunized with tropomyosin and cholera toxin. The mice from NG received cholera toxin in PBS. Subsequently, the mice from EG received *B. lactis*. CD4$^+$ T cells were gated by CD4 expression and forward scatter characteristics. The statistical difference was significant if $P < 0.05$.

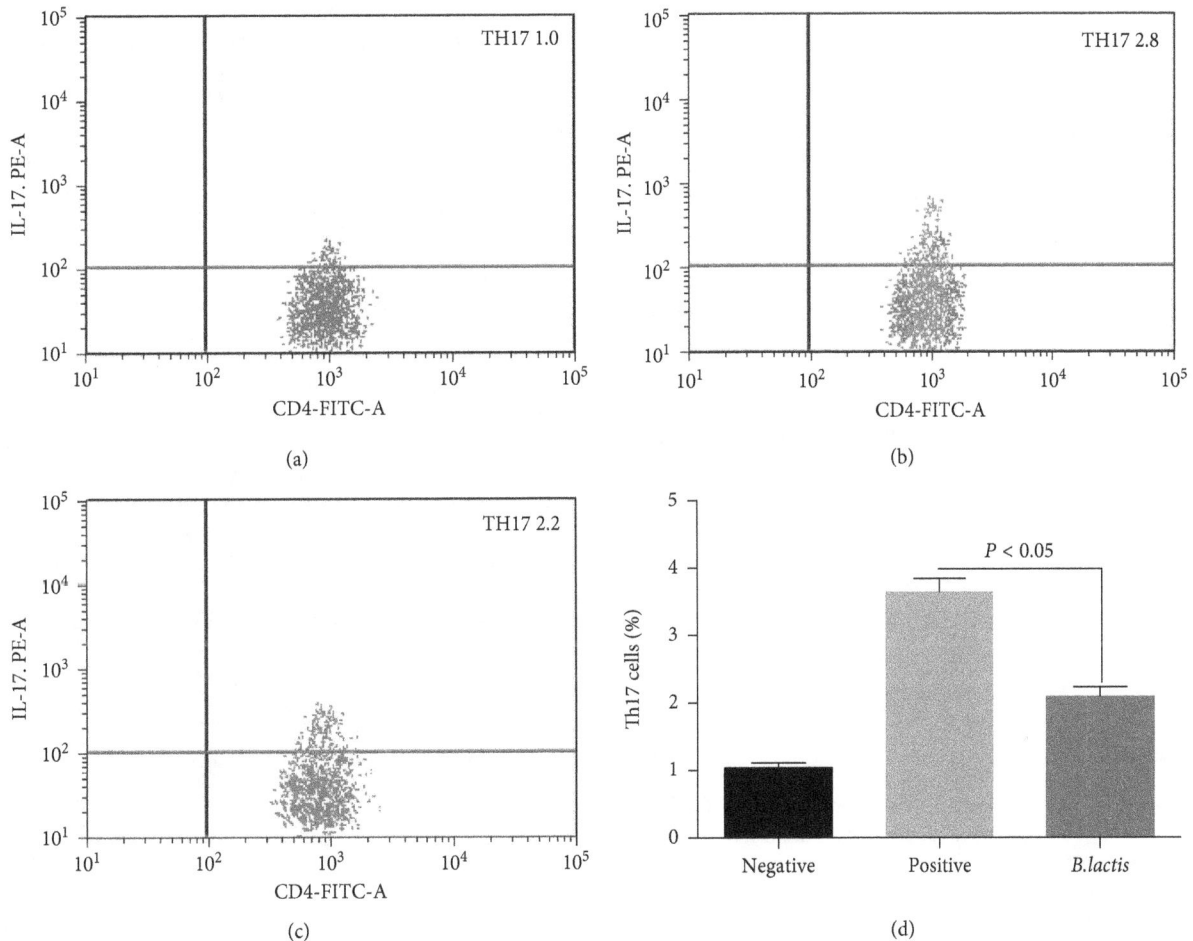

(a)   (b)

(c)   (d)

FIGURE 7: The effects of *B. lactis* on the percentage of Th17 cells in mouse allergy models. (a) The percentage of Th17 cells in the NG. (b) The percentage of Th17 cells in the PG. (c) The percentage of Th17 ells in the EG. (d) The effects of *B. lactis* on the percentage of Th17 cells. BALB/c mice were randomly divided into 3 groups ($n = 8$ in each group): negative control group (NG), positive control group (PG), and experiment group (EG). The mice from PG and EG were individually immunized with tropomyosin and cholera toxin. The mice from NG received cholera toxin in PBS. Subsequently, the mice from EG received *B. lactis*. $n = 8$ for each group. CD4$^+$ T cells were gated by CD4 expression and forward scatter characteristics. The statistical difference was significant if $P < 0.05$.

induction of Th1-type immunity and enhanced the regulatory lymphocyte [39].

There are some limitations for the present work. To maintain the insignificant difference of statistical data between two groups, the both groups were not advised to avoid certain food based on anamnesis and diagnostic test results. Furthermore, the lack of change in scores in the control group did not mean that no effective treatment was offered. The comparison of two groups showed that *B. lactis* treatment would be more effective than control group. The levels of transcription factor FoxP3 and cytokines TGF-β, IL-17A, and IL-23 were not measured in the children with food allergy. The work was limited because most patients did not agree to obtain small splenic biopsy by using an invasive surgery. Serum cytokine can be measured simply by using ELISA kits, and the results were unstable with time increasing. The food from different places will result in different allergic symptoms, and the problems were not explored in the present work. The detail components were not analyzed in different kinds of food and can be a main issue affecting the final results. Therefore, further research is highly demanded to address these problems in the future work.

5. Conclusion

B. lactis can effectively alleviate allergic reactions on food-specific IgE of food in children [73], and its related molecular mechanism may be involved with the balance of the Treg/Th17 cells. *B. lactis* treatment significantly increased the expression of FoxP3 and TGF-β related to Treg cells and reduced the expression of IL-17A and IL-23 related to Th17 cells. The probiotics consumption increased the ratio of Treg/Th17 cells to suppress the occurrence of allergic reactions. However, its specific mechanism of action is not yet clear and further study is still needed.

References

[1] R. Sinitkul, W. Manuyakorn, W. Kamchaisatian et al., "De novo food allergy in pediatric liver transplantation recipients," *Asian Pacific Journal of Allergy and Immunology*, vol. 36, no. 3, pp. 166–174, 2018.

[2] N. Lomidze and M. Gotua, "Prevalence of self-reported food allergy in different age groups of Georgian population," *Georgian Medical News*, vol. 241, pp. 40–44, 2015.

[3] R. Jiménez-Saiz, D. K. Chu, T. S. Mandur et al., "Lifelong memory responses perpetuate humoral T H 2 immunity and anaphylaxis in food allergy," *Journal of Allergy and Clinical Immunology*, vol. 140, no. 6, pp. 1604–1615.e5, 2017.

[4] C. A. Carter and P. A. Frischmeyer-Guerrerio, "The genetics of food allergy," *Current Allergy and Asthma Reports*, vol. 18, no. 1, p. 2, 2018.

[5] Z. F. Ma, N. A. Majid, Y. Yamaoka, and Y. Y. Lee, "Food allergy and *Helicobacter pylori* infection: a systematic review," *Frontiers in Microbiology*, vol. 7, p. 368, 2016.

[6] J. A. Lieberman, M. Greenhawt, and A. Nowak-Wegrzyn, "The environment and food allergy," *Annals of Allergy, Asthma and Immunology*, vol. 120, no. 5, pp. 455–457, 2018.

[7] M. Usui, A. Harada, S. Yasumoto et al., "Relationship between the risk for a shrimp allergy and freshness or cooking," *Bioscience, Biotechnology, and Biochemistry*, vol. 79, no. 10, pp. 1698–1701, 2015.

[8] H. Broekman, A. C. Knulst, G. de Jong et al., "Is mealworm or shrimp allergy indicative for food allergy to insects?," *Molecular Nutrition and Food Research*, vol. 61, no. 9, article 1601061, 2017.

[9] R. Misnan, S. Murad, Z. H. M. Yadzir et al., "Identification of the major allergens of Charybdis feriatus (red crab) and its cross-reactivity with Portunus pelagicus (blue crab)," *Asian Pacific Journal of Allergy and Immunology*, vol. 30, no. 4, p. 285, 2012.

[10] A. Purohit, J. Shao, J. M. Degreef et al., "Role of tropomyosin as a cross-reacting allergen in sensitization to cockroach in patients from Martinique (French Caribbean island) with a respiratory allergy to mite and a food allergy to crab and shrimp," *European Annals of Allergy and Clinical Immunology*, vol. 39, no. 3, pp. 85–88, 2007.

[11] L. Farioli, L. M. Losappio, M. G. Giuffrida et al., "Mite-induced asthma and IgE levels to shrimp, mite, tropomyosin, arginine kinase, and der p 10 are the most relevant risk factors for challenge-proven shrimp allergy," *International Archives of Allergy and Immunology*, vol. 174, no. 3-4, pp. 133–143, 2017.

[12] D.-X. Fei, Q.-M. Liu, F. Chen et al., "Assessment of the sensitizing capacity and allergenicity of enzymatic cross-linked arginine kinase, the crab allergen," *Molecular Nutrition and Food Research*, vol. 60, no. 7, pp. 1707–1718, 2016.

[13] X. Sun, H.-T. Mao, and W.-X. Yang, "Gene expression pattern of myosin Va during spermatogenesis of Chinese mitten crab, *Eriocheir sinensis*," *Gene*, vol. 508, no. 1, pp. 78–84, 2012.

[14] M. Guo, S. Liu, M. Ismail et al., "Changes in the myosin secondary structure and shrimp surimi gel strength induced by dense phase carbon dioxide," *Food Chemistry*, vol. 227, pp. 219–226, 2017.

[15] M. G. Giuffrida, D. Villalta, G. Mistrello et al., "Shrimp allergy beyond tropomyosin in Italy: clinical relevance of arginine kinase, Sarcoplasmic calcium binding protein and hemocyanin," *European Annals of Allergy and Clinical Immunology*, vol. 46, no. 5, pp. 172–177, 2014.

[16] M.-J. Hu, G.-Y. Liu, Y. Yang et al., "Cloning, expression, and the effects of processing on sarcoplasmic-calcium-binding protein: an important allergen in mud crab," *Journal of Agricultural and Food Chemistry*, vol. 65, no. 30, pp. 6247–6257, 2017.

[17] S. H. Sicherer, A. Muñoz-Furlong, and H. A. Sampson, "Prevalence of seafood allergy in the United States determined by a random telephone survey," *Journal of Allergy and Clinical Immunology*, vol. 114, no. 1, pp. 159–165, 2004.

[18] A. L. Lopata, R. E. O'Hehir, and S. B. Lehrer, "Shellfish allergy," *Clinical and Experimental Allergy*, vol. 40, no. 6, pp. 850–858, 2010.

[19] P. Licona-Limón, L. K. Kim, N. W. Palm, and R. A. Flavell, "TH2, allergy and group 2 innate lymphoid cells," *Nature Immunology*, vol. 14, no. 6, pp. 536–542, 2013.

[20] M. Klatka, E. Grywalska, M. Partyka, M. Charytanowicz, E. Kiszczak-Bochynska, and J. Rolinski, "Th17 and Treg cells in adolescents with Graves' disease. Impact of treatment with methimazole on these cell subsets," *Autoimmunity*, vol. 47, no. 3, pp. 201–211, 2014.

[21] C. B. Schmidt-Weber, "Th17 and treg cells innovate the TH1/TH2 concept and allergy research," *Chemical Immunology and Allergy*, vol. 94, pp. 1–7, 2008.

[22] J. Peng, Z. Yu, L. Xue et al., "The effect of foxp3-overexpressing Treg cells on non-small cell lung cancer cells," *Molecular Medicine Reports*, vol. 17, no. 4, pp. 5860–5868, 2018.

[23] M. Zhao, H. Zhang, X. Liu et al., "The effect of TGF-β on treg cells in adverse pregnancy outcome upon toxoplasma gondii infection," *Frontiers in Microbiology*, vol. 8, p. 901, 2017.

[24] H. Bai, X. Gao, L. Zhao et al., "Respective IL-17A production by $\gamma\delta$ T and Th17 cells and its implication in host defense against chlamydial lung infection," *Cellular and Molecular Immunology*, vol. 14, no. 10, pp. 850–861, 2016.

[25] J. R. Fernandes, T. K. Berthoud, A. Kumar, and J. B. Angel, "IL-23 signaling in Th17 cells is inhibited by HIV infection and is not restored by HAART: implications for persistent immune activation," *PLoS One*, vol. 12, no. 11, Article ID e0186823, 2017.

[26] L. Zhang, J. Yan, B. Yang et al., "IL-23 activated $\gamma\delta$ T cells affect Th17 cells and regulatory T cells by secreting IL-21 in children with primary nephrotic syndrome," *Scandinavian Journal of Immunology*, vol. 87, no. 1, pp. 36–45, 2017.

[27] S. Sakaguchi, N. Sakaguchi, M. Asano et al., "Immunological self-tolerance maintained by activated T-cells expressing il-2 receptor alpha-chains (Cd25) - breakdown of a single mechanism of self-tolerance causes various autoimmune-diseases," *Journal of Immunology*, vol. 155, no. 3, pp. 1151–1164, 1995.

[28] C. T. Weaver, L. E. Harrington, P. R. Mangan, M. Gavrieli, and K. M. Murphy, "Th17: an effector CD4 T cell lineage with regulatory T cell ties," *Immunity*, vol. 24, no. 6, pp. 677–688, 2006.

[29] M. L. Shinohara, J.-H. Kim, V. A. Garcia, and H. Cantor, "Engagement of the type I interferon receptor on dendritic cells inhibits T helper 17 cell development: role of intracellular osteopontin," *Immunity*, vol. 29, no. 1, pp. 68–78, 2008.

[30] H. Kopf, G. M. de la Rosa, O. M. Z. Howard, and X. Chen, "Rapamycin inhibits differentiation of Th17 cells and promotes generation of FoxP3+ T regulatory cells," *International Immunopharmacology*, vol. 7, no. 13, pp. 1819–1824, 2007.

[31] R. He, M. K. Oyoshi, H. Jin, and R. S. Geha, "Epicutaneous antigen exposure induces a Th17 response that drives airway inflammation after inhalation challenge," *Proceedings of the National Academy of Sciences*, vol. 104, no. 40, pp. 15817–15822, 2007.

[32] R. H. Wilson, G. S. Whitehead, H. Nakano, M. E. Free, J. K. Kolls, and D. N. Cook, "Allergic sensitization through the airway primes Th17-dependent neutrophilia and airway hyperresponsiveness," *American Journal of Respiratory and Critical Care Medicine*, vol. 180, no. 8, pp. 720–730, 2009.

[33] Z.-H. Shen, C.-X. Zhu, Y.-S. Quan et al., "Relationship between intestinal microbiota and ulcerative colitis: mechanisms and clinical application of probiotics and fecal microbiota transplantation," *World Journal of Gastroenterology*, vol. 24, no. 1, pp. 5–14, 2018.

[34] N. A. N. Mohd Nor, S. Abbasiliasi, M. N. Marikkar et al., "Defatted coconut residue crude polysaccharides as potential prebiotics: study of their effects on proliferation and acidifying activity of probiotics in vitro," *Journal of Food Science and Technology*, vol. 54, no. 1, pp. 164–173, 2016.

[35] G. W. Shu, Y. X. He, N. Lei et al., "Cellulase-assisted extraction of polysaccharides from white hyacinth bean: characterization of antioxidant activity and promotion for probiotics proliferation," *Molecules*, vol. 22, no. 10, p. 1764, 2017.

[36] L.-C. Lew and M.-T. Liong, "Bioactives from probiotics for dermal health: functions and benefits," *Journal of Applied Microbiology*, vol. 114, no. 5, pp. 1241–1253, 2013.

[37] L. Fu, J. Song, C. Wang et al., "Bifidobacterium infantis potentially alleviates shrimp tropomyosin-induced allergy by tolerogenic dendritic cell-dependent induction of regulatory T cells and alterations in gut microbiota," *Frontiers in Immunology*, vol. 8, p. 1536, 2017.

[38] T. P. Tan, Z. Ba, M. E. Sanders et al., "Safety of bifidobacterium animalis subsp. lactis (B. Lactis) strain BB-12-Supplemented yogurt in healthy children," *Journal of Pediatric Gastroenterology and Nutrition*, vol. 64, no. 2, pp. 302–309, 2017.

[39] J. Y. Kim, Y. O. Choi, and G. E. Ji, "Effect of oral probiotics (Bifidobacterium lactis AD011 and Lactobacillus acidophilus AD031) administration on ovalbumin-induced food allergy mouse model," *Journal of Microbiology and Biotechnology*, vol. 18, no. 8, pp. 1393–1400, 2008.

[40] S. Podder, S. K. Gupta, and G. K. Saha, "Incrimination of Blomia tropicalis as a potent allergen in house dust and its role in allergic asthma in Kolkata Metropolis, India," *World Allergy Organization Journal*, vol. 3, no. 5, pp. 182–187, 2010.

[41] D. Gislason and T. Gislason, "IgE-mediated allergy toLepidoglyphus destructorin an urban population-an epidemiologic study," *Allergy*, vol. 54, no. 8, pp. 878–883, 1999.

[42] R. X. Foong, G. Roberts, A. T. Fox et al., "Pilot study: assessing the clinical diagnosis of allergy in atopic children using a microarray assay in addition to skin prick testing and serum specific IgE," *Clinical and Molecular Allergy*, vol. 14, no. 1, p. 8, 2016.

[43] A. Lakshman, M. Modi, G. Prakash et al., "Evaluation of bortezomib-induced neuropathy using total neuropathy score (reduced and clinical versions) and NCI CTCAE v4.0 in newly diagnosed patients with multiple myeloma receiving bortezomib-based induction," *Clinical Lymphoma Myeloma and Leukemia*, vol. 17, no. 8, pp. 513–519, 2017.

[44] R. Chopra, P. P. Vakharia, R. Sacotte et al., "Severity strata for eczema area and severity index (EASI), modified EASI, scoring atopic dermatitis (SCORAD), objective SCORAD, atopic dermatitis severity index and body surface area in adolescents and adults with atopic dermatitis," *British Journal of Dermatology*, vol. 177, no. 5, pp. 1316–1321, 2017.

[45] S. S. Clark, "Electrolyte disturbance associated with jejunal conduit," *Journal of urology*, vol. 112, no. 1, pp. 42–47, 1974.

[46] S. M. Lee, S.-E. Park, Y.-S. Nam et al., "Analgesic effectiveness of nerve block in shoulder arthroscopy: comparison between interscalene, suprascapular and axillary nerve blocks," *Knee Surgery, Sports Traumatology, Arthroscopy*, vol. 20, no. 12, pp. 2573–2578, 2012.

[47] F. Long, X. Yang, R. Wang, X. Hu, and F. Chen, "Effects of combined high pressure and thermal treatments on the allergenic potential of shrimp (Litopenaeus vannamei) tropomyosin in a mouse model of allergy," *Innovative Food Science and Emerging Technologies*, vol. 29, pp. 119–124, 2015.

[48] X.-M. Li, B. H. Schofield, C.-K. Huang, G. I. Kleiner, and H. A. Sampson, "A murine model of IgE-mediated cow's milk

hypersimulativity," *Journal of Allergy and Clinical Immunology*, vol. 103, no. 2, pp. 206–214, 1999.

[49] A. Arocho, B. Chen, M. Ladanyi, and Q. Pan, "Validation of the 2-????Ct calculation as an alternate method of data analysis for quantitative PCR of BCR-ABL P210 transcripts," *Diagnostic Molecular Pathology*, vol. 15, no. 1, pp. 56–61, 2006.

[50] M. Ben-Shoshan, L. Soller, D. W. Harrington et al., "Eczema in early childhood, sociodemographic factors and lifestyle habits are associated with food allergy: a nested case-control study," *International Archives of Allergy and Immunology*, vol. 166, no. 3, pp. 199–207, 2015.

[51] J. H. Hu, N. P. Li, Y. Lv et al., "Investigation on indoor air pollution and childhood allergies in households in six Chinese cities by subjective survey and field measurements," *International Journal of Environmental Research and Public Health*, vol. 14, no. 9, p. 979, 2017.

[52] N. R. More and N. S. Pradhan, "Contribution of my faculty in food protein allergy," *Ayurlog: National Journal of Research in Ayurved Science*, vol. 6, no. 01, pp. 1–4, 2018.

[53] S. E. Ashley, H.-T. T. Tan, R. Peters et al., "Genetic variation at the Th2 immune gene IL13 is associated with IgE-mediated paediatric food allergy," *Clinical and Experimental Allergy*, vol. 47, no. 8, pp. 1032–1037, 2017.

[54] M. Worm, I. Reese, B. Ballmer-Weber et al., "Guidelines on the management of IgE-mediated food allergies," *Allergo Journal International*, vol. 24, no. 7, pp. 256–293, 2015.

[55] S. Benedé, A. B. Blázquez, D. Chiang, L. Tordesillas, and M. C. Berin, "The rise of food allergy: environmental factors and emerging treatments," *EBioMedicine*, vol. 7, pp. 27–34, 2016.

[56] S. C. Diesner, C. Bergmayr, B. Pfitzner et al., "A distinct microbiota composition is associated with protection from food allergy in an oral mouse immunization model," *Clinical Immunology*, vol. 173, pp. 10–18, 2016.

[57] N. R. Schellpfeffer, H. L. Leo, M. Ambrose, and A. N. Hashikawa, "Food allergy trends and epinephrine autoinjector presence in summer camps," *The Journal of Allergy and Clinical Immunology: In Practice*, vol. 5, no. 2, pp. 358–362, 2017.

[58] K. Jeong, J. Kim, K. Ahn et al., "Age-based causes and clinical characteristics of immediate-type food allergy in Korean children," *Allergy, Asthma and Immunology Research*, vol. 9, no. 5, pp. 423–430, 2017.

[59] M. Fazlollahi, Y. Chun, A. Grishin et al., "Early-life gut microbiome and egg allergy," *Allergy*, vol. 73, no. 7, pp. 1515–1524, 2018.

[60] M. P. C. Neto, J. de Souza Aquino, L. de Fatima Romao da Silva et al., "Gut microbiota and probiotics intervention: a potential therapeutic target for management of cardiometabolic disorders and chronic kidney disease?," *Pharmacological Research*, vol. 130, pp. 152–163, 2018.

[61] A. Lee, Y. J. Lee, H. J. Yoo et al., "Consumption of dairy yogurt containing lactobacillus paracasei ssp. paracasei, bifidobacterium animalis ssp. lactis and heat-treated lactobacillus plantarum improves immune function including natural killer cell activity," *Nutrients*, vol. 9, no. 6, pp. 1–9, 2017.

[62] J. Saavedra, A. Abi-Hanna, N. Moore, and R. Yolken, "Effect of long term consumption of infant formulas with bifidobacteria (B) and S. thermophilus (ST) on stool patterns and diaper rash in infants," *Journal of Pediatric Gastroenterology and Nutrition*, vol. 27, no. 4, p. 483, 1998.

[63] I. H. Ismail, R. J. Boyle, P. V. Licciardi et al., "Early gut colonization byBifidobacterium breveandB. catenulatumdifferentially modulates eczema risk in children at high risk of developing allergic disease," *Pediatric Allergy and Immunology*, vol. 27, no. 8, pp. 838–846, 2016.

[64] S. Faber, "Treatment of abnormal gut flora improves symptoms in patients with irritable bowel syndrome," *The American Journal of Gastroenterology*, vol. 95, no. 9, p. 2533, 2000.

[65] G. Boehm, M. Lidestri, P. Casetta et al., "Supplementation of a bovine milk formula with an oligosaccharide mixture increases counts of faecal bifidobacteria in preterm infants," *Archives of Disease in Childhood-Fetal and Neonatal Edition*, vol. 86, no. 3, pp. F178–F181, 2002.

[66] N. Takahashi, H. Kitazawa, T. Shimosato et al., "An immunostimulatory DNA sequence from a probiotic strain ofBifidobacterium longuminhibits IgE productionin vitro," *FEMS Immunology and Medical Microbiology*, vol. 46, no. 3, pp. 461–469, 2006.

[67] A. M. DeWitt, L. Mattsson, I. Lauer, G. Reese, and J. Lidholm, "Recombinant tropomyosin fromPenaeus aztecus (rPen a 1) for measurement of specific immuno-globulin E antibodies relevant in food allergy to crustaceans and other invertebrates," *Molecular Nutrition and Food Research*, vol. 48, no. 5, pp. 370–379, 2004.

[68] L. Fu, J. Peng, S. Zhao et al., "Lactic acid bacteria-specific induction of CD4(+)Foxp3(+)T cells ameliorates shrimp tropomyosin-induced allergic response in mice via suppression of mTOR signaling," *Scientific Reports*, vol. 7, no. 1, 1987 pages, 2017.

[69] F. Capobianco, C. Butteroni, B. Barletta et al., "Oral sensitization with shrimp tropomyosin induces in mice allergen-specific IgE, T cell response and systemic anaphylactic reactions," *International Immunology*, vol. 20, no. 8, pp. 1077–1086, 2008.

[70] K. Oboki, T. Ohno, H. Saito, and S. Nakae, "Th17 and allergy," *Allergology International*, vol. 57, no. 2, pp. 121–134, 2008.

[71] M. L. Manni, M. E. Clay, K. J. McHugh et al., *C31. Experimental Asthma Therapies*, American Thoracic Society, New York, NY, USA, 2016.

[72] G. Rai, S. Das, M. A. Ansari et al., "Phenotypic and functional profile of Th17 and Treg cells in allergic fungal sinusitis," *International Immunopharmacology*, vol. 57, pp. 55–61, 2018.

[73] H. A. Sampson, "Utility of food-specific IgE concentrations in predicting symptomatic food allergy," *Journal of Allergy and Clinical Immunology*, vol. 107, no. 5, pp. 891–896, 2001.

11

Isolation of Extended-Spectrum β-lactamase- (ESBL-) Producing *Escherichia coli* and *Klebsiella pneumoniae* from Patients with Community-Onset Urinary Tract Infections in Jimma University Specialized Hospital, Southwest Ethiopia

Mengistu Abayneh (ID),[1] **Getnet Tesfaw,**[2] **and Alemseged Abdissa**[2]

[1]*School of Medical Laboratory Sciences, Mizan-Tepi University, Mizan Aman, Ethiopia*
[2]*School of Medical Laboratory Sciences, Institute of Health Sciences, Jimma University, P.O. Box 378, Jimma, Ethiopia*

Correspondence should be addressed to Mengistu Abayneh; menge.abay@gmail.com

Guest Editor: Alberto Antonelli

Background. Klebsiella pneumoniae and *Escherichia coli* are the major extended-spectrum β-lactamase- (ESBL-) producing organisms increasingly isolated as causes of complicated urinary tract infections and remain an important cause of failure of therapy with cephalosporins and have serious infection control consequence. *Objective.* To assess the prevalence and antibiotics resistance patterns of ESBL-producing *Escherichia coli* and *Klebsiella pneumoniae* from community-onset urinary tract infections in Jimma University Specialized hospital, Southwest Ethiopia, 2016. *Methodology.* A hospital-based cross-sectional study was conducted, and a total of 342 urine samples were cultured on MacConkey agar for the detection of etiologic agents. Double-disk synergy (DDS) methods were used for detection of ESBL-producing strains. A disc of amoxicillin + clavulanic acid (20/10 μg) was placed in the center of the Mueller–Hinton agar plate, and cefotaxime (30 μg) and ceftazidime (30 μg) were placed at a distance of 20 mm (center to center) from the amoxicillin + clavulanic acid disc. Enhanced inhibition zone of any of the cephalosporin discs on the side facing amoxicillin + clavulanic acid was considered as ESBL producer. *Results.* In the current study, ESBL-producing phenotypes were detected in 23% ($n = 17$) of urinary isolates, of which *Escherichia coli* accounts for 76.5% ($n = 13$) and *K. pneumoniae* for 23.5% ($n = 4$). ESBL-producing phenotypes showed high resistance to cefotaxime (100%), ceftriaxone (100%), and ceftazidime (70.6%), while both ESBL-producing and non-ESBL-producing isolates showed low resistance to amikacin (9.5%), and no resistance was seen with imipenem. In the risk factors analysis, previous antibiotic use more than two cycles in the previous year (odds ratio (OR), 6.238; 95% confidence interval (CI), 1.257–30.957; $p = 0.025$) and recurrent UTI more than two cycles in the last 6 months or more than three cycles in the last year (OR, 7.356; 95% CI, 1.429–37.867; $p = 0.017$) were found to be significantly associated with the ESBL-producing groups. *Conclusion.* Extended-spectrum β-lactamases- (ESBL-)producing strain was detected in urinary tract isolates. The occurrence of multidrug resistance to the third-generation cephalosporins, aminoglycosides, fluoroquinolones, trimethoprim-sulfamethoxazole, and tetracyclines is more common among ESBL producers. Thus, detecting and reporting of ESBL-producing organisms have paramount importance in the clinical decision-making.

1. Introduction

Drug-resistant microbes of all kinds can move among people and animals, from one country to another without notice. Since 21st century, it is thought that the emergence of extended-spectrum β-lactamase- (ESBL-) producing bacteria may present an increasing risk of transmission of resistant strains in humans and animals. They is a worrying global public health issue as infections caused by such enzyme-producing organisms are associated with a higher morbidity and mortality and greater fiscal burden. The problem is clearly severe in developing countries where studies on this subject, drug availability, and its appropriate use were limited and resistance rate was high [1, 2].

ESBL-producing organisms are capable of hydrolyzing penicillin, broad-spectrum cephalosporins, and mono-bactams, but they do not affect the cephamycins or carbapenems, and their activity is inhibited by clavulanic acid. In addition, ESBL-producing organisms are frequently exhibiting resistance to other antimicrobial classes such as fluoroquinolones, aminoglycosides, and trimethoprim-sulfamethoxazole due to associated resistance mechanisms, which may be either chromosomally or plasmid-encoded [3–6]. The widespread use of third-generation cephalosporin was believed to be the major cause of mutations in these enzymes that leads to the emergence of plasmid-encoded ESBLs. These ESBLs were transferred between bacteria by plasmids, which were in turn spread by clonal distribution between hospitals and countries through patient mobility [7].

The presence of ESBLs complicates antibiotic selection, especially in patients with serious infections, such as bacteremia. The reason for this is that ESBL-producing bacteria, including those originating in the community, are often multiresistant to various antibiotics; an interesting feature of isolates that produce CTX-M (CTX stands for cefotaximases and M for Munich) is the coresistance to the fluoroquinolones. Type CTX-M ESBLs have been described as an enzyme preferentially hydrolyzing cefotaxime over ceftazidime and also hydrolyzing cefepime with high efficiency [8, 9].

The spread and the burden of ESBL-producing bacteria are greater in developing countries. Findings of a recent review showed that pooled prevalence of healthcare-associated infections in resource-limited settings (15.5%) was twice the average prevalence in Europe (7.1%). Some plausible reasons for this difference include the following conditions that are prevalent in low-income countries: crowded hospitals, more extensive self-treatment and use of nonprescription antimicrobials, poorer hygiene in general and particularly in hospitals, and less effective infection control [10–12].

In comparison with the rest of the world, there is generally a lack of comprehensive data regarding ESBL-producing Enterobacteriaceae in African countries. The real situation of antibiotic resistance is also not clear since ESBL-producing organisms as well as non-ESBL producers are not routinely cultured and their resistance to antibiotics cannot be tested. Therefore, this study was conducted to determine the prevalence and antimicrobial resistance pattern of ESBL-producing *Escherichia coli* and *Klebsiella pneumoniae* isolated from community-onset UTI patients at Jimma University Specialized Hospital, Southwest Ethiopia.

2. Materials and Methods

2.1. Study Area and Period. The study was conducted at Jimma University Specialized Hospital (JUSH) in Jimma town from March to June, 2016. Jimma University specialized hospital is located southwest of Addis Ababa, capital city of Ethiopia, and currently it is the only more than

300-bedded teaching hospitals in the Southwestern part of the country.

2.2. Study Design and Study Participants. A cross-sectional study was conducted to evaluate the prevalence and antimicrobial resistance pattern of ESBL-producing *E. coli* and *K. pneumoniae* among community-onset UTI infections in Jimma University Specialized hospital (JUSH), Southwest Ethiopia. All outpatients with age groups of ≥15 years and who are suspected of symptoms of urinary tract infections as diagnosed clinically within 48 hours of admission and those coming from outpatient departments for laboratory diagnosis of urine were taken as study participants. Written informed consent was obtained from the patients or guardians of the patient before data collection. The patients who were suspected of symptoms of UTI were identified by communicating with the physicians as he/she put "UTI" on the laboratory request forms as identification numbers for those patients suspected of UTI as diagnosed clinically and requested to laboratory for urinalysis tests. Patients who received antibiotics within the past 2 weeks were excluded.

2.3. Definitions. Community-onset infections are defined infections that have an onset within 48 hours of hospital admission or that present in the outpatient setting [13]. Such infections can be divided into two groups. The first group is associated with healthcare institutions and includes patients receiving intravenous treatment or specialized care, those received hemodialysis treatment or antineoplastic chemotherapy, those who have attended at any hospital clinic within the previous 30 days, those who have been admitted in an acute care center two days within the previous 90 days, and residents of nursing homes or long-term care centers. The second group represents truly community-acquired infections in patients who do not meet the above mentioned criteria.

2.4. Data Collection

2.4.1. Sociodemographic and Clinical Data. Sociodemographic and other clinical data such as age, sex, previous antibiotic use more than two cycles per year, previous intravenous therapy at home or any clinics and repeated outpatient visits at hospital in the last 30 days, previous hospitalization in an acute care center 2 or more days in the 90 days, previous invasive procedures of the urinary tract, previous wound care by specialized nursing or family within 30 days, presence of diabetes mellitus, and recurrent urinary tract infections were collected by face-to-face interviewing of the patient or guardian of the patient by using a well-structured questionnaire before laboratory sample collection.

2.4.2. Laboratory Data Collection. A total of 342 midstream urine samples were collected with a sterile, wide mouthed, and leak proof containers. A 10 μl (0.01 ml) well-mixed urine sample was inoculated into MacConkey agar (Oxoid, UK)

and incubated at 37°C for 24 hours. The colony count with at least 10^5 CFU/ml for single midstream urine was taken as positive urine culture as described previously [14]. All the isolates were preliminarily screened by their colony morphology, pigment production (pink to colorless flat or mucoid colonies), and Gram-staining techniques (Gram-negative rods, nonsporing, and noncapsulated). Further identifications of isolates were made by conformation of motility and other relevant biochemical tests. For example, an isolate was considered as *E. coli* when it is indole (dark pink ring) and methyl-red positive, citrate negative (no change or remained green) and urea negative, gas and acid producer, and motile and were considered as *K. pneumoniae* when it is indole and methyl-red negative, citrate positive, urea slow producing, and nonmotile. In case of delay, the isolated bacteria were kept at 2–8°C in the nutrient broth for not more than 24 hrs until the antimicrobial sensitivity test was done.

2.5. ESBL Detection Methods.
ESBL-producing *E. coli and K. pneumonia* were first screened for ESBL production by the phenotypic method and then will be confirmed by the phenotypic confirmatory test as per Clinical and Laboratory Standards Institute (CLSI) guidelines 2014 [15].

2.5.1. Phenotypic Screening for ESBL Production.
The ESBL screening test was performed by the standard disk diffusion method by using ceftazidime (30 μg), cefotaxime (30 μg), and ceftriaxone (30 μg) (Oxoid, UK). More than one antibiotic disc were used for screening to improve the sensitivity of ESBLs detection, as recommended by CLSI guidelines 2014 [15]. Freshly grown colonies were suspended into normal saline, and the turbidity of the suspension was adjusted at 0.5 McFarland's standard. This suspension was inoculated onto Mueller–Hinton agar (Oxoid, UK) with sterile cotton swab, and then all the above three antibiotics discs were placed at a gap of 20 mm and incubated at 35 ± 2°C for 16–18 hours. The isolates with reduced susceptibility to cefotaxime (zone diameter of ≤27 mm), ceftazidime (zone diameter of ≤22 mm), and ceftriaxone (zone diameter of ≤25 mm) around the disks were suspected as ESBLs producers [15].

2.5.2. Phenotypic Confirmation of ESBL Producers.
Confirmation of suspected ESBLs producers was done by using the double-disk approximation or double-disk synergy (DDS) method on Mueller–Hinton agar, as recommended by CLSI guidelines 2014 [15]. A disc of amoxicillin + clavulanic acid (20/10 μg) was placed in the center of the Mueller–Hinton Agar plate, and then cefotaxime (30 μg) and ceftazidime (30 μg) were placed at a distance of 20 mm (center to center) from the amoxicillin+ clavulanic acid disc on the same plate. The plate was incubated at 37°C for 24 hours and examined for an enhancement or expansion of inhibition zone of the oxyimino-β-lactam caused by the synergy of the clavulanate in the amoxicillin-clavulanate disk which was interpreted as positive for ESBL production.

2.6. Antimicrobial Susceptibility Testing.
The antimicrobial susceptibility testing was done by using Kirby–Bauer disc-diffusion technique on Mueller–Hinton agar according to the CLSI guidelines 2014 [15] for the following antimicrobial discs: amoxicillin/clavulanic acid (20/10 μg), cefotaxime (30 μg), ceftriaxone (30 μg), ceftazidime (30 μg), ampicillin (10 μg), cephalothin (30 μg), ciprofloxacin (5 μg), nalidixic acid (30 μg), norfloxacin (10 μg), gentamycin (10 μg), amikacin (30 μg), tetracycline (30 μg), trimethoprim-sulfamethoxazole (1.25/23.75 μg), imipenem (30 μg), and chloramphenicol (30 μg) (Oxoid; UK). The selections of antimicrobial agents depend on the availability and recommendations from CLSI 2014 [15]. After overnight incubation of the Mueller–Hinton agar plate with antimicrobial discs at 37°C, the zone of inhibition was measured by using a ruler and interpreted by comparing the Kirby–Bauer chart. Control strains (*K. pneumoniae* ATCC 700603 and *Escherichia coli* ATCC 25922) were used to monitor quality of antibiotic discs during antimicrobial susceptibility testing and during ESBL detection methods.

Multidrug resistance (MDR) is defined as resistance to three or more classes of antibiotics [16].

2.7. Data Analysis.
The data were analyzed by using SPSS version 16.0. The difference in categorical variables and susceptibility pattern between ESBL producer and non-ESBL-producing groups were analyzed statistically by using chi-squared (Fisher's exact) test. Odds ratios (ORs) and their 95% confidence intervals (CIs) were calculated, and p value < 0.05 was regarded as statistically significant. The findings were presented in tables.

3. Results

3.1. Clinical Specimens and Isolates Recovered.
In the current study, about 74 (21.6%) of urine samples were confirmed as positive urine culture, of which 63 (85.1%) were *E. coli* and 11 (14.9%) were *K. pneumoniae*. Out of 74 positive urine cultures, 17 (23.0%) were confirmed as positive for ESBL production. *E. coli* accounts for large number of urinary isolates as well as higher proportion of ESBL production (13 (76.5%)) than *K. pneumoniae* (4 (23.5%)). The maximum bacterial isolates and higher proportion of ESBL-producing strains were isolated from females (12 (70.6%)) than male (5 (29.4%)). The mean age of patients from which ESBL producers was detected is 35.07 years (±13.30 SD). From the total ESBL producers, 9 (52.9%) were isolated from patients older than 50 years of age (Table 1).

Patients in the ESBL group were further divided into healthcare-associated and community-acquired groups, and 9 (52.9%) of ESBL isolates were isolated from individuals who have no history of healthcare contact (community acquisition), with a higher proportion of *E. coli*, 8 (61.5%) (Table 1).

3.2. Risk Factors for Isolations of ESBL-Producing Strains.
In the current study, different types of possible risk factors were analyzed but only any antibiotic use more than two

TABLE 1: Distribution of ESBL-producing and non-ESBL-producing *E. coli* and *K. pneumoniae* isolated from community-onset urinary tract infections in JUSH, Southwest Ethiopia, 2016.

Characteristics		Total isolate N (%)	ESBLs-positive ($n = 17$)	ESBLs-negative ($n = 57$)	p value
Age and sex groups					
Age	15–49	51 (68.9%)	8 (47.1%)	43 (75.4%)	0.130
	≥50	23 (31.1%)	9 (52.9%)	14 (24.6%)	
Sex	Female	53 (71.6%)	12 (70.6%)	41 (71.9%)	0.874
	Male	21 (28.4%)	5 (29.4%)	16 (28.1%)	
Organisms					
E. coli		63 (85.1%)	13 (76.5%)	50 (87.7%)	0.263
K. pneumoniae		11 (14.9%)	4 (23.5%)	7 (12.3%)	
Distribution					
Community-acquired		49 (66.2%)	9 (52.9%)	40 (70.2%)	0.192
Healthcare-associated		25 (33.8%)	8 (47.1%)	17 (29.8%)	

cycles in the previous year (OR = 6.238; 95% CI = 1.257–30.957; p = 0.025) and recurrent UTI more than two cycles in the last 6 months or more than three cycles in the last year (OR = 7.356; 95% CI = 1.429–37.867; p = 0.017) were identified as an independent risk factors for acquisition of ESBL-producing strains (Table 2).

3.3. Resistance Profile of ESBL-Producing and Non-ESBL-Producing Isolates.
In the current study, ESBL-producing isolates showed higher resistance not only towards third-generation cephalosporins but also towards other antimicrobial agents tested (p = 0.001). Resistance rates to cefotaxime, ceftriaxone, and ceftazidime are 100%, 100%, and 70.6%, respectively. All ESBL-producing and non-ESBL-producing isolates were resistant to ampicillin (Table 3).

3.4. Resistance Profiles of Isolates from Healthcare-Associated versus Community-Acquired.
The current study finding showed that there are no differences in resistance profiles of isolates from patients who have history of healthcare-associated infections and those isolates from pure community-acquired infections for most of antimicrobial agents tested ($p > 0.05$) (Table 4).

3.5. Multidrug Resistance Pattern of E. coli and K. pneumoniae.
In this study, multidrug resistance (≥3 antibiotic classes) pattern was more prevalent among the ESBL-producing isolates. In our finding, 82.4% of ESBL-producing isolates were showed cross-resistance against both co-trimoxazole and tetracycline, with 52.9% coresistant to tetracycline, fluoroquinolones, co-trimoxazole, aminoglycosides, and chloramphenicol classes of antibiotics plus beta-lactam groups of antibiotics. Coexistence of ESBL phenotype with 5, 6, and 7 types of non-β lactam antibiotics were 11 (64.7%), 9 (51.9%), and 4 (23.5%), respectively (Table 5).

4. Discussion

Until recently, ESBL-producing organisms were viewed as hospital-acquired or healthcare-associated pathogens, i.e., affecting patients who had typically been in hospitals or

other healthcare facilities. However, in recent years, ESBL-producing Enterobacteriaceae isolates have shifted from the hospital to the community or have been recognized in community patients who had no prior contact with the healthcare system [17].

In our study, the ESBL-producing phenotype were detected in 23% (17/74) of the urinary isolates, which was slightly higher than a result obtained in Taiwan (20.7%) [18] and higher than previous study finding in the same area, in which the proportions of ESBL producers from outpatients were 14.3% [19]. The higher finding in our study may be related with the more distributions of ESBL from time to time in the study area.

In contrast, the proportions of ESBLs observed in our study are lower than that in previous reports in Saudi Arabia (42.38%) [20] and in Tanzania (45.2%) [21]. The reasons for this decline observed in our study may be explained by the inclusion of only single specimens from outpatient only. This reason supported by the fact that hospital environment played a role for maintenance of ESBL-producing organism [22]. Moreover, higher rate of fecal carriage of ESBLs producers among inpatients were also observed elsewhere in Saudi Arabia [23], which support the notions that hospital acquired isolates are more likely to become ESBL producer.

Although advanced molecular methods for species identifications and characterizations of ESBL typing were not conducted in our study, *Escherichia coli* accounts for a large number of urinary isolates as well as higher numbers of ESBL production 76.5% than *K. pneumoniae* 23.5%. Our finding was correlated with the previous study finding in the same area, in which three (75%) of the four ESBL producers from outpatients were *E. coli* [19]. Another study finding in Israel also showed that higher prevalence of ESBL-producing isolates from outpatients was for *E. coli* (57.8%) [8].

A community-origin explaining this rise of ESBLs has been observed in many surveys, but in our setting it is difficult to ascertain accurately, as faecal colonization surveys among humans without direct or indirect hospital exposure are scarce. Accordingly, the gut plays a prominent role in the development of antibiotic resistance and the emergence of resistant microorganisms which may be subsequent agents of urinary infection in vulnerable patients

TABLE 2: Characteristics of patients infected with ESBLs-producing and non-ESBLs-producing *E. coli* and *K. pneumoniae* among community-onset urinary tract infections in JUSH, Southwest Ethiopia, 2016.

Variables	Category	ESBLs-positive	ESBLs-negative	OR (95% CI)	p value
Age groups	15–49	8 (47.1%)	43 (75.4%)		0.130
	≥50	9 (52.9%)	14 (24.6%)		
Sex	Female	12 (70.6%)	41 (71.9%)		0.874
	Male	5 (29.4%)	16 (28.1%)		
Healthcare-associated risk factors					
Any antibiotic use more than two cycles in the previous year	Yes	13 (76.5%)	27 (47.37%)	6.238 (1.257–30.957)	0.025*
	No	4 (23.5%)	30 (52.63%)		
Prior intravenous therapy at home or any clinic within 30 days	Yes	3 (17.6%)	7 (12.3%)		0.608
	No	14 (82.4%)	50 (87.7%)		
Repeated outpatient visit or attendant at hospital within 30 days	Yes	2 (11.76%)	10 (17.5%)		0.829
	No	15 (88.23%)	47 (82.5%)		
Previous hospitalization in an acute care center >2 days within 90 days	Yes	1 (5.9%)	1 (1.8%)		0.532
	No	16 (94.1%)	56 (98.2%)		
History of invasive procedure of the urinary tract within the previous year	Yes	0	1 (1.8%)		0.966
	No	17 (100%)	56 (98.2%)		
Previous wound or specialized nursing care within 30 days	Yes	1(5.9%)	1 (1.8%)		0.495
	No	16 (94.1%)	56 (98.2%)		
Underlying diseases					
Presence of diabetes mellitus	Yes	5 (29.4%)	9 (15.8%)		0.815
	No	12 (70.6%)	48 (84.2%)		
Recurrent UTI >two cycle in the last 6 months or > three cycles in the last year	Yes	7 (41.2%)	8 (14.0%)	7.356 (1.429–37.867)	0.015*
	No	10 (58.8%)	49 (86.0%)		

OR: odds ratio, CI: confidence interval, * p value less than 0.05.

TABLE 3: Resistance profiles of ESBL-producing and non-ESBL-producing *Escherichia coli* and *Klebsiella pneumoniae* isolates in JUSH, Southwest of Ethiopia.

Antibiotics	Total R (N%)	ESBL-positive (n = 17) (N%)		ESBL-negative (n = 57) (N%)		p value
	R	R	S	R	S	
Cefotaxime	18 (24.3%)	17 (100%)	0	1(1.8%)	56 (98.2%)	0.001
Ceftriaxone	17 (23.0%)	17 (100%)	0	0	57 (100%)	0.001
Ceftazidime	16 (21.6%)	12 (70.6%)	5 (29.4%)	4 (7.0%)	53 (93.0%)	0.001
AMC	27 (36.5%)	14 (82.4%)	3 (17.6%)	13 (22.8%)	44 (77.2%)	0.001
Cephalothin	53 (71.6%)	17 (100%)	0	36 (63.2%)	21 (36.8%)	0.051
Ampicillin	74 (100%)	17 (100%)	0	57 (100%)	0	—
Gentamicin	17 (23%)	11 (64.7%)	6 (35.3%)	6 (10.5%)	51(89.5%)	0.001
Amikacin	7 (9.5%)	4 (23.5%)	13 (76.5%)	3 (5.3%)	54 (94.7%)	0.024
NA	38 (51.4%)	13 (76.5%)	4 (23.5%)	25 (43.9%)	32 (56.1%)	0.001
CIP	24 (32.4%)	13 (76.5%)	4 (23.5%)	11 (19.3%)	46 (80.7%)	0.001
Norfloxacin	23 (31.1%)	13 (76.5%)	4 (23.5%)	10 (17.5%)	47 (82.5%)	0.001
SXT	41 (55.4%)	14 (82.4%)	3(17.6%)	27 (47.4%)	30 (52.6%)	0.001
Tetracycline	45 (60.8%)	14 (82.4%)	3 (17.6%)	31 (54.4%)	26 (45.6%)	0.021
C	30 (40.5%)	12 (70.6%)	5 (29.4%)	18 (31.6%)	39 (68.4%)	0.004
Imipenem	0	0	17 (100%)	0	57 (100%)	—

R: resistant, S: sensitive, AMC: amoxicillin-clavulanic acid, NA: nalidixic acid, CIP: ciprofloxacin, SXT: trimethoprim-sulfamethoxazole, C: chloramphenicol.

[24, 25]. A recent report from Cameroon [26] showed 16% fecal carriage of ESBLs isolates with the majority (over 80%) of these being *E. coli*, and in Saudi Arabia 12.7% isolates were ESBLs producers, of which 95.6% were *E. coli* and 4.4% were *K. pneumoniae* [27]. Therefore, in patients admitted to the hospital with community-acquired UTIs, the risk factors for acquiring ESBL-producing organisms should be considered before initiating treatment.

In our study, 52.9% of ESBL-producing isolates were isolated from individuals who have no history of healthcare contact (community-acquisition), with a higher proportion

of *E. coli*, 61.5%. This finding is in agreement with the previous report done in Switzerland [28], where 64% patients with ESBL-producing *E. coli* had community-acquired and 36% had healthcare-associated UTIs, and in Spain 68% had community-acquired and 32% cases comprised healthcare-associated cases [29].

The data concerning risk factors for the development of infection with ESBL-producing bacteria among outpatients are very scarce in our settings. In the our study, any antibiotic use more than two cycles in the previous year (OR = 6.238; 95% CI =1.257–30.957; $p = 0.025$) and recurrent UTI more

TABLE 4: Resistance profiles of isolates from healthcare-associated versus true community-acquired in JUSH, Southwest of Ethiopia.

Antibiotics	Total R (N%)	Healthcare-associated		Community-acquired		p value
	R	R	S	R	S	
Cefotaxime	18 (24.3%)	9 (36%)	16 (64%)	9 (18.4%)	40 (81.6%)	0.168
Ceftriaxone	17 (23.0%)	9 (36%)	16 (64%)	9 (18.4%)	40 (81.6%)	0.168
Ceftazidime	16 (21.6%)	9 (36%)	16 (64%)	7 (14.3%)	42 (85.7%)	0.041
AMC	27 (36.5%)	10 (40%)	15 (60%)	17 (36.7%)	32 (65.3%)	0.799
Cephalothin	53 (71.6%)	18 (72%)	7 (28%)	35 (71.4%)	14 (28.6%)	1.000
Ampicillin	74 (100%)	25(100%)	0	49 (100%)	0	—
Gentamicin	17 (23%)	9 (36%)	16 (64%)	8 (16.3%)	41(83.7%)	0.080
Amikacin	7 (9.5%)	4 (16%)	21 (84%)	3 (6.1%)	46 (93.9%)	0.217
NA	38 (51.4%)	14 (56%)	11 (44%)	24 (49%)	25 (51%)	0.628
CIP	24 (32.4%)	9 (36%)	16 (64%)	15 (30.6%)	34 (69.4%)	0.793
Norfloxacin	23 (31.1%)	9 (36%)	16 (64%)	14 (28.6%)	35 (71.4%)	0.793
SXT	41 (55.4%)	15 (60%)	10 (40%)	26 (53.1%)	23 (46.9%)	1.000
Tetracycline	45 (60.8%)	14 (56%)	11 (44%)	31 (54.4%)	18 (45.6%)	0.610
C	30 (40.5%)	14 (56%)	11 (44%)	16 (32.6%)	33 (67.4%)	0.079
Imipenem	0	0	25 (100%)	0	49 (100%)	—

R: resistant, S: sensitive, AMC: amoxicillin-clavulanic acid, NA: nalidixic acid, CIP: ciprofloxacin, SXT: trimethoprim-sulfamethoxazole, C: chloramphenicol.

TABLE 5: Frequency of multidrug resistance pattern of ESBL-producing isolates from community-onset UTI patients in JUSH, Southwest of Ethiopia.

Antibiotic classes	MDR rate (N (%))
Beta-lactams + SXT, T	14 (82.4%)
Beta-lactams + SXT, T, NA	13 (76.5%)
Beta-lactams + SXT, T, NA, CIP, GEN	11 (64.7%)
Beta-lactams + SXT, T, NA, CIP, GEN, C	9 (52.9%)
Beta-lactams + SXT, T, NA, CIP, GEN, AK, C	4 (23.5%)

Beta-lactams: (ampicillin, cephalothin, amoxicillin-clavulanic acid, cefotaxime, ceftazidime, and ceftriaxone), GEN: gentamicin, AK: amikacin, CIP: ciprofloxacin, SXT: trimethoprim-sulfamethoxazole, T: tetracycline, NA: nalidixic acid, C: chloramphenicol.

than two cycles in the last 6 months, or more than three cycles in the last year (OR = 7.356; 95% CI =1.429–37.867; $p = 0.017$) were identified as independent risk factors for development or acquisition of ESBL-producing organisms. Our finding is also correlated with the previous studies in Israel [8]. This may suggest that the greater exposure to antibiotics may lead to development of selection pressures.

In our study finding, 82.4% of ESBL-producing isolates showed multidrug resistance to different families of antibiotics such as SXT and tetracycline. This finding is correlated with other studies in developing countries such as Tanzania [21], and in Guinea-Bissau [30], nearly all ESBL-producing E. coli isolates in the community were multidrug-resistant.

Multidrug resistance nature of these isolates may be explained by the fact that ESBLs are plasmid-mediated enzymes which are carrying multiresistant genes by plasmid, transposon, and integron and also they are readily transferred to other bacteria, not necessarily of the same species, and bacteria with multiple resistances to antibiotics are widely distributed in hospitals and increasingly being isolated from community [31]. This fact supported by recent surveys from Canada [32] and Spain [33] has illustrated an alarming trend of associated resistance among ESBL-

producing organisms isolated from community sites, especially those producing CTX-M types, which exhibited coresistance to SXT, tetracycline, gentamicin, and ciprofloxacin. Thus, our study results well support the fact that ESBL producers confer high levels of resistance to not only third-generation cephalosporins but also to other non-β lactams group of antibiotics.

This study also revealed that all ESBL-producing and non-ESBL-producing isolates showed resistance to ampicillin. Our finding correlated with the fact that β-lactamase-negative isolates may be resistant to ampicillin by other mechanisms. In contrast, better susceptibility was noticed to amikacin and no resistance was observed with imipenem. Better susceptibility to amikacin was also noticed in previous study in our study area [19]. This may be explained by the absence of routine use of amikacin as empirical therapy and its absence of considerable cross-resistance with β-lactam groups of antibiotics.

Although MIC determination of resistant strains was not conducted in our study, further analysis of the antimicrobial resistance pattern among isolates from infections associated with healthcare institutions and those from "true" community-acquired infections showed that there are no differences between the two groups in the resistance pattern ($p \geq 0.05$). The similarity in resistance pattern between healthcare associated isolates and "true" community-acquired isolates may be related to frequent use and misuse of non-prescribed antibiotics in the community as well as in healthcare facilities especially in private healthcare sectors and the time to time spreads of resistant strains from healthcare institutions to the community in our setting. Therefore, this finding gives an attention from health policymakers to promote rational use of antibiotics in healthcare settings as well as in the community.

5. Conclusion

The data obtained in our study indicate that ESBL-positive phenotypes were prevalent not only patients who had typically been in hospitals or other healthcare facilities but also in community patients. Coresistance to other classes of antimicrobial agents such as aminoglycosides, fluoroquinolones, co-trimoxazole, and tetracyclines was also more common among ESBLs positive phenotypes. Any antibiotic use more than two cycles in the previous year and recurrent UTI was identified as independent risk factors for acquisition of ESBL-producing organisms. Thus, our finding gives an attention to promote rational use of antibiotics in healthcare settings and surveillance studies in order to monitor the changes in the antimicrobial resistance pattern.

5.1. Limitations of the Study. Advanced molecular methods for species identification and characterization of ESBL typing and MIC determination of resistant strains were not conducted due to lack of availability.

Authors' Contributions

MA, GT, and AA participated in the study design, were responsible for the laboratory analyses, drafted the manuscript, and approved the final version. MA was responsible for recruitment and sampling and analyzed the data.

Acknowledgments

We would like to thank Jimma University, Institute of Health, for material support. We also thank all the study participants for their participation in this study and the staff of JUSH for their support in facilitating specimen collection and patient information.

References

[1] J. D. D. Pitout, P. Nordmann, K. B. Laupland, and L. Poirel, "Emergence of Enterobacteriaceae producing extended-spectrum β-lactamases (ESBLs) in the community," *Journal of Antimicrobial Chemotherapy*, vol. 56, no. 1, pp. 52–59, 2005.

[2] D. K. Byarugaba, *Antimicrobial Resistance in Developing Countries*, Springer, New York, NY, USA, 2009.

[3] A. Önnberg, P. Mölling, J. Zimmermann, and B. Söderquist, "Molecular and phenotypic characterization of *Escherichia coli* and *Klebsiella pneumoniae* producing extended-spectrum β-lactamases with focus on CTX-M in a low-endemic area in Sweden," *APMIS*, vol. 119, no. 4-5, pp. 287–295, 2011.

[4] EFSA, "Scientific opinion on the public health risks of bacterial strains producing extended-spectrum β-lactamases and/or AmpC β-lactamases in food and food producing strains," *EFSA Journal*, vol. 9, no. 8, pp. 1–95, 2011.

[5] N. Shayanfar, M. Rezaei, M. Ahmadi, and F. Ehsanipour, "Evaluation of extended-spectrum β-lactamases (ESBLs)-positive strains of *Klebsiella pneumoniae* and *Escherichia coli* in bacterial cultures," *Iranian Journal of Pathology*, vol. 5, no. 1, pp. 34–39, 2010.

[6] R. H. Dhillon and J. Clark, *ESBLs: A Clear and Present Danger?*, Hindawi Publishing Corporation, Cairo, Egypt, 2012.

[7] C. G. Giske, D. L. Monnet, C. Otto et al., "Clinical and economic impact of common multidrug-resistant," *Antimicrobial Agents and Chemotherapy*, vol. 52, no. 3, pp. 813–821, 2008.

[8] R. Colodner, W. Rock, B. Chazan et al., "Risk factors for the development of extended-spectrum β-lactamases (ESBLs)-producing bacteria in non-hospitalized patients," *European Journal of Clinical Microbiology and Infectious Diseases*, vol. 23, no. 3, pp. 163–167, 2004.

[9] R. Bonnet, "Growing group of extended-spectrum β-lactamases (ESBLs): the CTX-M enzymes," *Antimicrobial Agents and Chemotherapy*, vol. 48, no. 1, pp. 1–14, 2004.

[10] M. V. Villegas, J. N. Kattan, M. G. Quinteros, and J. M. Casellas, "Prevalence of extended-spectrum β-lactamases (ESBLs) in South America, European Society of Clinical Microbiology and Infectious Diseases," *Clinical Microbiology and Infection*, vol. 14, pp. 154–158, 2008.

[11] P. M. Hawkey, "Prevalence and clonality of extended-spectrum β-lactamases (ESBLs) in Asia," *Clinical Microbiology and Infection*, vol. 14, pp. 159–165, 2008.

[12] J. Tham, E. Melander, M. Walder, P. J. Edquist, and I. Odenholt, "Prevalence of faecal *ESBLs* carriage in the community and in a hospital setting in a county of Southern Sweden," *European Journal of Clinical Microbiology and Infectious Diseases*, vol. 30, no. 10, pp. 1159–1162, 2011.

[13] N. D. Friedman, "Health care-associated blood stream infections in adults: a reason to change the accepted definition of community-acquired infections," *Annals of Internal Medicine*, vol. 137, no. 10, p. 791, 2002.

[14] CDC/HICPAC, *Urinary Tract Infection (UTI) Event for Long-Term Care Facilities*, CDC, Atlanta, GA, USA, 2009.

[15] Clinical and Laboratory Standards Institute, *Performance Standards for Antimicrobial Susceptibility Testing; Twenty-Fourth Informational Supplement. CLSI document M100-S24*, Clinical and Laboratory Standards Institute, Wayne, PA, USA, 2014.

[16] A. Magiorakos, A. Srinivasan, R. B. Carey et al., "Bacteria: an international expert proposal for interim standard definitions for acquired resistance," *Clinical Microbiology and Infection*, vol. 18, pp. 268–281, 2011.

[17] Y. Doi, *ESBLs-producing Escherichia coli in the community: an emerging public health threat*, 2009.

[18] Y. S. Yang, C. H. Ku, J. C. Lin et al., "Impact of extended-spectrum β-lactamase (ESBLs)-producing *Escherichia coli* and *Klebsiella pneumoniae* on the outcome of community-onset bacteremic urinary tract infections," *J Microbiol Immunol Infect. Taiwan Society of Microbiology*, vol. 43, no. 3, pp. 194–199, 2010.

[19] S. M. Siraj, S. Ali, and B. Wondafrash, "Extended-spectrum β-lactamase (ESBLs)-production in *Klebsiella pneumoniae* and *Escherichia coli* at Jimma University Specialized Hospital, South-West Ethiopia," *BioPublisher*, vol. 5, no. 1, pp. 1–9, 2015.

[20] T. A. El-kersh, M. A. Marie, Y. A. Al-sheikh, and S. A. Al-kahtani, "Prevalence and risk factors of community-acquired urinary tract infections due to *ESBLs*-producing Gram negative bacteria in an Armed Forces Hospital in Southern Saudi Arabia," *Global Advanced Research Journal of Medicine and Medical Science*, vol. 4, no. 7, pp. 321–330, 2015.

[21] S. J. Moyo, S. Aboud, M. Kasubi, E. F. Lyamuya, and S. Y. Maselle, "Antimicrobial resistance among producers and non-producers of extended spectrum β-lactamases (ESBLs) in urinary isolates at a tertiary Hospital in Tanzania," *BMC Research Notes*, vol. 3, no. 1, p. 348, 2010.

[22] S.-H. K. Kang, Ji-W. H.-B. K. Bang, E.-C. K. Nam-Joong Kim et al., "Community-acquired versus nosocomial *Klebsiella pneumoniae* bacteremia : clinical features, treatment outcomes, and clinical implication of antimicrobial resistance," *Journal of Korean Medical Science*, vol. 12, no. 5, pp. 816–822, 2006.

[23] A. A. Kader, A. Kumar, and K. A. Kamath, "Fecal carriage of extended-spectrum β-lactamase (ESBLs)-producing *Escherichia coli* and *Klebsiella pneumoniae* in patients and asymptomatic healthy individuals," *Infection Control and Hospital Epidemiology*, vol. 28, no. 9, pp. 1114–1116, 2007.

[24] J. Rodríguez-Baño, L. López-Cerero, M. D. Navarro, P. Díaz de Alba, and A. Pascual, "Faecal carriage of extended-spectrum β-lactamases (ESBLs)-producing *Escherichia coli*: prevalence, risk factors and molecular epidemiology," *Journal of Antimicrobial Chemotherapy*, vol. 62, no. 5, pp. 1142–1149, 2008.

[25] A. A. Kader and K. A. Kamath, "Faecal carriage of extended-spectrum β-lactamase (ESBLs)-producing bacteria in the community," *Eastern Mediterranean Health Journal*, vol. 15, no. 6, pp. 1365–1370, 2009.

[26] C. M. Lonchel, C. Meex, J. Gangoué-Piéboji et al., "Proportion of extended-spectrum β-lactamases (ESBLs)-producing *Enterobacteriaceae* in community setting in Ngaoundere, Cameroon," *BMC Infectious Diseases*, vol. 12, no. 1, p. 53, 2012.

[27] M. Niki, I. Hirai, A. Yoshinaga et al., "Extended-Spectrum β-lactamases (ESBLs)-producing *Escherichia coli* strains in the feces of carriers contribute substantially to urinary tract infections in these patients," *Infection*, vol. 39, no. 5, pp. 467–471, 2011.

[28] S. Meier, R. Weber, R. Zbinden, C. Ruef, and B. Hasse, "Extended-spectrum β-lactamase-producing Gram-negative pathogens in community-acquired urinary tract infections: an increasing challenge for antimicrobial therapy," *Infection*, vol. 39, no. 4, pp. 333–340, 2011.

[29] J. Rodríguez-Baño, J. C. Alcalá, J. M. Cisneros et al., "Community infections caused by extended-spectrum β-lactamases (ESBLs)-producing *Escherichia coli*," *Archives of Internal Medicine*, vol. 168, no. 17, pp. 1897–1902, 2008.

[30] A. Rodrigues, C. G. Giske, and P. Naucle, "Fecal carriage of *ESBLs*-producing *E. coli* and *K. pneumoniae* in children in Guinea-Bissau : a hospital-based cross-sectional study," *PLoS One*, vol. 7, no. 12, Article ID e51981, 2012.

[31] G. A. Jacoby and A. A. Medeiros, "More extended-spectrum β-lactamases," *Antimicrobial Agents and Chemotherapy*, vol. 35, no. 9, pp. 1697–1704, 1991.

[32] J. D. D. Pitout, N. D. Hanson, D. L. Church, and K. B. Laupland, "Population-based laboratory surveillance for *Escherichia coli*-producing extended-spectrum β-lactamases (ESBLs): importance of community isolates with blaCTX-M genes," *Clinical Infectious Diseases*, vol. 38, no. 12, pp. 1736–1741, 2004.

[33] J. Rodríguez-baño, M. D. Navarro, L. Martínez-martínez et al., "Epidemiology and clinical features of infections caused by extended-spectrum β-lactamases (ESBLs)-producing *Escherichia coli* in non-hospitalized patients," *Journal of Clinical Microbiology*, vol. 42, no. 3, pp. 1089–1094, 2004.

12

Oral Yeast Colonization and Fungal Infections in Peritoneal Dialysis Patients

Liliana Simões-Silva,[1,2,3] Sara Silva,[4] Carla Santos-Araujo,[5,6] Joana Sousa,[4]
Manuel Pestana,[1,2,5,7] Ricardo Araujo,[1,8,9] Isabel Soares-Silva,[1,2]
and Benedita Sampaio-Maia[1,2,4]

[1]i3S-Instituto de Investigação e Inovação em Saúde, Universidade do Porto, Porto, Portugal
[2]INEB-Instituto de Engenharia Biomédica, Universidade do Porto, Rua Alfredo Allen 208, 4200-180 Porto, Portugal
[3]Faculty of Medicine, University of Porto, Porto, Portugal
[4]Faculty of Dental Medicine, University of Porto, Porto, Portugal
[5]Department of Nephrology, São João Hospital Center, EPE, Porto, Portugal
[6]Department of Physiology and Cardiothoracic Surgery, Cardiovascular R&D Center, Faculty of Medicine, University of Porto, Porto, Portugal
[7]Department of Renal, Urological and Infectious Diseases, Faculty of Medicine, University of Porto, Porto, Portugal
[8]Ipatimup, Institute of Molecular Pathology and Immunology of the University of Porto, Porto, Portugal
[9]Department of Medical Biotechnology, School of Medicine, Flinders University, Adelaide, SA 5042, Australia

Correspondence should be addressed to Benedita Sampaio-Maia; bmaia@fmd.up.pt

Academic Editor: Jorge Garbino

Peritonitis and exit-site infections are important complications in peritoneal dialysis (PD) patients that are occasionally caused by opportunistic fungi inhabiting distant body sites. In this study, the oral yeast colonization of PD patients and the antifungal susceptibility profile of the isolated yeasts were accessed and correlated with fungal infection episodes in the following 4 years. Saliva yeast colonization was accessed in 21 PD patients and 27 healthy controls by growth in CHROMagar-Candida® and 18S rRNA/ITS sequencing. PD patients presented a lower oral yeast prevalence when compared to controls, namely, *Candida albicans*. Other species were also isolated, *Candida glabrata* and *Candida carpophila*. The antifungal susceptibility profiles of these isolates revealed resistance to itraconazole, variable susceptibility to caspofungin, and higher MIC values of posaconazole compared to previous reports. The 4-year longitudinal evaluation of these patients revealed *Candida parapsilosis* and *Candida zeylanoides* as PD-related exit-site infectious agents, but no correlation was found with oral yeast colonization. This pilot study suggests that oral yeast colonization may represent a limited risk for fungal infection development in PD patients. Oral yeast isolates presented a variable antifungal susceptibility profile, which may suggest resistance to some second-line drugs, highlighting the importance of antifungal susceptibility assessment in the clinical practice.

1. Introduction

Peritoneal dialysis (PD) is a home-based and widely used renal replacement therapy for patients with end-stage renal disease (ESRD). In PD patients, infectious complications, namely, peritonitis and exit-site infections, account for a significant percentage of catheter loss, transfer to haemodialysis, prolonged hospitalization, or even death, making prevention of infection a critical step to the success of a PD program [1]. Although a rare event, fungal peritonitis is associated with significant morbidity and mortality in PD patients [2]. Fungal exit-site infections are more frequent than peritonitis, but more easily resolved, although they may potentiate the development of a subsequent peritonitis [3]. Fungal infections are primarily caused by opportunistic fungal pathogens, such as *Candida* species, that take advantage of a locally or systemically debilitated immune system to proliferate in the human host and cause disease. In a recent study where fungal exit-site infections of PD patients were evaluated, the most frequently isolated species were *Candida parapsilosis* (67%), followed by *Candida glabrata* (10%), *Candida famata* (7%), and *Candida zeylanoides* (7%) [4].

Factors that influence the occurrence of PD-related infections are still not completely understood. Some authors have highlighted the importance of the oral microbiome as a starting point for dissemination of pathogens to distant body sites [5, 6]. Despite the association between oral pathology and adverse outcomes of renal patients [7], so far, existing studies have neither evaluated the oral yeast colonization of PD patients nor evaluated its relation with the development of fungal infections. This topic is particularly relevant when considering the opportunistic character of *Candida* species, a frequent colonizer of the oral cavity [6] and the immune impairment of ESRD patients and knowing that chronic kidney disease itself, and PD therapy in particular, alters significantly the oral milieu [8].

Therefore, in the present study, the oral yeast colonization and the oral health of PD patients were characterized and compared with a healthy population. The antifungal susceptibility profile of yeasts isolated from the oral cavity was also assessed. Additionally, the clinical history of fungal infections was evaluated and related with the oral yeast colonization of PD patients.

2. Material and Methods

Patients followed up for at least 1 month in the PD outpatient clinic of the Nephrology Department of "Centro Hospitalar de S. João," over 18 years of age and with no recent history of infection (less than 1 month) were invited to participate in the study. A convenience sample was obtained related with the attendance of patients to the outpatient clinic during a period of 6 months. A group of 21 PD patients accepted to participate and were included in the study. The control group consisted of 27 adult healthy subjects, including 10 PD family members (in order to select individuals living in similar environment and conditions as the patients) and 17 nonfamily members of PD patients. The exclusion criteria were: inability to give informed consent, pregnancy, and severe acute illness. The study protocol was approved by the Ethics Committee for Health and Institutional Review Board of "Centro Hospitalar de S. João," and all recruited patients and controls were asked to give their written informed consent. This work is constituted by a cross-sectional study, regarding the comparison of *Candida* oral colonization in PD patients and controls, followed by a longitudinal study, in which the history of *Candida* spp. infections was analysed during 4 years to establish a comparison between the *Candida* species present in the oral cavity and the *Candida* species responsible for subsequent PD-related fungal infections. Regarding the longitudinal evaluation of PD-related fungal infections, the study began with 21 patients, and due to PD technique dropout, 20, 19, 14, and 11 patients remained at the end of the first, second, third, and fourth follow-up year, respectively.

Patients' clinical information was gathered including age, gender, smoking habits, blood pressure, aetiology of renal disease, residual renal function, PD vintage, infectious complications during PD, and PD-related fungal infection episodes and agents. Demographic information was gathered for control population, namely, age, gender, and smoking habits.

A noninvasive intraoral examination was performed in both groups in order to evaluate the oral hygiene by visible plaque index (VPI) in four sites of each tooth (mesiobuccal, midbuccal, distobuccal, and midlingual); the percentage of the examined sites with visible plaque ranged from 0% to 100%. Whole saliva was collected in both groups before oral examination for microbial analysis and pH evaluation. The patients were instructed not to eat, drink, and perform the normal mouth hygiene at least two hours before the procedure. Samples of nonstimulated saliva were collected in one time point for each patient under resting conditions. The patients were asked to spit the whole-mouth saliva after 5 min. The volume was quantified gravimetrically, and the salivary flow rate was determined (mL min^{-1}). The pH of saliva was determined immediately after collection using pH strips (5.0–8.0, Duotest, Germany). The saliva was mixed 1 : 1 in Brain Heart Infusion with 20% glycerol and cryopreserved at −80°C until microbial analysis.

Saliva samples were unfrozen for yeast isolation and quantification. The samples were serially diluted with 0.9% sterile NaCl solution and plated in triplicate in a selective and differential culture medium, CHROMagar-Candida. Plates were incubated aerobically for 48 h at 37°C. Total number of colonies was determined, and quantification results were expressed in logarithmic scale of colony forming units per ml of saliva (Log_{10} CFU mL^{-1}). Identification of *Candida albicans* was possible due to the specific colour of the colonies. Isolates were identified by 18S rDNA and internal transcribed spacer (ITS) region DNA sequencing approach as previously described [9]. PCR amplification was performed using a group of specific primers: EF3 (5′-TCCTCTAAATGACCAAGTTTG-3′), EF4 (5′-GGAAGGG[G/A]TGTATTTATTAG-3′), fung5 (5′-GTAAAAGTCCTGGTTCCCC-3′), ITS1 (5′TCCGTAGGTGAACCTTGCGG-3′), and ITS4 (5′-TCCTCCGCTTATTGATATGC-3′) in a Thermo-Hybaid-PX2 thermal cycler. Amplification products were visualized in a polyacrilamide gel followed by silver-staining. Sequence analysis was performed in a genetic analyser ABI-Prism-3100 (Applied Biosystems). Genomic data were compared with a database that comprises a large collection of yeast sequences of 18S rDNA and ITS regions obtained from GenBank.

Antifungal susceptibility testing was performed by the determination of minimum inhibitory concentration (MIC) and according to clinical breakpoints (CBP) defined in the M27-A3 and M27-S4 protocols of the Clinical and Laboratory Standards Institute (CLSI) (http://clsi.org/). Due to the loss of viability of some isolates, antifungal susceptibility was performed in 2 isolates from the PD group and 4 out of 10 from the controls. The following antifungals were tested: voriconazole (Pfizer, Groton, CT), posaconazole (Schering-Plough, Summit, NJ), fluconazole (Pfizer, Groton, CT), amphotericin B (Bristol-Myers Squibb, New York, NY, USA), caspofungin (Merck, Rahway, NJ, USA), anidulafungin (Pfizer, Groton, CT, USA), and micafungin (Astellas Pharma, Inc., Tokyo, Japan). For species whose clinical breakpoints are not defined, the phenotype was characterized based on epidemiological cutoff values (ECVs) according to Pfaller and Diekema [10].

Saliva biochemical parameters were quantified by an automatic analyser, Pentra C200 (Horiba ABX Diagnostics, Switzerland). In brief, phosphate was detected by UV using phosphomolybdate, whereas α-amylases were detected by an enzymatic photometric test, using the substrate 4,6-ethylidene-(G7)-p-nitrophenyl-(G1)-α-D6 maltoheptaoside (EPS-G7). In addition, salivary IgA was determined by immunoturbidimetry and urea by enzymatic UV test (method "Urease–GLDH").

Statistical analyses were performed using IBM® SPSS® version 23.0 (Statistical Package for Social Sciences). The categorical variables were described through relative frequencies (%) and analysed by the chi-square independence test or Fisher exact test when more than 1 cell had expected counts less than 5. The normality test was performed with Shapiro-Wilk. When normally distributed, continuous variables were described using mean ± standard deviation (SD) and analysed by student's t-test, whereas when not normally distributed, continuous variables were described using median (min, max) and analysed by the Mann–Whitney U test. $P < 0.05$ was assumed to denote a significant difference.

3. Results

PD patients and controls presented similar demographic characteristics (Table 1).

The clinical history of PD patients, such as the most prevalent aetiologies of chronic kidney disease, and the most relevant clinical data, such as PD vintage, residual renal function, and blood pressure determined at the day of sample collection, are presented in Table 2. Additionally, this table also presents the prevalence of patients on specific medication reported to be associated with altered susceptibility to fungal infections, namely, calcium channel blockers, statins, vitamin D, and iron supplementation [11–14].

The study was initiated by an oral clinical evaluation and saliva collection. At this point, the average time on PD therapy was 15.5 ± 16.9 months, ranging from 1 to 72 months (Table 2).

PD patients presented a lower prevalence of yeasts in saliva compared to the healthy controls; however, the difference did not attain statistical significance (Table 3). Three *Candida* species were identified, namely, *C. albicans* and *C. glabrata* in PD patients and *C. albicans* and *C. carpophila* in controls. The prevalence of *C. albicans* was significantly lower in PD patients than in controls. One control was colonized by two different species: *C. albicans* and *C. glabrata*. Despite the low oral yeast prevalence in PD patients, the quantification of total yeast number (Log_{10} CFU mL^{-1}) in individuals colonized with yeast did not differ between PD patients and the control group (Table 3).

TABLE 1: Age and sex of peritoneal dialysis (PD) patients and controls.

	PD patients ($n = 21$)	Controls ($n = 27$)	P value
Age (years)	46.8 ± 9.7	43.2 ± 11.9	0.273
Sex (male, %)	42.9%	18.5%	0.066

Results are shown in prevalence (%) or mean ± SD. PD, peritoneal dialysis.

TABLE 2: Aetiology of chronic kidney disease (CKD), time on peritoneal dialysis, residual renal function, and blood pressure of peritoneal dialysis (PD) patients.

	PD patients ($n = 21$)
Aetiology of CKD	
Glomerular disease	52.3%
Diabetic nephropathy	19.0%
Other glomerular disease	33.3%
Tubulointerstitial disease	23.8%
Autosomal dominant polycystic kidney disease	14.3%
Other tubulointerstitial disease	9.5%
Unknown	23.8%
PD vintage (months)	15.5 ± 16.9
Residual renal function (mL min^{-1})	7.0 ± 4.5
Blood pressure	
Systolic	130.2 ± 19.7
Diastolic	78.3 ± 11.0
Therapy	
Calcium channel blockers	47.6%
Statins	57.1%
Vitamin D supplementation	71.4%
Iron supplementation	90.5%

Results are shown in prevalence (%). CKD, chronic kidney disease; PD, peritoneal dialysis.

TABLE 3: Prevalence and quantification of yeast colonizers in peritoneal dialysis (PD) patients and controls.

	PD patients ($n = 21$)	Controls ($n = 27$)	P value
Yeast prevalence	9.6% (2/21)	33.3% (9/27)	0.083
Yeasts (Log_{10} CFU mL^{-1})	2.39 ± 0.80	2.55 ± 0.82	0.803
Species prevalence			
Candida albicans	4.8% (1/21)	33.3% (9/27)	0.029*
Candida glabrata	0%	3.7% (1/27)	>0.999
Candida carpophila	4.8% (1/21)	0%	0.438

Results are prevalence (%) or mean ± SD. PD, peritoneal dialysis; CFU, colony-forming units. *$P < 0.05$.

Six *Candida* isolates from the oral cavity were analysed for antifungal susceptibility profile: 4 isolates from controls (3 *C. albicans*, and 1 *C. glabrata*) and 2 isolates from PD patients (1 *C. albicans*, and 1 *C. carpophila*). All the isolates were resistant to itraconazole (MIC > 1 μg mL^{-1}); presented a non-wild type phenotype regarding posaconazole (NWT, MIC > 2 μg mL^{-1}); and were susceptible to anidulafungin (MIC < 0.125 μg mL^{-1}), voriconazole (MIC < 0.125 μg mL^{-1}),

TABLE 4: Smoking habits, oral hygiene, and saliva biochemistry of peritoneal dialysis (PD) patients and controls.

	PD patients	Controls	P value
Smoking habits			
Past (%)	58.3%	40.9%	0.331
Present (%)	16.7%	22.7%	>0.999
Visual plaque index (%)	56 (16, 100)	69 (14, 100)	0.489
Saliva biochemistry			
Flow rate (mL min^{-1})	0.41 (0.05, 1.06)	0.26 (0.10, 1.04)	0.432
pH	8.0 (6.5, 8.0)	6.8 (6.2, 8.0)	<0.001*
Urea (mg dL^{-1})	110.41 ± 36.64	47.85 ± 23.88	<0.001*
Phosphorus (mg dL^{-1})	22.76 ± 8.19	18.58 ± 16.86	0.486
IgA (mg dL^{-1})	143.0 (126.0, 178.0)	136.5 (30.0, 167.0)	0.361
Amylase (U L^{-1})	309.45 (127.40, 757.50)	562.6 (312.90, 571.10)	0.310

Results are prevalence (%), median (min, max) or mean ± SD; PD, peritoneal dialysis. *$P < 0.05$.

and fluconazole (MIC < 4 μg mL^{-1}). A similar susceptibility profile was obtained for all isolates regarding amphotericin B (MIC = 1 μg mL^{-1}) and flucytosine (MIC = 0.125 μg mL^{-1}). *Candida glabrata* isolated from the control group was the only *Candida* isolate resistant to micafungin (MIC = 0.5 μg mL^{-1}). A variable susceptibility to caspofungin (MIC ranging from 0.25 to 1 μg mL^{-1}) was observed for the *Candida* isolates. The susceptibility epidemiological cutoffs for antifungals are still not defined for *C. carpophila*; nevertheless, the susceptibility values were 0.125 μg mL^{-1} for flucytosine, 0.25 μg mL^{-1} for voriconazole, 0.5 μg mL^{-1} for amphotericin B, 1 μg mL^{-1} for caspofungin and micafungin, 2 μg mL^{-1} for posaconazole, and 4 μg mL^{-1} for fluconazole, itraconazole, and anidulafungin.

Table 4 depicts the oral factors that can play a role on yeast growth in the oral cavity. Saliva pH and urea levels were higher in PD patients when compared to the control group.

Regarding PD-related fungal infections, clinical records of this group of PD patients were analysed. In the period previous to sample collection, no peritonitis of fungal origin was recorded, and only one exit-site infection episode was recorded from fungal origin, namely, due to *C. parapsilosis*. This patient, however, did not present yeast oral colonization at the time of the study (approximately one year after the infection).

Moreover, concerning the longitudinal evaluation, PD-related infections of fungal origin were recorded during the 4 years following sample collection. During this period, 4 exit-site fungal infection episodes were recorded, 2 of them in the same patient. These 2 episodes occurred with a time difference of more than 5 months and were caused by *Candida parapsilosis*, although in one of the episodes bacterial agents were also isolated. Other two patients presented infections either by *Candida parapsilosis* or

Candida zeylanoides. No peritonitis of fungal origin was recorded for these patients within this time frame.

A comparison between the *Candida* species identified in saliva of PD patients and fungal infectious agents responsible for the exit-site infections did not reveal the existence of common species (Figure 1).

In addition, none of the patients that presented oral yeast colonization developed PD-related fungal infections. Also, no relationship was found between PD-related fungal infectious agents and oral colonization of family controls.

4. Discussion

PD-related infections from fungal origin are important complications in PD patients, and the opportunistic fungi inhabiting distant body sites may represent a major source of infection. According to our results, oral yeast colonization constitutes a limited risk for fungal infections in PD patients, due to the lack of relationship between fungal oral colonizers and PD infectious agents. Additionally, PD patients presented a lower prevalence of oral yeasts, in particular *C. albicans*, in comparison to a healthy population.

Interestingly, non-*Candida albicans* species were also found to be normal colonizers of saliva, namely, *C. carpophila* in PD patients and *C. glabrata* in controls. To our knowledge, this is the first study to detect the yeast *C. carpophila* in human saliva. It is possible that the modified oral environment of PD patients results in a shift of yeast prevalence compared with the healthy population resulting in the emergence of rare yeasts, such as *C. carpophila*.

Several factors may contribute to the altered prevalence of yeasts in the oral cavity of PD patients, in particular regarding *C. albicans*. *C. albicans* is the most prevalent fungal specie in the oral cavity, being described as more sensitive than other *Candida* species to potential combined environmental factors present in the oral cavity [15]. Thus, the lower oral *C. albicans* colonization of PD patients could be justified not only by a higher exposure to antifungal therapy, recommended during an antibiotic course [16, 17], but also by alterations of the oral environment secondary to systemic ESRD effects, PD therapy, and medication. Regarding the antifungal therapy, the protocol followed in our department consists in the prescription of fluconazole (100 mg day^{-1}) whenever a patient starts antibiotic therapy after the first use without success. However, since none of our patients had an infectious episode in the month previous to sample collection, this may not be the reason for a lower level of *Candida albicans* colonization. Regarding the medication of these patients, several molecules are reported to be associated with altered susceptibility to fungal infections and can influence yeast colonization in this population. 47.6% of the PD patients were on calcium channel blockers therapy, described to have an inhibitory effect on oxidative stress response of *Candida albicans* [11]; 57.1% were prescribed with statins, 3-hydroxy-3-methylglutaryl-CoA (HMG-CoA) reductase inhibitors, used to lower patients' cholesterol but that also affects ergosterol levels exhibiting antifungal properties [12]; 71.4% were supplemented with vitamin D known to affect fungal growth in

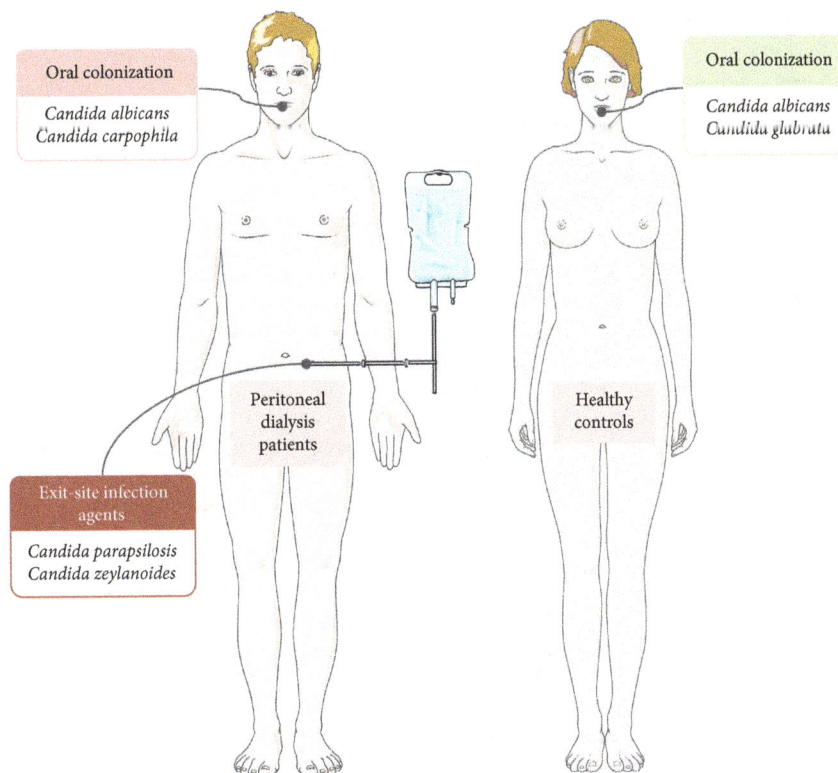

FIGURE 1: Oral *Candida* colonization of PD patients and healthy controls and *Candida* agents responsible for PD-related infections. Figure was produced using Servier Medical Art, http://www.servier.com/Powerpoint-image-bank.

a dose-dependent manner [13]; and 90.5% had iron supplementation, an essential element for microbial growth and known to influence host susceptibility to *C. albicans* infections [14].

In order to investigate other possible causes for the reduced oral *C. albicans* colonization of PD patients, we further evaluated specific oral parameters such as oral hygiene, smoking habits, and saliva biochemistry, given that previous studies found relevant changes in the oral status of chronic kidney disease patients undergoing PD [18]. In accordance to previous studies, saliva pH and urea levels were significantly altered in PD patients in comparison with controls [8, 19]. The high urea levels may contribute in part to the higher salivary pH, due to the ammonia production as a result of urea hydrolysis [8, 19]. This altered oral pH may have an impact on *Candida* growth, given that oral *Candida* isolates have been shown to be more adapted to acidic conditions [20]. It is known that neutral to alkaline pH can cause severe stress to *C. albicans* including impaired nutrient acquisition, as a consequence of a disrupted proton gradient, and malfunctioning of pH-sensitive proteins [21]. In addition, changes in the oral pH may be the major ecological factor that alters the oral commensal microbiome, leading to shifts in its natural diversity [22]. Recent advances on bacterial–fungal interkingdom communication have shown a negative correlation between the *Candida* load and the diversity of the salivary microbiome [22]. This suggests that, globally, the oral microbiome of PD patients may be altered; the impact of these changes on PD-related infections deserves to be further clarified.

Despite the limited number of isolates tested for antifungal susceptibility profile, we verified that all were resistant to itraconazole and presented a non-wild type phenotype regarding posaconazole. Also, the MIC values of posaconazole for *C. albicans* and *C. glabrata* isolates are higher than the previously reported values for wild-type strains [23]. This resistance profile may not be associated to the frequent prophylactic antifungal therapy prescription during an antibiotic course [16, 17], given that oral nystatin and fluconazole are the common choices [1]. However, itraconazole and posaconazole susceptibility profiles in oral *Candida* isolates are a matter of concern since both these drugs are second-line agents for the treatment of oropharyngeal candidiasis [24]. Also, we observed variable susceptibility profiles of *Candida* isolates to caspofungin. Taking into account that itraconazole, posaconazole, and caspofungin are prescribed for the treatment of systemic fungal infections [25] and that previous studies report the existence of antifungal resistance to itraconazole and caspofungin [26], we consider it relevant to determine the susceptibility to these antifungals in all clinical isolates.

This study presents some limitations, particularly the limited number of patients analysed and the methodology for yeast isolation (direct spread plate technique), which is associated with limited sensitivity [27]. However, it is important to highlight that the percentage of *Candida* that we obtained is similar to other studies that used the same methodology [28]. On the other hand, it is important to highlight that 10 elements of the control group were family members of the PD patients. This is a relevant aspect since the oral microbial colonization is strongly correlated to the diet, oral hygiene, and familial predisposition.

In conclusion, oral yeast colonization may represent a limited risk for fungal infections in PD patients, given that in this pilot study there is an absence of relationship between patients with oral yeast colonization and the development of PD-related fungal infections; the *Candida* species found in oral cavity are different from the ones identified as PD-related fungal infectious agents; and also, PD patients present a low prevalence of oral yeast colonization, namely, *C. albicans*. Despite the low number of oral *Candida* isolates, the antifungal susceptibility profile revealed a possible resistance to some second-line drugs, suggesting the need for the assessment of antifungal susceptibilities in clinical practice. Further studies are still necessary to fully characterize the oral yeast colonization in this population.

Acknowledgments

The authors thank the nurse Maria João Sousa, Department of Nephrology, São João Hospital Center, EPE, for the help with sample collection and Margarida Tabaio from Faculty of Dental Medicine for helping with the oral evaluation. This work was financed by FEDER–Fundo Europeu de Desenvolvimento Regional funds through the COMPETE 2020–Operational Programme for Competitiveness and Internationalisation (POCI), Portugal 2020, and by Portuguese funds through FCT–Fundação para a Ciência e a Tecnologia/Ministério da Ciência, Tecnologia e Inovação in the framework of the project "Institute for Research and Innovation in Health Sciences" (POCI-01-0145-FEDER-007274); by the project NORTE-01-0145-FEDER-000012, supported by Norte Portugal Regional Operational Programme (NORTE 2020), under the Portugal 2020 Partnership Agreement, through the European Regional Development Fund (ERDF); and by IJUP projects, University of Porto. Liliana Simões-Silva is supported by SFRH/BD/84837/2012, and Isabel Soares-Silva is supported by SFRH/BPD/101016/2014 from FCT/QREN–POPH/FSE.

References

[1] D. J. Campbell, D. W. Johnson, D. W. Mudge, M. P. Gallagher, and J. C. Craig, "Prevention of peritoneal dialysis-related infections," *Nephrology Dialysis Transplantation*, vol. 30, no. 9, pp. 1461–1472, 2015.

[2] R. Miles, C. M. Hawley, S. P. McDonald et al., "Predictors and outcomes of fungal peritonitis in peritoneal dialysis patients," *Kidney International*, vol. 76, no. 6, pp. 622–628, 2009.

[3] M. A. Kleinpeter, "Successful treatment of *Candida* infections in peritoneal dialysis patients: case reports and review of the literature," *Advances in Peritoneal Dialysis*, vol. 20, pp. 58–61, 2004.

[4] S. Coelho, A. Beco, A. Oliveira, C. Santos, and M. Pestana, "Exit-site fungal infections: experience of a Peritoneal Dialysis Unit," *Portuguese Journal of Nephrology & Hypertension*, vol. 30, no. 4, pp. 277–282, 2016.

[5] X. Li, K. M. Kolltveit, L. Tronstad, and I. Olsen, "Systemic diseases caused by oral infection," *Clinical Microbiology Reviews*, vol. 13, no. 4, pp. 547–558, 2000.

[6] B. Sampaio-Maia, I. M. Caldas, M. L. Pereira, D. Perez-Mongiovi, and R. Araujo, "The oral microbiome in health and its implication in oral and systemic diseases," *Advances in Applied Microbiology*, vol. 97, pp. 171–210, 2016.

[7] A. V. Kshirsagar, R. G. Craig, K. L. Moss et al., "Periodontal disease adversely affects the survival of patients with end-stage renal disease," *Kidney International*, vol. 75, no. 7, pp. 746–751, 2009.

[8] G. Bayraktar, I. Kurtulus, R. Kazancioglu et al., "Oral health and inflammation in patients with end-stage renal failure," *Peritoneal Dialysis International*, vol. 29, no. 4, pp. 472–479, 2009.

[9] F. Monteiro-da-Silva, R. Araujo, and B. Sampaio-Maia, "Interindividual variability and intraindividual stability of oral fungal microbiota over time," *Medical Mycology*, vol. 52, no. 5, pp. 498–505, 2014.

[10] M. A. Pfaller and D. J. Diekema, "Progress in antifungal susceptibility testing of *Candida* spp. by use of Clinical and Laboratory Standards Institute broth microdilution methods, 2010 to 2012," *Journal of Clinical Microbiology*, vol. 50, no. 9, pp. 2846–2856, 2012.

[11] Q. Yu, C. Xiao, K. Zhang et al., "The calcium channel blocker verapamil inhibits oxidative stress response in *Candida albicans*," *Mycopathologia*, vol. 177, no. 3-4, pp. 167–177, 2014.

[12] P. W. Bergman and L. Bjorkhem-Bergman, "Is there a role for statins in fungal infections?," *Expert Review of Anti-Infective Therapy*, vol. 11, no. 12, pp. 1391–1400, 2013.

[13] J. H. Lim, S. Ravikumar, Y. M. Wang et al., "Bimodal influence of vitamin D in host response to systemic *Candida* infection-vitamin D dose matters," *Journal of Infectious Diseases*, vol. 212, no. 4, pp. 635–644, 2015.

[14] R. S. Almeida, D. Wilson, and B. Hube, "*Candida albicans* iron acquisition within the host," *FEMS Yeast Research*, vol. 9, no. 7, pp. 1000–1012, 2009.

[15] D. Kaloriti, A. Tillmann, E. Cook et al., "Combinatorial stresses kill pathogenic *Candida* species," *Medical Mycology*, vol. 50, no. 7, pp. 699–709, 2012.

[16] W. K. Lo, C. Y. Chan, S. W. Cheng, J. F. Poon, D. T. Chan, and I. K. Cheng, "A prospective randomized control study of oral nystatin prophylaxis for *Candida* peritonitis complicating continuous ambulatory peritoneal dialysis," *American Journal of Kidney Diseases*, vol. 28, no. 4, pp. 549–552, 1996.

[17] C. Restrepo, J. Chacon, and G. Manjarres, "Fungal peritonitis in peritoneal dialysis patients: successful prophylaxis with

fluconazole, as demonstrated by prospective randomized control trial," *Peritoneal Dialysis International*, vol. 30, no. 6, pp. 619–625, 2010.

[18] C. P. Bots, J. H. Poorterman, H. S. Brand et al., "The oral health status of dentate patients with chronic renal failure undergoing dialysis therapy," *Oral Diseases*, vol. 12, no. 2, pp. 176–180, 2006.

[19] A. Al-Nowaiser, G. J. Roberts, R. S. Trompeter, M. Wilson, and V. S. Lucas, "Oral health in children with chronic renal failure," *Pediatric Nephrology*, vol. 18, no. 1, pp. 39–45, 2003.

[20] T. Klinke, S. Kneist, J. J. de Soet et al., "Acid production by oral strains of *Candida albicans* and lactobacilli," *Caries Research*, vol. 43, no. 2, pp. 83–91, 2009.

[21] F. L. Mayer, D. Wilson, and B. Hube, "*Candida albicans* pathogenicity mechanisms," *Virulence*, vol. 4, no. 2, pp. 119–128, 2013.

[22] E. A. Kraneveld, M. J. Buijs, M. J. Bonder et al., "The relation between oral *Candida* load and bacterial microbiome profiles in Dutch older adults," *PLoS One*, vol. 7, no. 8, p. e42770, 2012.

[23] M. A. Pfaller, L. Boyken, R. J. Hollis et al., "Wild-type MIC distributions and epidemiological cutoff values for posaconazole and voriconazole and *Candida* spp. as determined by 24-hour CLSI broth microdilution," *Journal of Clinical Microbiology*, vol. 49, no. 2, pp. 630–637, 2011.

[24] S. Patil, R. S. Rao, B. Majumdar, and S. Anil, "Clinical appearance of oral *Candida* infection and therapeutic strategies," *Frontiers in Microbiology*, vol. 6, p. 1391, 2015.

[25] U. Allen, "Antifungal agents for the treatment of systemic fungal infections in children," *Paediatrics and Child Health*, vol. 15, no. 9, pp. 603–615, 2010.

[26] K. Zomorodian, A. Bandegani, H. Mirhendi, K. Pakshir, N. Alinejhad, and A. Poostforoush Fard, "In vitro susceptibility and trailing growth effect of clinical isolates of *Candida* species to azole drugs," *Jundishapur Journal of Microbiology*, vol. 9, no. 2, p. e28666, 2016.

[27] L. P. Samaranayake, T. W. MacFarlane, P. J. Lamey, and M. M. Ferguson, "A comparison of oral rinse and imprint sampling techniques for the detection of yeast, coliform and *Staphylococcus aureus* carriage in the oral cavity," *Journal of Oral Pathology and Medicine*, vol. 15, no. 7, pp. 386–388, 1986.

[28] R. Rio, L. Simões-Silva, S. Garro, M. J. Silva, A. Azevedo, and B. Sampaio-Maia, "Oral yeast colonization throughout pregnancy," *Medicina Oral Patología Oral y Cirugia Bucal*, vol. 22, no. 2, pp. e144–e148, 2017.

13

The Relationship between Colonization by *Moraxella catarrhalis* and Tonsillar Hypertrophy

Mirela C. M. Prates,[1] Edwin Tamashiro,[1] José L. Proenca-Modena,[2,3,4] Miriã F. Criado,[2] Tamara H. Saturno,[1] Anibal S. Oliveira,[2] Guilherme P. Buzatto,[1] Bruna L. S. Jesus,[2] Marcos G. Jacob,[1] Lucas R. Carenzi,[1] Ricardo C. Demarco,[1] Eduardo T. Massuda,[1] Davi Aragon,[5] Fabiana C. P. Valera,[1] Eurico Arruda,[2,3] and Wilma T. Anselmo-Lima (iD)[1]

[1]Department of Ophthalmology, Otorhinolaryngology, Head and Neck Surgery, Ribeirao Preto Medical School,
 University of São Paulo, Ribeirao Preto, SP 14049-900, Brazil
[2]Department of Cell Biology, Ribeirao Preto Medical School, University of São Paulo, Ribeirao Preto, SP 14049-900, Brazil
[3]Virology Research Center, Ribeirao Preto Medical School, University of São Paulo, Ribeirao Preto, SP 14049-900, Brazil
[4]Department of Genetics, Evolution and Bioagents, Institute of Biology, University of Campinas, Campinas, SP 13083-970, Brazil
[5]Department of Pediatrics, Ribeirao Preto Medical School, University of São Paulo, Ribeirao Preto, SP 14049-900, Brazil

Correspondence should be addressed to Wilma T. Anselmo-Lima; wtalima@fmrp.usp.br

Academic Editor: Maria L. Tornesello

We sought to investigate the prevalence of potentially pathogenic bacteria in secretions and tonsillar tissues of children with chronic adenotonsillitis hypertrophy compared to controls. Prospective case-control study comparing patients between 2 and 12 years old who underwent adenotonsillectomy due to chronic adenotonsillar hypertrophy to children without disease. We compared detection of *Streptococcus pneumoniae*, *Haemophilus influenzae*, *Staphylococcus aureus*, *Pseudomonas aeruginosa*, and *Moraxella catarrhalis* by real-time PCR in palatine tonsils, adenoids, and nasopharyngeal washes obtained from 37 children with and 14 without adenotonsillar hypertrophy. We found high frequency (>50%) of *Haemophilus influenzae*, *Streptococcus pneumoniae*, *Moraxella catarrhalis*, and *Pseudomonas aeruginosa* in both groups of patients. Although different sampling sites can be infected with more than one bacterium and some bacteria can be detected in different tissues in the same patient, adenoids, palatine tonsils, and nasopharyngeal washes were not uniformly infected by the same bacteria. Adenoids and palatine tonsils of patients with severe adenotonsillar hypertrophy had higher rates of bacterial coinfection. There was good correlation of detection of *Moraxella catarrhalis* in different sampling sites in patients with more severe tonsillar hypertrophy, suggesting that *Moraxella catarrhalis* may be associated with the development of more severe hypertrophy, that inflammatory conditions favor colonization by this agent. *Streptococcus pneumoniae*, *Staphylococcus aureus*, *Haemophilus influenzae*, and *Moraxella catarrhalis* are frequently detected in palatine tonsils, adenoids, and nasopharyngeal washes in children. Simultaneous detection of *Moraxella catarrhalis* in adenoids, palatine tonsils, and nasopharyngeal washes was correlated with more severe tonsillar hypertrophy.

1. Introduction

Chronic tonsillar diseases have great impact in general health worldwide, particularly in children [1]. Chronic inflammation and hypertrophy of the tonsils may be associated with complications such as chronic rhinosinusitis, auditory tube dysfunction, otitis media, obstructive sleep apnea, periodontal problems, and alterations in orofacial and behavioral development in children [2–4]. Despite the great public health importance of chronic adenotonsillar hypertrophy, little is known of its pathogenesis.

Multiple factors are involved in host colonization by microorganisms [5]. The human microbiota creates a microenvironment that allows for interactions between different microorganisms [6], and evidence suggests that infections by different combinations of microorganisms may lead to increased adenotonsillar sizes [7–9].

Bacteria such as *Streptococcus pneumoniae* (*S. pneumoniae*), *Haemophilus influenzae* (*H. influenzae*), *Staphylococcus aureus* (*S. aureus*), and *Moraxella catarrhalis* (*M. catarrhalis*) are commonly detected in the upper respiratory tract of healthy individuals and also in acute upper respiratory diseases [10–13], but it is still unclear if they have any pathogenic role in chronic adenotonsillitis. These bacteria can potentially interact with each other in biofilms and stimulate chronic tonsillar inflammation [14, 15]. One study evaluated the possible effect of biofilm-producing bacteria (BPB) in tonsillar specimens in clinical features of 22 children, and they observed a significant correlation of BPB presence with intensity of tonsillar hyperplasia, being *S. aureus* the most frequent pathogen.

In the present study, the presence of genomic DNA of five bacteria commonly detected in respiratory infections was associated with symptoms and signs of chronic adenotonsillar disease.

2. Material and Methods

2.1. Study Design. In this cross-sectional case-control study, the frequency of detection of bacterial genomes was compared between children with chronic adenotonsillar hypertrophy and controls. The study was conducted between May 2010 and August 2012, with children 2–12 years old (mean of 6 years) who were treated at the Otorhinolaryngology Division of the University Hospital, Medical School of Ribeirao Preto, University of São Paulo.

The study group consisted of children who underwent adenotonsillectomy due to chronic adenotonsillar hypertrophy. Before surgery, all children were assessed with a full otorhinolaryngological examination, including flexible nasal endoscopy. Inclusion criteria were the presence of sleep apnea, tonsillar hypertrophy grade ≥3 (both palatine tonsils (PT) occupied 50% or more of the oropharynx width), and the adenoid (AD) occupied 70% or more of the nasopharynx at endoscopy.

The control group consisted of children who underwent cochlear implantation, in the absence of symptoms of adenotonsillar disease or hypertrophy, palatine tonsils graded ≤2 (both PT occupied 50% or less of the oropharynx width), and AD occupied 50% or less of the nasopharynx at endoscopy.

Exclusion criteria for both groups were the presence of symptoms and signs of acute infection of the upper respiratory airways at the time of surgery, antibiotic use 4 weeks prior to surgery, past history of adenotonsillar or sinonasal surgery, genetic syndromes, a history suggestive of primary ciliary dyskinesia, cystic fibrosis, or immunodeficiencies.

During adenotonsillectomy under general anesthesia, three samples were collected from every patient: (a) nasopharyngeal wash (NPW): saline flushed into both nasal cavities and collected at the nasopharynx using a sterile syringe; (b) fragment of adenoid tissue (AD), collected with a conventional Beckman curette for adenoidectomy; and (c)

fragment of palatine tonsil (PT) collected with a cold-knife scalpel. From control patients, during surgery for cochlear implant, a mouth-opener was placed and small tissue fragments were obtained with punch biopsy from adenoid and palatine tonsil tissues, apart from NPW.

Tissue samples from PT and AD were placed in Eagle's minimal essential medium (MEM) supplemented with 10% fetal bovine serum and 15% antibiotic-antimycotic solution (penicillin-streptomycin 20,000 U/ml and amphotericin B 200 mg/mL, both from Gibco (Grand Island, NY, USA)) and transported on ice within a maximum of 4 hours for further processing in the laboratory. Tissue samples were washed twice with MEM to remove debris and blood clots, and then minced in TRIzol® reagent (Invitrogen, Carlsbad, CA, USA) for subsequent extraction of total nucleic acids. NPW samples were distributed in several aliquots, including one of 250 μL added to 750 μL of TRIzol®. All samples were frozen at −70°C until further testing.

2.2. Detection of Bacterial DNA. The bacterial genome was detected by real-time PCR using TaqMan probes (Applied Biosystems®, Foster City, CA, USA) after DNA extraction with TRIzol®. Primers and probes were designed to detect *S. aureus*, *S. pneumoniae*, *H. influenzae*, *M. catarrhalis*, and *Pseudomonas aeruginosa* (*P. aeruginosa*) (Table 1). Each real-time PCR assay was done with 1 μL of extracted DNA (approximately 100 ng), 0.25 μL of specific *primers* (10 pmol/μL), 0.125 μL of probe (10 pmol/μL), and 5 μL of TaqMan® Universal PCR Master Mix (Applied Biosystems®, Foster City, CA, USA). Cycling parameters were 50°C for 2 minutes, 95°C for 10 minutes, followed by 45 cycles of 95°C for 15 seconds and 60°C for 1 minute. Quantification of bacterial DNA was done by comparison with a standard curve generated for each bacterial strain, diluted in a 10-fold series (*S. aureus*, *S. pneumoniae*, *H. influenzae*, *M. catarrhalis*, and *P. aeruginosa*), thus allowing for determination of bacterial loads.

2.3. Statistical Analysis. Comparisons between groups were made by Fisher's exact test, and agreement among the three specimens (AD, PT, and NPW) was assessed by kappa coefficients. In all analyses, $p < 0.05$ was considered statistically significant.

2.4. Ethics Statement. All legal guardians signed informed consent forms. The study was performed in accordance with the Declaration of Helsinki and approved by the Ethics Committee of the University Hospital, Medical School of Ribeirão Preto, file number 10466/2008.

3. Results

3.1. Demographic Data. A total of 51 children were enrolled: 37 in the tonsillectomy group and 14 in the cochlear implant control group. In both groups, children ages were 2 to 12 years, with mean ages of 6 years and 4.1 years, respectively, in the tonsillectomy and control groups.

TABLE 1: Primers and probes used for bacterial detection.

Bacteria	Primers	Probes	References
S. pneumoniae	5'TGCAGAGCGTCCTTTGGTCTAT3' (FORWARD) 5'CTCTTACTCGTGGTTTCCAACTTGA3' (REVERSE)	FAM 5'TGGCGCCCATAAGCAACACTCGAA-Tamra 3' TAMRA	Corless et al., [16]
S. aureus	5'GTTGCTTAGTGTTAACTTTAGTTGTA 3' (FORWARD) 5'AATGTCGCAGGTTCTTTATGTAATTT 3' (REVERSE)	5'-VIC-AAGTCTAAGTAGCTCAGCAAATGCA-MGB-3'	Kilic et al., [17]
P. aeruginosa	5'CGAGTACAACATGGCTCTGG 3' (FORWARD) 5'ACCGGACGCTCTTTACCATA 3' (REVERSE)	5'-FAM-CCTGCAGCACCAGGTAGCGC-Tamra-3'	Feizabadi et al., [18]
H. influenzae	5'CCAGCTGCTAAAGTATTAGTAGAAG 3' (FORWARD) 5'TTCACCGTAAGATACTGTGCC 3' (REVERSE)	5'-VIC-CAGATGCAGTTGAAGGTTATTTAG-MGB-3'	Abdeldaim et al., [19]
M. catarrhalis	5'GTCAAACAGCTGGAGGTATTGC 3' (FORWARD) 5'GACATGATGCTCACCTGCTCTA 3' (REVERSE)	5'-NED-ATCGCAATTGCAACTTT-MGB-3'	Heiniger et al., [20]

S. pneumonia: Streptococcus pneumoniae; S. aureus: Staphylococcus aureus; P. aeruginosa: Pseudomonas aeruginosa; H. influenzae: Haemophilus influenzae; M. catarrhalis: Moraxella catarrhalis.

TABLE 2: Detection rates of bacteria in tonsillar tissues and nasopharyngeal washes from patients with adenotonsillar hypertrophy and controls.

Bacteria	Palatine tonsils		Adenoids		NPW		Total	
	Controls n (%)	ATH n (%)	Controls n (%)	ATH n (%)	Controls n (%)	ATH n (%)	Controls n (%)	ATH n (%)
S. aureus	0 (0)	3 (8.1)	2 (14.2)	1 (2.7)	0 (0)	4 (10.8)	2 (14.2)	6 (16.2)
S. pneumoniae	4 (28.6)	19(51.3)	9 (64.2)	21(56.7)	11 (78.5)	26 (70.2)	12 (85.7)	29 (78.3)
H. influenzae	8 (57.1)	24(64.8)	9 (64.2)	16(43.2)	10 (71.4)	26(70.2)	12 (85.7)	30 (81)
P. aeruginosa	4 (28.6)	6 (16.2)	2 (14.2)	8 (21.6)	2 (14.2)	9 (24.3)	6 (42.8)	17 (45.9)
M. catarrhalis	3 (21.4)	6 (16.2)	4 (28.5)	15(40.5)	7 (50)	20 (54)	7 (50)	21 (56.7)

NPW: nasopharyngeal washes; ATH: adenotonsillar hypertrophy. S. aureus: $p > 1.00$; S. pneumoniae: $p > 0.70$; H. influenzae: $p > 1.00$; P. aeruginosa: $p > 1.00$; M. catarrhalis: $p > 0.75$. S. pneumonia: Streptococcus pneumoniae; S. aureus: Staphylococcus aureus; H. influenzae: Haemophilus influenzae; P. aeruginosa: Pseudomonas aeruginosa; M. catarrhalis: Moraxella catarrhalis.

3.2. Bacterial Detection by Real-Time PCR.

The overall rates of bacterial detection in all sampling sites (PT, AD, and NPW) were similar between patients with chronic adenotonsillitis and controls (Table 2). H. influenzae and S. pneumoniae were the most frequently detected bacteria in both groups, with frequencies around 80%. P. aeruginosa and M. catarrhalis were also similarly detected in both groups, approximately 50% of the patients. The least frequent bacterium in all samples was S. aureus, detected in approximately 15% in both groups.

3.3. Comparison of Bacteria Detection Rates and Bacterial Loads between Different Sampling Sites.

To assess the agreement in bacteria rates between the different sample sites, kappa test was used (Table 3).

In the control group, the correlation between AD and PT was good for H. influenzae (kappa: 0.6829), but only moderate for M. catarrhalis (kappa: 0.4324). Correlations between NPW and AD (kappa: 0.5714) or PT (kappa = 0.4286) were also moderate for M. catarrhalis.

There was lack of agreement between different sampling sites with regard to all other bacteria in this group of patients.

In the group of patients with chronic adenotonsillitis, kappa analyses revealed no correlation between bacteria rates in PT and AD (Table 3). Comparison between NPWs and PT revealed only moderate correlation for M. catarrhalis (kappa: 0.6273) and S. pneumoniae (0.5325), but not for the other bacteria. Similarly, comparisons between NPWs and AD revealed moderate correlations for S. aureus (0.5277) and S. pneumoniae (0.4873).

To further probe into differences in the magnitudes of bacterial colonization of different sites, quantitative values of bacterial loads were compared among those sites for both groups of patients (Table 4). No significant differences in bacterial loads were detected, what may be partially due to restricted sizes of some subgroups.

3.4. Bacteria Detection and Intensity of Tonsillar Hypertrophy.

Bacteria detection rates in different sampling sites were finally compared only among the 22 (59.4%) patients who had

Table 3: Analyses of agreement of bacteria detection rates among different specimens collected from patients with chronic adenotonsillitis, severe adenotonsillar hypertrophy, and controls.

Bacteria	Specimens	Patients	Kappa coefficient	95% CI
S. aureus	Adenoid × palatine tonsil	Control	0	(1.04; 1.04)
		Chronic adenotonsillitis	−0.0435	(−0.1098; 0.0228)
		Severe adenotonsillar hypertrophy	−0.0769	(−0.1958; 0.0419)
	Palatine tonsil × nasopharyngeal wash	Control	0	(−1.04; 1.04)
		Chronic adenotonsillitis	−0.0465	(−0.1218; 0.0287)
		Severe adenotonsillar hypertrophy	−0.0769	(−0.1958; 0.0419)
	Adenoid × nasopharyngeal wash	Control	0	(−1.04; 1.04)
		Chronic adenotonsillitis	0.5277	(0.0599; 0.9954)
		Severe adenotonsillar hypertrophy	0.614	(0.1266; 1.0000)
S. pneumoniae	Adenoid × palatine tonsil	Control	−0.1455	(−0.5712; 0.2802)
		Chronic adenotonsillitis	0.132	(−0.1858; 0.4497)
		Severe adenotonsillar hypertrophy	0.0833	(−0.3336; 0.5003)
	Palatine tonsil × nasopharyngeal wash	Control	0.3171	(−0.1899; 0.8241)
		Chronic adenotonsillitis	0.5325	(0.2658; 0.7991)
		Severe adenotonsillar hypertrophy	0.5299	(0.1836; 0.8763)
	Adenoid × nasopharyngeal wash	Control	0.1967	(−0.0539; 0.4473)
		Chronic adenotonsilliti	0.4873	(0.2219; 0.7528)
		Severe adenotonsillar hypertrophy	0.5299	(0.1836; 0.8763)
H. influenza	Adenoid × palatine tonsil	Control	0.6829	(0.2996; 1.0000)
		Chronic adenotonsillitis	0.2725	(−0.0046; 0.5495)
		Severe adenotonsillar hypertrophy	0.3937	(0.0567; 0.7307)
	Palatine tonsil × nasopharyngeal wash	Control	0.4179	(−0.1244; 0.9602)
		Chronic adenotonsillitis	0.2825	(0.0243; 0.5408)
		Severe adenotonsillar hypertrophy	0.1538	(−0.1936; 0.5013)
	Adenoid × nasopharyngeal wash	Control	0.087	(−0.4156; 0.5895)
		Chronic adenotonsillitis	0.3854	(0.0724; 0.6984)
		Severe adenotonsillar hypertrophy	0.5217	(0.1575; 0.8859)
P. aeruginosa	Adenoid × palatine tonsil	Control	−0.2353	(−0.4760; 0.0054)
		Chronic adenotonsillitis	0.2986	(−0.0725; 0.6696)
		Severe adenotonsillar hypertrophy	0.2281	(−0.3034; 0.7646)
	Palatine tonsil × nasopharyngeal wash	Control	−0.1667	(−0.3277; −0.0056)
		Chronic adenotonsillitis	0.0082	(−0.3152; 0.3317)
		Severe adenotonsillar hypertrophy	0.0494	(−0.3519; 0.4507)
	Adenoid × nasopharyngeal wash	Control	0.1765	(−0.3573; 0.7103)
		Chronic adenotonsillitis	−0.0761	(−0.3555; 0.2034)
		Severe adenotonsillar hypertrophy	−0.2222	(−0.4076; −0.0369)
M. catarrhalis	Adenoid × palatine tonsil	Control	0.4324	(−0.1001; 0.9649)
		Chronic adenotonsillitis	0.3183	(0.0437; 0.5928)
		Severe adenotonsillar hypertrophy	0.4086	(−0.0008; 0.8180)
	Palatine tonsil × nasopharyngeal wash	Control	0.5714	(0.1830; 0.9598)
		Chronic adenotonsillitis	0.6273	(0.3876; 0.8671)
		Severe adenotonsillar hypertrophy	0.7179	(0.4334; 1.0000)
	Adenoid × nasopharyngeal wash	Control	0.4286	(0.0402; 0.8170)
		Chronic adenotonsillitis	0.2825	(0.0761; 0.4890)
		Severe adenotonsillar hypertrophy	0.4211	(0.0989; 0.7432)

S. pneumonia: Streptococcus pneumoniae; S. aureus: Staphylococcus aureus; H. influenzae: Haemophilus influenzae; P. aeruginosa: Pseudomonas aeruginosa; M. catarrhalis: Moraxella catarrhalis.

severe tonsillar hypertrophy (Brodsky index ≥3). H. influenzae was detected in palatine tonsils from 12 of those 22 patients (54.5%) and S. pneumoniae was detected in 11 (50%) patients (Figure 1(a)). The AD of highly hypertrophic patients were also frequently infected with S. pneumoniae and H. influenza (resp, 50% and 31.8%) (Figure 1(b)).

The frequencies of bacteria codetections were especially high in patients with more severe tonsillar hypertrophy (Figures 1(c) and 1(d)). More than one of the bacteria tested, and sometimes all four of them were codetected in 41% of tissue samples from PT and AD from patients with tonsillar hypertrophy (Figures 1(c) and 1(d)).

Kappa analyses were also performed considering only patients with severe tonsillar hypertrophy (Table 3). Remarkably, there was a good correlation (0.7179) between AD and NPW and moderate correlations between AD and PT (0.4086) and between PT and NPW (0.4211) with regard to detection of M. catarrhalis. With regard to S. aureus, S.

TABLE 4: Descriptive statistics for bacterial loads by group and tissue.

Tissue	Bacteria	Mean	Standard deviation	Minimum	1° Quartile	Median	3° Quartile	Maximum
Adenotonsillitis								
	S. aureus	16.64	0.56	15.89	16.28	16.7	16.99	17.25
	S. pneumoniae	17.82	1.9	13.31	16.87	17.84	19.15	21.28
	H. influenza	10.65	2.31	5.95	9.34	10.86	12.44	14.33
	P. aeruginosa	8.95	1.12	7.01	8.54	9.05	9.99	10.05
Adenoid	*M. catarrhalis*	11.59	0.95	10.88	11.02	11.16	11.95	13.36
	S. aureus	17.58		17.58	17.58	17.58	17.58	17.58
	S. pneumoniae	18.13	1.95	12.61	16.95	18.47	19.11	21.31
	H. influenza	10.41	1.59	7.29	9.04	10.47	11.53	13.36
	P. aeruginosa	7.7	0.6	6.66	7.2	7.9	8.23	8.24
	M. catarrhalis	13.05	1.68	10.67	11.26	13.38	14.05	16.6
	S. aureus	14.87	0.51	14.11	14.57	15.09	15.17	15.18
Palatine tonsil	*S. pneumoniae*	17.62	6	6.49	14.14	17.44	19.59	39.47
	H. influenza	10.31	2.37	3.91	8.76	10.47	11.83	14.21
	P. aeruginosa	4.77	1.37	1.24	4.92	5	5.19	5.85
	M. catarrhalis	12.97	3.36	7.38	9.77	13.53	15.36	18.85
	S. aureus	*	*	*	*	*	*	*
Nasopharyngeal washes	*S. pneumoniae*	21.99	4.57	19.48	19.55	19.82	24.43	28.84
	H. influenza	11.33	2.22	8.06	9.76	11.31	12.67	15.07
	P. aeruginosa	8.62	1.33	6.82	7.72	8.81	9.51	10.02
	M. catarrhalis	14.91	1.07	13.74	13.74	15.18	15.82	15.82
	S. aureus	17.51	0.52	17.14	17.14	17.51	17.87	17.87
Adenoid	*S. pneumoniae*	20.83	5.22	15.07	16.78	20.86	22.36	31.61
	H. influenza	11.3	2.43	9.01	9.71	10.63	12.15	16.8
	P. aeruginosa	7.05	3.09	4.86	4.86	7.05	9.23	9.23
	M. catarrhalis	13.88	1.88	12.43	12.62	13.24	15.13	16.59
	S. aureus	*	*	*	*	*	*	*
Palatine tonsil	*S. pneumoniae*	18.04	3.74	12.81	14.71	18.1	20.54	24.63
	H. influenza	9.8	2.82	4.02	9.01	9.82	11.22	13.9
	P. aeruginosa	4.89	0.3	4.67	4.67	4.89	5.1	5.1
Controls								
Nasopharyngeal washes	*M. catarrhalis*	14.28	5.21	8.09	10.36	11.51	19.38	21.31

*The bacteria were not detected in the specific sample. *S. pneumonia*: *Streptococcus pneumoniae*; *S. aureus*: *Staphylococcus aureus*; *H. influenzae*: *Haemophilus influenzae*; *P. aeruginosa*: *Pseudomonas aeruginosa*; *M. catarrhalis*: *Moraxella catarrhalis*.

pneumoniae and *H. influenzae*, the level of concordance between detection in severely hypertrophic palatine tonsils and in NPW was moderate.

4. Discussion

Chronic tonsillitis is characterized by chronic or recurrent infections of the tonsils and adenoids that can lead to tissue enlargement. Tonsillar hypertrophy is one of the most common diseases found in children and its etiology is still obscure. Its treatment is based on the administration of antibiotics and adeno/tonsillectomy, which is one of the most common surgical procedures performed worldwide. Many studies have reported that adeno/tonsillectomy leads to a reduction in the number of episodes of throat pain in children in the first year after surgery compared to non-surgical treatment [1, 21–24].

Many studies have shown that the tonsils of patients with recurrent tonsillitis are colonized by a large number of bacteria, both pathogenic and nonpathogenic, showing that these agents possibly may play a role in the development of chronic tonsillar disease [1, 7, 21, 25]. In patients undergoing adenoidectomy, for instance, there is a decrease in the detection of pathogenic agents in the nasopharyngeal region [26].

There is evidence that large numbers of bacteria make up surface biofilms of the adenoids [27], supported by research 16s RNAs indicating that the tonsils are reservoirs of pathogens [28] hosting very diverse microbial communities, some of them potentially pathogenic. Confirming these data, Winther et al. observed a large number of bacteria located in adenoids, more specifically in the mucus that lines the surface of this tissue. In addition, bacterial biofilms were present in 8 of 9 adenoids and were more common in the caudal region of this tissue [27].

Pathogenic bacteria such as *Neisseria* sp., *Streptococcus* sp., *Haemophilus influenzae*, *Staphylococcus aureus*, *Actinomyces*, *Bacteroides*, *Prevotella*, *Porphyromonas*, *Peptostreptococcus*, and *Fusobacterium* sp. are often isolated from the nasopharynx, both from healthy and sick children [29]. Other studies, although the results were contradictory, some of the bacteria most commonly detected in the upper respiratory tract were also found in AD and PT of children with tonsillar hypertrophy, including *H. influenzae*, *M. catarrhalis*, and *S. pneumoniae* [11, 13, 15].

In the present study, detection and loading frequencies of genomic DNA were determined by real-time PCR for five of the most common bacteria of the nasopharyngeal microbiota, namely: *H. influenzae*, *M. catarrhalis*,

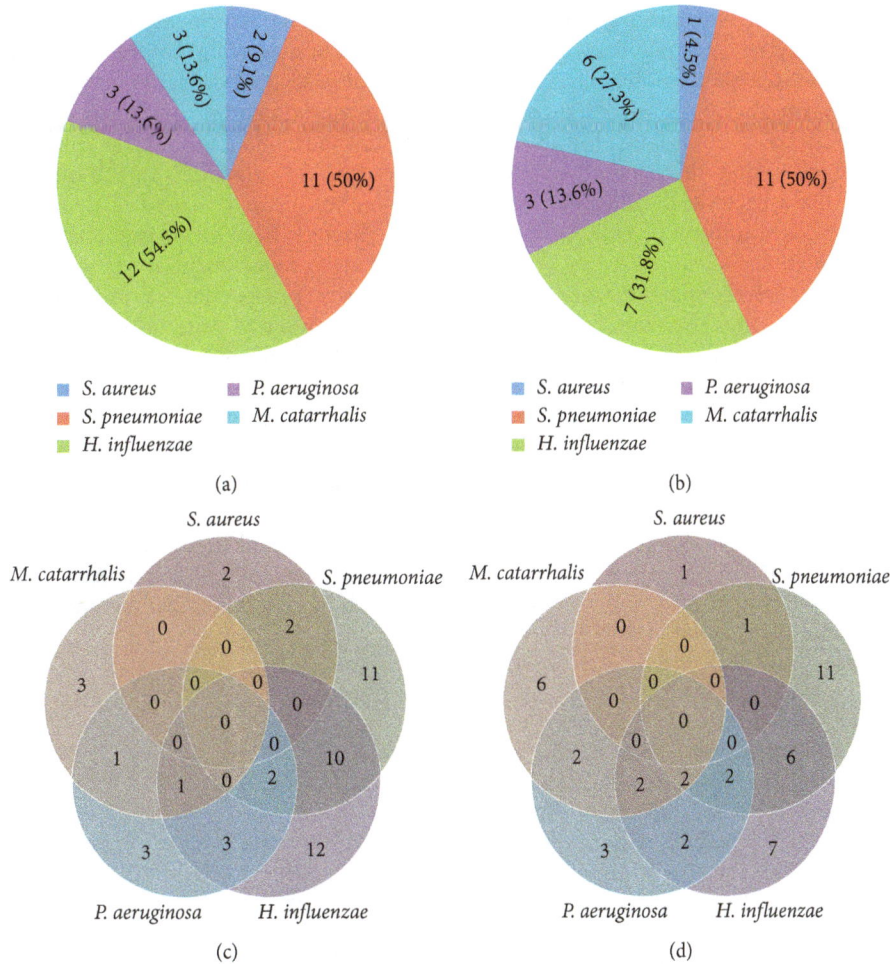

FIGURE 1: Bacterial detection in tonsils of patients with higher hypertrophy. The graph shows the frequency of bacterial detection in tonsils (a) and in adenoids (b). The graph shows the patients who presented bacterial codetection in the (c) tonsils and in adenoids (d).

S. pneumoniae, *P. aeruginosa*, and *S. aureus*. It is important to note that the tests were done on tissue fragments of both AD and PT, as well as on NPWs, which cannot distinguish the exact niche where these microbial genomic DNA were found. There is some evidence that points out that the microbiome of tonsils and adenoids may vary according to the microniche analyzed. Using *in situ* hybridization technique, for instance, Swidsinski et al. demonstrated in asymptomatic individuals that, depending on the type of bacteria, these microbes are mainly found either infiltrating the adenoid and tonsils, in the surface covered by a thick slime of inflammatory cells or within tissue macrophages [30].

Regardless of the state of tonsillar hypertrophy, the highest detection rates of *H. influenzae* and *S. pneumoniae* were found in approximately 80% of the patients, while *M. catarrhalis* and *P. aeruginosa* were found in almost 50% of the children, and *S. aureus* in only 15%. These results are in agreement with previously published data [31, 32], and corroborate with the findings that *H. influenzae*, *M. catarrhalis*, *S. pneumoniae*, and *P. aeruginosa* colonize the upper respiratory tract of a large proportion of children. In addition, the genome load for different bacteria varied significantly in the same tissue, suggesting that potentially pathogenic bacteria may vary widely in tonsillar biofilms.

The lack of uniform association of specific bacteria with tonsil hypertrophy is not surprising and suggests that the role of these bacteria in the development of tonsillar hypertrophy is far from clear and probably not due to a direct effect.

The sampling sites and methods used for bacterial detection are critical in this type of study. Pathogenic and anaerobic bacteria are easily detected in the nuclei of the tonsils, while commensal aerobic bacteria are found on the surface of these tissues [33, 34]. In addition, bacterial cultures detect only viable microorganisms, while molecular methods can detect scarce quantities of noncultured bacteria [35]. Also, molecular analyses based on sequencing and pirosequencing of 16S ribosomal RNA have been used with the objective to determine the microbiota localized on the surface and inside the adenoid tissue [36].

In the present study, different types of clinical samples were tested for five potentially pathogenic bacteria by a sensitive molecular assay, the real-time PCR assay. Nasopharyngeal lavages allowed the detection of planktonic bacteria, while fragments of tonsillar tissue provided direct association with sessile biofilms. No differences were observed in bacterial frequency or bacterial loads between control children and patients with adenotonsillar hypertrophy. We should emphasize that bacterial detection was widely different between adenoids and palatine tonsils in all patient groups. This suggests that there may be tissue-specific colonization by these bacteria in different tonsils, rather than a homogenous distribution of planktonic biofilm microorganisms in all tissues.

Several studies indicate that *H. influenzae* may be associated with tonsillar hypertrophy. For example, although Van Staaij and colleagues found similar rates of detection of *H. influenzae* in patients with and without chronic adenotonsillar disease, this bacterium was significantly more frequent in patients with more severe tonsillar hypertrophy. This result was in agreement with other published studies [37–39]. In addition, Brodsky et al. [32] found in *H. influenzae* a significant positive association between high bacterial load and tonsil weight.

In the present study, kappa analysis compared the detection of a bacterium at different sampling sites of different patient groups to assess whether extensive infection by certain bacteria could be associated with amygdala hypertrophy. In the control group, represented by the children as ATH group, despite the difference of slits in the middle ages, a good correlation was found between the detection of *H. influenzae* in the tonsils and in the adenoids, but the agreement was only moderate or poor for the detection of between other sampling sites and the other groups.

The rates of detection of *M. catarrhalis* were higher in patients with severe adenotonsillar hypertrophy, and there was good agreement between the detection of this bacterium in NPW, adenoids, and palatine tonsils of these patients. Perhaps *M. catarrhalis* infection may be relevant to the development of adenotonsillar hypertrophy or, alternatively, the involvement of *M. catarrhalis* in the normal nasopharynx microbiota is favored by tonsillar hypertrophy. In fact, the presence of MCR_1483, a protein generally expressed during inflammation of the respiratory tract, may facilitate colonization by *M. catarrhalis* [40].

The role of colonizing bacteria in the development of tonsillar hypertrophy is currently unknown. In our study, we evaluated a single facet of a complex interaction between the microbiota and the host. The influence of other factors, including the individual characteristics of each patient's immune system, coinfection, and other nonmicrobial agents, could eventually interfere with the results [41–43]. A particularly useful example of mutual cross protection in complex populations of bacteria was that *H. influenzae* could be protected from death mediated by complement by *M. catarrhalis* [41].

5. Conclusions

In summary, in the present study, a high proportion of children with chronic tonsillar inflammation and hypertrophy had detectable potentially pathogenic bacteria in tonsillar tissues, as well as in the control patients. Importantly, in patients with more severe tonsillar hypertrophy,

there was good agreement between sites for detection of *M. catarrhalis*, suggesting that this bacterium may be associated with more severe tonsillar hypertrophy or, alternatively, the microenvironment of chronically inflamed hypertrophic tonsils can facilitate colonization by *M. catarrhalis*. The roles played by *M. catarrhalis* in the biofilm of severely hypertrophic tonsils may well be related to protection of certain other bacteria from innate immunity factors, in a way similar to what was documented for *H. influenzae*. More comprehensive prospection of tonsillar microbiomes are required in order to better assess the roles that bacteria may play in adenotonsillar hypertrophy.

Acknowledgments

The authors thank Maria Cecília Onofre for secretarial assistance. This study was supported by São Paulo Research Foundation–FAPESP, CAPES, and CNPq.

References

[1] J. L. Proenca-Modena, F. C. P. Valera, M. G. Jacob et al., "High rates of detection of respiratory viruses in tonsillar tissues from children with chronic adenotonsillar disease," *PLoS One*, vol. 7, no. 8, Article ID e42136, 2012.

[2] L. H. Endo, J. Vassallo, E. Sakano, and P. Brousset, "Detection of Epstein-Barr virus and subsets of lymphoid cells in adenoid tissue of children under 2 years of age," *International Journal of Pediatric Otorhinolaryngology*, vol. 66, no. 3, pp. 223–226, 2002.

[3] P. Kurnatowski, L. Putynski, M. Lapienis, and B. Kowalska, "Physical and emotional disturbances in children with adenotonsillar hypertrophy," *Journal of Laryngology and Otology*, vol. 122, no. 9, pp. 931–935, 2008.

[4] U. L. Demir, B. Cetinkaya, S. Karaca, and D. Sigirli, "The impacts of adenotonsillar hypertrophy on periodontal health in children: a prospective controlled pilot study," *American Journal of Otolaryngology*, vol. 34, no. 5, pp. 501–504, 2013.

[5] H. Faden, L. Duffy, A. Williams, D. A. Krystofik, and J. Wolf, "Epidemiology of nasopharyngeal colonization with nontypeable *Haemophilus influenzae* in the first 2 years of life," *Journal of Infectious Diseases*, vol. 172, no. 1, pp. 132–135, 1995.

[6] M. M. Pettigrew, J. F. Gent, R. B. Pyles, A. L. Miller, J. Nokso-Koivisto, and T. Chonmaitree, "Viral-bacterial interactions and risk of acute otitis media complicating upper respiratory tract infection," *Journal of Clinical Microbiology*, vol. 49, no. 11, pp. 3750–3755, 2011.

[7] Y. J. Moghaddam, M. Rafeey, and R. Radfar, "Comparative assessment of *Helicobacter pylori* colonization in children tonsillar tissues," *International Journal of Pediatric Otorhinolaryngology*, vol. 73, no. 9, pp. 1199–1201, 2009.

[8] P. Brandtzaeg, "Immunology of tonsils and adenoids: everything the ENT surgeon needs to know," *International Journal of Pediatric Otorhinolaryngology*, vol. 67, no. 1, pp. S69–S76, 2003.

[9] P. Hellings, M. Jorissen, and J. L. Ceuppens, "The Waldeyer's ring," *Acta Oto-Rhino-Laryngologica Belgica*, vol. 54, no. 3, pp. 237–241, 2000.

[10] D. Bogaert, R. de Groot, and P. W. H. Hermans, "Streptococcus pneumoniae colonisation: the key to pneumococcal disease," *The Lancet Infectious Diseases*, vol. 4, no. 3, pp. 144–154, 2004.

[11] J. A. García-Rodríguez and M. J. F. Martinez, "Dynamics of nasopharyngeal colonization by potential respiratory pathogens," *Journal of Antimicrobial Chemotherapy*, vol. 50, no. 3, pp. 59–74, 2002.

[12] K. A. Brogden, J. M. Guthmiller, and C. E. Taylor, "Human polymicrobial infections," *The Lancet*, vol. 365, no. 9455, pp. 253–255, 2005.

[13] G. A. Mackenzie, A. J. Leach, J. R. Carapetis, J. Fisher, and P. S. Morris, "Epidemiology of nasopharyngeal carriage of respiratory bacterial pathogens in children and adults: cross-sectional surveys in a population with high rates of pneumococcal disease," *BMC Infectious Diseases*, vol. 10, p. 310, 2010.

[14] A. A. T. M. Bosch, G. Biesbroek, K. Trzcinski, E. A. M. Sanders, and D. Bogaert, "Viral and bacterial interactions in the upper respiratory tract," *PLoS Pathogens*, vol. 9, no. 1, article e1003057, 2013.

[15] S. Torretta, L. Drago, P. Marchisio et al., "Recurrences in chronic tonsillitis substained by tonsillar biofilm-producing bacteria in children. Relationship with the grade of tonsillar hyperplasy," *International Journal of Pediatric Otorhinolaryngology*, vol. 77, no. 2, pp. 200–204, 2013.

[16] C. E. Corless, M. Guiver, R. Borrow, V. Edwards-Jones, A. J. Fox, and E. B. Kaczmarski, "Simultaneous detection of Neisseria meningitidis, Haemophilus influenzae, and Streptococcus pneumoniae in suspected cases of meningitis and septicemia using real-time PCR," *Journal of Clinical Microbiology*, vol. 39, no. 4, pp. 1553–1558, 2001.

[17] A. Kilic, K. L. Muldrew, Y.-W. Tang, and A. Celal Basustaoglu, "Triplex real-time polymerase chain reaction assay for simultaneous detection of Staphylococcus aureus and coagulase-negative staphylococci and determination of methicillin resistance directly from positive blood culture bottles," *Diagnostic Microbiology and Infectious Disease*, vol. 66, no. 4, pp. 349–355, 2010.

[18] M. M. Feizabadi, A. Majnooni, B. Nomanpour et al., "Direct detection of Pseudomonas aeruginosa from patients with healthcare associated pneumonia by real time PCR," *Infection, Genetics and Evolution*, vol. 10, no. 8, pp. 1247–1251, 2010.

[19] G. M. Abdeldaim, A. Majnooni, B. Nomanpour et al., "Detection of Haemophilus influenzae in respiratory secretions from pneumonia patients by quantitative real-time polymerase chain reaction," *Diagnostic Microbiology and Infectious Disease*, vol. 64, no. 4, pp. 366–373, 2009.

[20] N. Heiniger, V. Spaniol, R. Troller, M. Vischer, and C. Aebi, "A reservoir of Moraxella catarrhalis in human pharyngeal lymphoid tissue," *Journal of Infectious Diseases*, vol. 196, no. 7, pp. 1080–1087, 2007.

[21] O. N. Develioglu, H. D. Ipek, H. Bahar, G. Can, M. Kulekci, and G. Aygun, "Bacteriological evaluation of tonsillar microbial flora according to age and tonsillar size in recurrent tonsillitis," *European Archives of Oto-Rhino-Laryngology*, vol. 271, no. 6, pp. 1661–1665, 2014.

[22] K. Stelter, "Tonsillitis and sore throat in children," *GMS Current Topics in Otorhinolaryngology-Head and Neck Surgery*, vol. 13, no. 7, pp. 1–24, 2014.

[23] Q. Wang, J. Du, C. Jie, H. Ouyang, R. Luo, and W. Li, "Bacteriology and antibiotic sensitivity of tonsillar diseases in Chinese children," *European Archives of Oto-Rhino-Laryngology*, vol. 274, no. 8, pp. 3153–3159, 2017.

[24] H. El-Hakim, "Tonsillectomy or adenotonsillectomy versus non-surgical treatment for chronic/recurrent acute tonsillitis," *Paediatrics & Child Health*, vol. 22, no. 2, pp. 94-95, 2017.

[25] J. J. Johnston and R. Douglas, "Adenotonsillar microbiome: an update," *Postgraduate Medical Journal*, vol. 94, no. 1113, pp. 398–403, 2018.

[26] A. Rajeshwary, S. Rai, G. Somayaji, and V. Pai, "Bacteriology of symptomatic adenoids in children," *North American Journal of Medical Sciences*, vol. 5, no. 2, pp. 113–118, 2013.

[27] B. Winther, B. C. Gross, J. O. Hendley, and S.V. Early, "Location of bacterial biofilm in the mucus overlying the adenoid by light microscopy," *Archives of Otolaryngology-Head & Neck Surgery*, vol. 135, no. 12, pp. 1239–1245, 2009.

[28] T. Ren, D. U. Glatt, T. N. Nguyen et al., "16S rRNA survey revealed complex bacterial communities and evidence of bacterial interference on human adenoids," *Environmental Microbiology*, vol. 15, no. 2, pp. 535–547, 2013.

[29] I. Brook, "The role of anaerobic bacteria in tonsillitis," *International Journal of Pediatric Otorhinolaryngology*, vol. 69, no. 1, pp. 9–19, 2005.

[30] A. Swidsinski, O. Göktas, C. Bessler et al., "Spatial organisation of microbiota in quiescent adenoiditis and tonsillitis," *Journal of Clinical Pathology*, vol. 60, no. 3, pp. 253–260, 2006.

[31] B. K. Van Staaij, E. H. Van Den Akker, E. H. De Haas Van Dorsser et al., "Does the tonsillar surface flora differ in children with and without tonsillar disease?," *Acta Oto-Laryngologica*, vol. 123, no. 7, pp. 873–878, 2003.

[32] L. Brodsky, L. Moore, and J. Stanievich, "The role of *Haemophilus influenzae* in the pathogenesis of tonsillar hypertrophy in children," *The Laryngoscope*, vol. 98, no. 10, pp. 1055–1060, 1988.

[33] J. B. Surow, S. D. Handler, S. A. Telian, G. R. Fleisher, and C. C. Baranak, "Bacteriology of tonsil surface and core in children," *The Laryngoscope*, vol. 99, no. 3, pp. 261–266, 1989.

[34] I. Brook, K. Shah, and W. Jackson, "Microbiology of healthy and diseased adenoids," *The Laryngoscope*, vol. 110, no. 6, pp. 994–999, 2000.

[35] J. T. Keer and L. Birch, "Molecular methods for the assessment of bacterial viability," *Journal of Microbiological Methods*, vol. 53, no. 3, pp. 175–183, 2003.

[36] L. Nistico, R. Kreft, A. Gieseke et al., "Adenoid reservoir for pathogenic biofilm bacteria," *Journal of Clinical Microbiology*, vol. 49, no. 4, pp. 1411–1420, 2011.

[37] R. Lindroos, "Bacteriology of the tonsil core in recurrent tonsillitis and tonsillar hyperplasia-a short review," *Acta Oto-Laryngologica*, vol. 120, no. 543, pp. 206–208, 2000.

[38] J. H. Jeong, D. W. Lee, R. A. Ryu et al., "Bacteriologic comparison of tonsil core in recurrent tonsillitis and tonsillar hypertrophy," *The Laryngoscope*, vol. 117, no. 12, pp. 2146–2151, 2007.

[39] E. A. Trafny, O. Olszewska-Sosinska, M. Antos-Bielska et al., "Carriage of antibiotic-resistant *Haemophilus influenzae* strains in children undergoing adenotonsillectomy," *International Journal of Medical Microbiology*, vol. 304, no. 5-6, pp. 554–564, 2014.

[40] S. P. W. de Vries, M. J. Eleveld, P. W. M. Hermans, and H. J. Bootsma, "Characterization of the molecular interplay

between *Moraxella catarrhalis* and human respiratory tract epithelial cells," *PLoS One*, vol. 8, no. 8, Article ID e72193, 2013.

[41] T. T. Tong, M. Morgelin, A. Forsgren, and K. Riesbeck, "*Haemophilus influenzae* survival during complement-mediated attacks is promoted by *Moraxella catarrhalis* outer membrane vesicles," *Journal of Infectious Diseases*, vol. 195, no. 11, pp. 1661–1670, 2007.

[42] T. Marom, J. Nokso-Koivisto, and T. Chonmaitree, "Viral-bacterial interactions in acute otitis media," *Current Allergy and Asthma Reports*, vol. 12, no. 6, pp. 551–558, 2012.

[43] T. F. Murphy, A. L. Brauer, C. Kirkham et al., "Role of the zinc uptake ABC transporter of *Moraxella catarrhalis* in persistence in the respiratory tract," *Infection and Immunity*, vol. 81, no. 9, pp. 3406–3413, 2013.

14

Helicobacter pylori Infection and Its Risk Factors: A Prospective Cross-Sectional Study in Resource-Limited Settings of Northwest Ethiopia

Markos Negash [ID],[1] **Habtamu Wondifraw Baynes** [ID],[2] **and Demeke Geremew**[1]

[1]*Department of Immunology and Molecular Biology, School of Biomedical and Laboratory Sciences, College of Medicine and Health Sciences, University of Gondar, Gondar, Ethiopia*
[2]*Department of Clinical Chemistry, School of Biomedical and Laboratory Sciences, College of Medicine and Health Sciences, University of Gondar, Gondar, Ethiopia*

Correspondence should be addressed to Markos Negash; markosnegash@yahoo.com

Guest Editor: Teresa Fasciana

Background. Helicobacter pylori (H. pylori) is implicated for the causation of gastrointestinal tract infections including gastric cancer. Although the infection is prevalent globally, the impact is immense in countries with poor environmental and socioeconomic status including Ethiopia. Epidemiological study on the magnitude of H. pylori and possible risk factors has priceless implication. Therefore, in this study, we determined the prevalence and risk factors of H. pylori infection in the resource-limited area of northwest Ethiopia. *Methods.* A prospective cross-sectional study was conducted on northwest Ethiopia among 201 systematically selected dyspeptic patients. Data were collected using a structured and pretested questionnaire, and stool and serum samples were collected and analyzed by SD BIOLINE H. pylori Ag and dBest H. pylori Disk tests, respectively. Chi-square test was performed to see association between variables, and binary and multinomial regression tests were performed to identify potential risk factors. P values <0.05 were taken statistically significant. *Result.* Prevalence of H. pylori was found to be 71.1% (143/201) and 37.3% (75/201) using the dBest H. pylori Test Disk and SD BIOLINE H. pylori Ag test, respectively. H. pylori seropositivity, using dBest H. pylori Disk tests, is significantly associated in age groups <10 years ($P = 0.044$) and married patients ($P = 0.016$). In those patients with H. pylori (a positive result with either the Ab or Ag test), drinking water from well sources had 2.23 times risk of getting H. pylori infection ($P = 0.017$), and drinking coffee (1.51 (0.79–2.96, $P = 0.025$)) and chat chewing (1.78 (1.02–3.46, $P = 0.008$) are the common risk factors. *Conclusion.* The present study discovered considerable magnitude of H. pylori among the dyspeptic patients in the study area. H. pylori infection is frequent in individuals drinking water from well sources, and thus, poor sanitation and unhygienic water supply are contributing factors. Policies aiming at improving the socioeconomic status will reduce potential sources of infection, transmission, and ultimately the prevalence and incidence of H. pylori.

1. Background

Helicobacter pylori (H. pylori) was the first formally recognized bacterial carcinogen. It has been etiologically associated with gastritis, peptic ulcer disease, gastric adenocarcinoma, and primary gastric lymphoma [1, 2].

Helicobacter pylori (H. pylori) colonizes 70–90% of the population in developing countries, whereas it is around 50% in developed countries [3–5]. In developing countries, an early childhood acquisition of H. pylori (30–50%)

reaching over 90% during adulthood is the pattern of infection. Unless treated, colonization persists lifelong. H. pylori infection has been attributed to poor socioeconomic status, poor hygienic practice, and overcrowding condition [6, 7], a whole mark in developing countries.

The bacterium differs genetically, survives in harsh acidic gastric environment, and currently develops resistance for several antibiotics. Although epidemiological distribution of H. pylori varies globally, the magnitude of H. pylori has been shown to be 70.1% (Africa), 69.4% (South America), 66.6%

(Western Asia), 34.3% (Western Europe), and 37.1% (North America) [8–10].

The prevalence of *H. pylori* in the Ethiopian dyspeptic patients is similarly high to other developing countries because most Ethiopian population live in households with low socioeconomic status and hygiene [7, 11, 12]. Magnitude of *H. pylori* among the outpatient department (based on a test kit detecting Immunoglobulin G (IgG) antibodies) at the University of Gondar Hospital (UOG Hospital) was ranged between 65.7% and 85.6% [13, 14]. Besides, it is a common reason to seek primary healthcare service and accounts for 10% of hospital admissions [15, 16].

All previous prevalence researches in the study area were conducted using IgG and/or IgM antibody rapid tests which have questionable performance in detecting acute infection and distinguishing active infection from previous exposure. Hence, the current study was conducted with an aim to determine the prevalence of *H. pylori* infection among the dyspeptic patients attending the UOG hospital in northwest Ethiopia, using stool antigen as well as serum antibodies technique and assessing potential risk factors.

2. Methods

2.1. Study Design, Period, and Area. This is a facility-based cross-sectional study which was conducted on patients with dyspepsia from February to March 2016 at the University of Gondar Hospital, Gondar, Ethiopia. The University of Gondar Hospital is one of the pioneer teaching hospitals in Ethiopia conducting community-based researches, providing teaching and diagnostic services for more than 5 million inhabitants.

2.2. Study Participants and Clinical Data Collection. After informed consent was taken from the dyspeptic patients, who visited the hospital outpatient department, suspected of *H. pylori* infection, all relevant clinical and sociodemographic data were collected using a structured and pretested questionnaire by trained data collectors.

2.3. Specimen Collection and Processing. Stool and blood specimens were collected from each patient for *H. pylori* antigen and antibody tests, respectively. The blood was centrifuged until serum is separated and stored in −20°C. The stool specimens were also stored in −20°C until the tests were performed. For this study, we followed the methods of Negash et al. [17] which has been evaluated four *H. pylori* diagnostic tests in the study area.

2.3.1. SD Bioline H. pylori Ag Test (Standard Diagnostic, Inc., Korea). Principle: the SD BIOLINE *H. pylori* Ag rapid test kit result window has 2 precoated lines, "T" (Test Line) and "C" (Control Line). Both the Test Line and the Control Line in the result window are not visible before applying any samples. The "T"' window coated with monoclonal anti-*H. pylori* will form a line after the addition of the stool specimen (if there is *H. pylori* antigen). The Control window is used for

the procedural control, and a line should always appear if the test procedure is performed correctly, and the test reagents are working [17].

2.3.2. dBest H. pylori Test Disk (Ameritech Diagnostic Reagent Co., Ltd., Tongxiang, Zhejiang, China). Principle: this test contains a membrane strip, which is precoated with *H. pylori* capture antigen on the test band region. The *H. pylori* antigen-colloid gold conjugate and serum sample moves along the membrane chromatographically to the test region (T) and forms a visible line as the antigen-antibody-antigen gold particle complex forms. This test device has a letter of T and C as "Test Line" and "Control Line" on the surface of the case. Both the test line and control line in the result window are not visible before applying any samples. The control line is used for the procedural control. Control line should always appear if the test procedure is performed properly, and the test reagents of the control line are working [17].

2.4. Statistical Analysis. The data were cleaned and double entered on the excel spread sheet and transported to Statistical Package for Social Sciences (SPSS). The chi-square test was performed to see association between dependent and independent variables. Binary logistic regression and multinomial regression tests were performed to identify potential risk factors of *H. pylori* infection. P value less than 0.05 were considered statistically significant.

3. Result

3.1. Demographic Characteristics. A total of 201 dyspeptic patients were included in the study, and serum and stool samples were analyzed by dBest *H. pylori* Test Disk and SD BIOLINE *H. pylori* Ag tests, respectively. The mean ± SD (range) age of the participants was 29.5 ± 14.85 (7–85) years with a median of 23 years. The majority (140) of the study participants were male (69%), study subjects from the urban area (141) accounted 70%, and 69 (34.3%) of the participants were married. Of 201 participants, 104 (51%) were students, 38 (18.9%) were farmers, and 23 (11.4%) were house wives (Table 1). In this study, participants who were diagnosed as positive to the *H. pylori* stool antigen test were immediately commenced appropriate therapy.

3.2. Prevalence of H. pylori with respect to Sociodemography of Participants. Accordingly, the prevalence of *H. pylori* was found to be 71.1% (143/201) and 37.3% (75/201) using the dBest *H. pylori* Ab Test Disk (95% CI: 64.2–77.6) and SD BIOLINE *H. pylori* Ag test (95% CI: 30.3–44.3), respectively (Table 2). The highest prevalence of *H. pylori* infection was seen among the males than the females (98 vs 45 by Ab test and 79 vs 27 by Ag test), and *H. pylori* is more frequent in individuals living from the urban area than rural (101 vs 42 using the Ab test and 76 vs 30 using the Ag test), respectively. Regarding the occupational status, the students are the majority groups who come up positive for *H. pylori* (both in

TABLE 1: Prevalence of *H. pylori* infection among the dyspeptic patients across sociodemographic characteristics at the University of Gondar Hospital Outpatient Department, $N = 201$.

Sociodemographic characteristics		Positive for the Ab test, N (%)	Positive for the Ag test, N (%)	Total, N (%)
Sex	Male	98 (70)	79 (56.7)	140 (69.7)
	Female	45 (73.8)	27 (44.3)	61 (30.3)
Age (years)	<10	1 (50)*	1 (50)	2 (1)
	10–19	10 (55.6)	12 (66.7)	18 (9)
	20–29	82 (67.2)	68 (55.7)	122 (60.6)
	30–39	12 (66.7)	6 (33.3)	18 (9)
	40–49	13 (92.9)	9 (64.3)	14 (7)
	50–59	12 (92.3)	5 (38.5)	13 (6.4)
	≥60	13 (92.9)	5 (35.7)	14 (7)
Residence	Urban	101 (71.6)	76 (53.9)	141 (70.1)
	Rural	42 (70)	30 (50)	60 (29.9)
Occupation	Farmer	30 (78.9)	19 (50)	38 (18.9)
	Student	73 (70.2)	64 (61.5)	104 (51.7)
	Government	14 (63.6)	8 (36.4)	22 (11)
	House wife	17 (73.9)	9 (39.1)	23 (11.4)
	Merchant	7 (87.5)	4 (50)	8 (4)
	No jobs	2 (33.3)	2 (33.3)	6 (3)
Education	Illiterate	40 (80)	24 (48)	50 (24.9)
	Primary	12 (63.2)	8 (42.1)	19 (9.5)
	Secondary	15 (62.5)	10 (41.7)	24 (11.9)
	College	76 (70.4)	64 (49.3)	108 (53.7)
Marital status	Married	56 (81.2)**	34 (49.3)	69 (34.3)
	Single	87 (65.9)	72 (54.5)	132 (65.7)
Number of siblings	0	94 (67.1)	80 (57.1)	140 (69.7)
	1–4	29 (76.3)	15 (39.5)	38 (18.9)
	5–10	20 (87)	11 (47.8)	23 (11.4)

N = number; Ag = antigen; Ab = antibody. *P value = 0.044; **P value = 0.016.

TABLE 2: Prevalence of *H. pylori* infection among the dyspeptic patients attending the University of Gondar Hospital Outpatient Department, $N = 201$.

Serologic tests	Prevalence of *H. pylori*			
	N	Percent (%)	SE	95% CI
dBest *H. pylori* Ab rapid test	143	71.1	3.2	64.2–77.6
SD BIOLINE *H. pylori* Ag test	75	37.3	3.5	30.3–44.3

N = number; SE = standard error; CI = confidence interval; Ag = antigen; Ab = Antibody.

the Ab and Ag tests) than others, and meanwhile *H. pylori* seropositivity, using the dBest *H. pylori* Disk tests, is significantly associated with the age groups <10 years (P value = 0.044) and married patients (P value = 0.016) (Table 1).

3.3. H. pylori Infection across Clinical Parameters and Associated Risk Factors. Clinically, the patients with heartburn, abdominal fullness, and belching had come up with positive for the *H. pylori* tests, and likewise, belching is significantly associated ($P = 0.038$), in logistic regression, with the antibody test. In those patients with *H. pylori* (a positive result with either a Ab or Ag test), drinking water from well sources had 2.23 times risk of getting *H. pylori* infection ($P = 0.017$), and drinking coffee (1.51 (0.79–2.96, $P = 0.025$) and chat chewing (1.78 (1.02–3.46, $P = 0.008$) are the most common risk factors (Tables 3 and 4).

4. Discussion

A recent study demonstrated that 65.3% of the patients were positive for *H. pylori* IgG using the immunochromatographic method [13]. This shows that the current prevalence of *H. pylori* infection based on antibodies is much lower. The current 37.3% magnitude of *H. pylori*, using the SD BIOLINE *H. pylori* Ag test, is lower than a 52.3% and 53% of report from Ethiopia [18, 19] and studies from African and Asian countries [20–22]. The variation for these findings might be the difference in the socioeconomic factors, exposure for risk factors, study settings, and essentially the variability in the diagnostic methods.

The present study revealed that *H. pylori* seropositivity has been associated with age. In developing nations, where the majority of children are infected before the age of 10, the prevalence in adults peaks at more than 80% before age 50 [23–25]. While in developed countries, evidence of infection in children is unusual but becomes more common later on adulthood. In this study, the increment in serological positivity of *H. pylori* is seen starting from children through adulthood which reaches the peak on 18–30 age groups (68 (55.7%)), but cases are becoming lower as the age gets older and older. Within any age group, infection appears to be more common in blacks and Hispanics compared to the white population; these differences are probably in part related to socioeconomic factors [26, 27].

TABLE 3: Prevalence of *H. pylori* infection among the dyspeptic patients across risk factors at the University of Gondar Hospital Outpatient Department, $N = 201$.

Risk factors		Positive for the Ab test, N (%)	Positive for the Ag test, N (%)	Total, N (%)	Multivariate OR (95% CI)	P value
Water source	Pipeline	111 (69.4)	86 (53.8)	160 (79.6)		
	River	27 (77.1)	15 (42.9)	35 (17.4)	2.23 (1.26–4.46)	0.017
	Well	5 (83.3)	5 (83.3)	6 (3)		
Washing hands with soap		87 (73.1)	63 (52.9)	119 (59.2)	1.04 (0.39–2.9)	0.743
Using toilet		69 (73.4)	49 (52.1)	94 (46.8)	1.80 (0.62–6.48)	0.496
Drinking alcohol		40 (65.6)	34 (55.7)	61 (30.3)	1.02 (0.48–2.9)	0.949
Drinking coffee		69 (74.2)	51 (54.8)	93 (46.3)	1.51 (0.79–2.96)	0.025
Chat chewing		4 (80)	4 (80)	5 (2.5)	1.78 (1.02–3.46)	0.008

TABLE 4: Prevalence of *H. pylori* infection among the dyspeptic patients across clinical parameters at the University of Gondar Hospital Outpatient Department, $N = 201$.

Clinical parameters	Positive for the Ab test, N (%)	Positive for the Ag test, N (%)	Total, N (%)
Heartburn	139 (70.6)	104 (47.2)	197 (98)
Epigastric pain	139 (70.9)	103 (52.6)	196 (97.5)
Abdominal fullness	133 (70.4)	101 (53.4)	189 (94)
Vomiting	51 (72.9)	41 (58.6)	70 (34.8)
Nausea	106 (71.1)	83 (55.7)	149 (74.1)
Belching	110 (71.4)	75 (48.7)*	154 (76.6)
Melena	43 (71.7)	27 (45)	60 (29.9)
Bloody vomiting	14 (87.5)	12 (75)	16 (8)

N = number; Ab = antibody; Ag = antigen. *P value = 0.038.

The increased prevalence of infection with age was initially thought to represent a continuing rate of bacterial acquisition throughout one's lifetime. However, epidemiologic evidence now indicates most infections are acquired during childhood even in developed countries [24, 28]. Most infections were acquired before five years of age with a declining incidence thereafter in one report from Ireland [29]. Thus, the frequency of *H. pylori* infection for any age group in any locality reflects that particular cohort's rate of bacterial acquisition during childhood years [28]. The organisms can be cultured from vomitus or diarrheal stools suggesting the potential for transmission among family members during periods of illness [30, 31].

The risk of acquiring *H. pylori* infection is related to the socioeconomic status and living conditions early in life. Factors such as density of housing, overcrowding, number of siblings, sharing a bed, and lack of running water have all been linked to a higher acquisition rate of *H. pylori* infection [32–34]. Our study proved that risk factors for acquiring *H. pylori* infection are most prevalent in the patients with *H. pylori* infection. Moreover, studies in the developing countries continue to show that childhood hygiene practices, and family education determines the prevalence of *H. pylori* infection [35]. In this study, illiterate individual accounts the majority (40/143 were positive for *H. pylori* Ab, and 24/106 were positive for *H. pylori* Ag tests) of *H. pylori* cases next to those who visited college. The association of *H. pylori* infection with the level of education, income, and race/ethnicity is not unique to *H. pylori*, since similar associations have been described with other chronic infections including cytomegalovirus, *herpes simplex virus-1*, and

hepatitis B [36]. Studies indicated that declination of *H. pylori* infection has been attributed to economic progress and improvement in sanitation [37]. This study revealed that most (101/143 (antibody); 76/106 (antigen)) *H. pylori* positive cases are from the urban areas indicating that urbanization accompanied with poor sanitation.

The route by which infection occurs remains unknown, but multiple ways of transmission are reported [38, 39]. Person-to-person transmission of *H. pylori* through either fecal/oral or oral/oral seems most likely [31, 39]. Humans appear to be the major reservoir of infection; however, *H. pylorus has* been isolated from primates in captivity and from domestic cats [40, 41]. One report described the identification of *H. pylori* in milk and gastric tissue of sheep suggesting that sheep may be a natural host for the organism [42]. This may explain the higher infection rate that has been observed among shepherds compared to their siblings [43]. Similarly in our study, form the total *H. pylori* cases, farmers accounted the second highest proportion showing that close contact with domestic cattle may potentially result *H. pylori* transmission.

In addition to fecal/oral transmission of bacteria, contaminated water supplies in developing countries may serve as an environmental source of bacteria. In this study, majority (111/143 (antibody), 86/106 (antigen)) of *H. pylori* positive individuals use water sources from pipeline. The organism remains viable in water for several days and, using the polymerase chain reaction techniques, evidence of *H. pylori* can be found in most samples of municipal water from the endemic areas of infection [44–46]. Children who regularly swim in rivers, streams, and pools drink stream water, or eat uncooked vegetables are more likely to be infected [47]. *H. pylori* have been cultured from diarrheal stools of children in Gambia, West Africa, where almost all inhabitants are infected by five years of age [48].

Intrafamilial clustering of infection further supports person-to-person transmission. Infected individuals are more likely to have infected spouses and children than uninfected individuals [34, 49]. A study of children in Columbia found that the risk of infection correlated directly with the number of children aged 2 to 9 in the household, while younger children were more likely to be infected if older siblings were also infected [50]. Isolation of genetically identical strains of *H. pylori* from multiple family members [51] and custodial patients in the same institution [52] and further studies support transmission among persons sharing the same living environment. In addition to the familial type of transmission that occurs in developed and other nations, horizontal transmission between persons who do not belong to a core family also appears to take place in countries where the prevalence of infection is high [49]. As revealed by studies conducted on Ethiopia and Thailand [14, 53, 54], *H. pylori* infection is higher in married individuals demonstrating that cluster living environment has an impact on *H. pylori* transmission.

At last, it should be considered that the dyspeptic patients, other than the present serum antibody and stool antigen tests, did not undergo further confirmatory tests (endoscopy with biopsy for the histology culture and/or the very least urea breath test) due to economic constraints.

5. Conclusion

The present study discovered considerable magnitude of *H. pylori* in the study area. *H. pylori* infection is frequent in individuals drinking water from well sources, and thus, poor sanitation and unhygienic water supply are contributing factors. Policies aiming at improving the socioeconomic status will reduce potential sources of infection, transmission, and ultimately the prevalence and incidence of *H. pylori* infection.

Abbreviations

Ab: Antibody
Ag: Antigen
IgG: Immunoglobulin G
IgM: Immunoglobulin M
IRB: Institutional Review Board
SD: Standard deviation
SPSS: Statistical Package for Social Sciences
UOG: University of Gondar Hospital.

Ethical Approval

This project was ethically cleared by the Institutional Review Board (IRB) of the University of Gondar. Participation was voluntary, and informed verbal consent was taken from all adult participants and from the next of kin, caretakers, or guardians on behalf of the minors/children before inclusion to the study. Initially, the participants were briefly explained about the objectives of the study, risks, and benefits of the procedures and on voluntary participation and the right to withdraw at any stage of the study using their local language. Participants were then asked if they understood what has been explained to them. If and only if they understand the facts, implications, and future consequences of their action on themselves or their children, they would like to be part of the study. Written consent was not acquired because all the participants were recruited from the outpatient department laboratory of the Gondar University Hospital where all the participant patients were sent to undergo the *H. pylori* antibody test. The additional stool antigen test was a noninvasive procedure with minimal or no risk associated with it. Besides, the patients were benefited from the stool antigen test as it added further information on whether to commence eradication therapy by the attending physician. The result from the antibody test was collected from the laboratory record book. Official permission was also obtained from the University of Gondar Hospital before access to the record book and the conduct of the study. Therefore, considering all these facts, only the verbal agreement was acquired to be included in the study. The IRB has also evaluated the consent procedure and cleared it as sufficient. Participants who were diagnosed as positive to the *H. pylori* stool antigen test were immediately linked to the medical outpatient department of the University of Gondar Hospital for appropriate treatment and follow-up.

Authors' Contributions

MN, HWB, and DG conceived the study concept and designed the study. MN and DG carried out data collection and laboratory analysis. MN, HWB, and DG supervised the data collection and laboratory analysis. MN, HWB, and DG analyzed the data and prepared the first manuscript draft. MN and DG reviewed the draft. All authors read and approved the final manuscript. All the authors are currently working at the University of Gondar.

Acknowledgments

Our gratitude goes to the technical staffs, the University of Gondar Hospital, and the staff for the unreserved support during the study and all the study participants.

References

[1] J. G. Kusters, A. H. M. Van Vliet, and E. J. Kuipers, "Pathogenesis of *Helicobacter pylori* infection," *Clinical Microbiology Reviews*, vol. 19, no. 3, pp. 449–490, 2006.

[2] M. Safavi, R. Sabourian, and A. Foroumadi, "Treatment of *Helicobacter pylori* infection: current and future insights," *World Journal of Clinical Cases*, vol. 4, no. 1, pp. 5–19, 2016.

[3] B. A. Salih, "*Helicobacter pylori* infection in developing countries: the burden for how long?," *Saudi Journal of Gastroenterology*, vol. 15, no. 3, pp. 201–207, 2009.

[4] R. M. Patrick, S. R. Kenn, and A. P. Michel, *Medical Microbiology*, Elsevier, New York, NY, USA, 5th edition, 2005.

[5] Y. G. David, Y. C. Lee, and M. S. Wu, "Rational *Helicobacter pylori* therapy: evidence-based medicine rather than medicine-based evidence," *Clinical Gastroenterology and Hepatology*, vol. 12, no. 2, pp. 177.e3–186.e3, 2014.

[6] R. S. Mhaskar, I. Ricardo, A. Azliyati et al., "Assessment of risk factors of *Helicobacter pylori* infection and peptic ulcer disease," *Journal of Global Infectious Diseases*, vol. 5, no. 2, pp. 60–67, 2013.

[7] D. Asrat, I. Nilsson, Y. Mengistu et al., "Prevalence of *Helicobacter pylori* infection among adult dyspeptic patients in Ethiopia," *Annals of Tropical Medicine & Parasitology*, vol. 98, no. 2, pp. 181–189, 2004.

[8] T. N. A. Archampong, R. H. Asmah, E. K. Wiredu, R. K. Gyasi, K. N. Nkrumah, and K. Rajakumar, "Epidemiology of *Helicobacter pylori* infection in dyspeptic Ghanian patients," *Pan African Medical Journal*, vol. 20, p. 178, 2015.

[9] T. Fasciana, C. Calà, C. Bonura et al., "Resistance to clarithromycin and genotypes in *Helicobacter pylori* strains isolated in Sicily," *Journal of Medical Microbiology*, vol. 64, no. 11, pp. 1408–1414, 2015.

[10] J. K. Y. Hooi, W. Y. Lai, W. K. Ng et al., "Global prevalence of *Helicobacter pylori* infection: systematic review and meta-analysis," *Gastroenterology*, vol. 153, no. 2, pp. 420–429, 2017.

[11] K. Desta, D. Asrat, and F. Derbie, "Seroprevalence of *Helicobacter pylori* infection among healthy blood donors in Addis Ababa, Ethiopia," *Ethiopian Journal of Health Sciences*, vol. 12, pp. 109–115, 2002.

[12] T. Tesfahun, M. Yohannes, D. Kassu, and A. Daniel, "Seroprevalence of *Helicobacter pylori* infection in and its relationship with ABO blood groups," *Ethiopian Journal of Health Development*, vol. 19, no. 1, pp. 55–59, 2005.

[13] M. Biniam, M. Beyene, and D. Mulat, "Seroprevalence and trend of *Helicobacter pylori* infection in Gondar University hospital among dyspeptic patients, Gondar, North West Ethiopia," *BMC Research Notes*, vol. 6, no. 1, p. 346, 2013.

[14] M. Feleke, K. Afework, M. Getahun et al., "Seroprevalence of *Helicobacter pylori* in dyspeptic patients and its relationship with HIV infection, ABO blood groups and life style in a university hospital, Northwest Ethiopia," *World Journal of Gastroenterology*, vol. 12, no. 12, pp. 1957–1961, 2006.

[15] Y. Niv and T. Rokkas, "Recent advances in *Helicobacter pylori* eradication," *Annals of Gastroenterology*, vol. 28, no. 4, pp. 415–416, 2015.

[16] A. S. Doffou, K. A. Attia, M. F. Yao Bathaix et al., "The *Helicobacter pylori* eradication rate in a high prevalence area (West Africa): three triple therapy comparative study," *Open Journal of Gastroenterology*, vol. 5, no. 12, pp. 200–206, 2015.

[17] M. Negash, A. Kassu, B. Amare, G. Yismaw, and B. Moges, "Evaluation of SD BIOLINE *H. pylori* Ag rapid test against double ELISA with SD *H. pylori* Ag ELISA and EZ-STEP

[18] K. Dargaze, G. Baye, A. Agersew, and A. Zelalem, "*Helicobacter pylori* infection and its association with anemia among adult dyspeptic patients attending Butajira Hospital, Ethiopia," *BMC Infectious Diseases*, vol. 14, no. 1, p. 656, 2014.

[19] G. Taddesse, A. Habteselassie, K. Desta, S. Esayas, and A. Bane, "Association of dyspepsia symptoms and *Helicobacter pylori* infections in private higher clinic, Addis Ababa, Ethiopia," *Ethiopian Medical Journal*, vol. 49, pp. 109–116, 2011.

[20] H. Shmuely, S. Obure, J. D. Passaro et al., "Dyspepsia symptoms and *Helicobacter pylori* infection, Nakuru, Kenya," *Emerging Infectious Diseases*, vol. 9, no. 9, pp. 1103–1107, 2003.

[21] B. V. Oti, R. G. Pennap, O. Dennis, S. A. Ajegena, and P. M. Adoga, "Prevalence and predictors of *Helicobacter pylori* infection among patients attending a healthcare facility in North-Central Nigeria," *Asian Pacific Journal of Tropical Disease*, vol. 7, no. 6, pp. 352–355, 2017.

[22] L. Shokrzadeh, K. Baghaei, Y. Yamaoka et al., "Prevalence of *Helicobacter pylori* infection in dyspeptic patients in Iran," *Gastroenterology Insights*, vol. 4, no. 1, p. 8, 2012.

[23] M. Selgrad, A. Kandulski, and P. Malfertheiner, "Dyspepsia and *Helicobacter pylori*," *Digestive Disease*, vol. 26, no. 3, pp. 210–214, 2008.

[24] M. S. Pearce, D. I. Campbell, K. D. Mann, L. Parker, and J. E. Thomas, "Deprivation, timing of preschool infections and *H. pylori* seropositivity at age 49–51 years: the Newcastle thousand families' birth cohort," *BMC Infectious Diseases*, vol. 13, no. 1, p. 422, 2013.

[25] W. Jafri, J. Yakoob, S. Abid, S. Siddiqui, S. Awan, and S. Q. Nizami, "*Helicobacter pylori* infection in children: population-based age-specific prevalence and risk factors in a developing country," *Acta Paediatrica*, vol. 99, no. 2, pp. 279–282, 2010.

[26] U. C. Ghoshal, R. Chaturvedi, and P. Correa, "The enigma of *Helicobacter pylori* infection and gastric cancer," *Indian Journal of Gastroenterology*, vol. 29, no. 3, pp. 95–100, 2010.

[27] A. C. Hernando-Harder, N. Booken, S. Goerdt, M. V. Singer, and H. Harder, "*Helicobacter pylori* infection and dermatologic diseases," *European Journal of Dermatology*, vol. 19, no. 5, pp. 431–444, 2009.

[28] E. Chak, G. W. Rutherford, and C. Steinmaus, "The role of breast-feeding in the prevention of *Helicobacter pylori* infection: a systematic review," *Clinical Infectious Diseases*, vol. 48, no. 4, pp. 430–437, 2009.

[29] M. Rowland, L. Daly, M. Vaughan, A. Higgins, B. Bourke, and B. Drumm, "Age-specific incidence of *Helicobacter pylori*," *Gastroenterology*, vol. 130, no. 1, pp. 65–72, 2006.

[30] A. Vega, H. Silva, and T. Cortiñas, "Evaluation of a serum-free transport medium supplemented with cyanobacterial extract, for the optimal survival of *Helicobacter pylori* from biopsy samples and strains," *European Journal of Clinical Microbiology & Infectious Diseases*, vol. 31, no. 2, pp. 135–139, 2012.

[31] S. Perry, M. De La Luz Sanchez, S. Yang et al., "Gastroenteritis and transmission of *Helicobacter pylori* infection in households," *Emerging Infectious Diseases*, vol. 12, no. 11, pp. 1701–1708, 2006.

[32] S. I. Yokota, M. Konno, S. I. Fujiwara et al., "Intrafamilial, preferentially mother-to-child and intraspousal, *Helicobacter pylori* infection in Japan determined by mutilocus sequence typing and random amplified polymorphic DNA fingerprinting," *Helicobacter*, vol. 20, no. 5, pp. 334–342, 2015.

[33] R. Shi, S. Xu, H. Zhang et al., "Prevalence and risk factors for *Helicobacter pylori* infection in Chinese populations," *Helicobacter*, vol. 13, no. 2, pp. 157–165, 2008.

[34] M. Kivi, A. L. Johansson, M. Reilly, and Y. Tindberg, "*Helicobacter pylori* status in family members as risk factors for infection in children," *Epidemiology and Infection*, vol. 133, no. 4, pp. 645–652, 2005.

[35] M. Nouraie, S. Latifi-Navid, H. Rezvan et al., "Childhood hygienic practice and family education status determine the prevalence of *Helicobacter pylori* infection in Iran," *Helicobacter*, vol. 14, no. 1, pp. 40–46, 2009.

[36] A. Zajacova, J. B. Dowd, and A. E. Aiello, "Socioeconomic and race/ethnic patterns in persistent infection burden among U. S. adults," *Journals of Gerontology Series A: Biological Sciences and Medical Sciences*, vol. 64A, no. 2, pp. 272–279, 2009.

[37] F. Rasheed, T. Ahmad, and R. Bilal, "Prevalence and risk factors of *Helicobacter pylori* infection among Pakistani population," *Pakistan Journal of Medical Sciences*, vol. 28, no. 4, pp. 661–665, 2012.

[38] C. Dube, T. C. Nkosi, A. M. Clarke, N. Mkwetshana, E. Green, and R. N. Ndip, "*Helicobacter pylori* in an asymptomatic population of eastern Cape Province, South Africa: public health implication," *Reviews on Environmental Health*, vol. 24, no. 3, pp. 249–255, 2009.

[39] B. Stanström, A. Mendis, and B. Marshall, "*Helicobacter pylori* the latest in diagnosis and treatment," *Australian Family Physician*, vol. 37, no. 8, pp. 608–612, 2008.

[40] A. A. Mohamed and A. H. El-Gohari, "Epidemiological aspects of *Helicobacter pylori* infections as an emergence zoonotic disease: animal reservoirs and public health implications (a review article)," in *Proceedings of 7th International Scientific Conference*, pp. 17–25, Mansoura, Egypt, 2012.

[41] M. Tabatabaei, "Application of molecular and central cultural methods for identification of *Helicobacter* spp in different animal sources," *Global Veterinaria*, vol. 8, pp. 292–297, 2012.

[42] M. P. Dore, A. R. Sepulveda, H. El-Zimaity et al., "Isolation of *Helicobacter pylori* from sheep-implications for transmission to humans," *American Journal of Gastroenterology*, vol. 96, no. 5, pp. 1396–1401, 2001.

[43] M. P. Dore, M. Bilotta, D. Vaira et al., "High prevalence of *Helicobacter pylori* infection in shepherds," *Digestive Diseases and Sciences*, vol. 44, no. 6, pp. 1161–1164, 1999.

[44] N. C. Quaglia, A. Dambrosio, G. Normanno et al., "High occurrence of *Helicobacter pylori* in raw goat, sheep and cow milk inferred by glmM gene: a risk of food-borne infection?," *International Journal of Food Microbiology*, vol. 124, no. 1, pp. 43–47, 2008.

[45] N. R. Bellack, M. W. Koehoorn, Y. C. MacNab, and M. G. Morshed, "A conceptual model of water's role as a reservoir in *Helicobacter pylori* transmission: a review of the evidence," *Epidemiology and Infection*, vol. 134, no. 3, p. 439, 2006.

[46] N. Queralt, R. Bartolomé, and R. Araujo, "Detection of *Helicobacter pylori* DNA in human faeces and water with different levels of faecal pollution in the north-east of Spain," *Journal of Applied Microbiology*, vol. 98, no. 4, pp. 889–895, 2005.

[47] T. L. Cover and M. J. Blaser, "*Helicobacter pylori* in health and disease," *Gastroenterology*, vol. 136, no. 6, pp. 1863–1873, 2009.

[48] O. Secka, Y. Moodley, M. Antonio et al., "Population genetic analyses of *Helicobacter pylori* isolates from Gambian adults and children," *PLoS One*, vol. 9, no. 10, Article ID e109466, 2014.

[49] S. Schwarz, G. Morelli, B. Kusecek et al., "Horizontal versus familial transmission of *Helicobacter pylori*," *PLoS Pathogens*, vol. 4, no. 10, article e1000180, 2008.

[50] K. J. Goodman and P. Correa, "Transmission of *Helicobacter pylori* among siblings," *The Lancet*, vol. 355, no. 9201, pp. 358–361, 2000.

[51] T. Falsafi, N. Sotoudeh, M. M. Feizabadi, and F. Mahjoub, "Analysis of genomic diversity among *Helicobacter pylori* strains isolated from iranian children by pulsed field gel electrophoresis," *Iranian Journal of Pediatrics*, vol. 24, no. 6, pp. 703–709, 2014.

[52] B. Linz, C. R. R. Vololonantenainab, A. Seck et al., "Population genetic structure and isolation by distance of *Helicobacter pylori* in Senegal and Madagascar," *PLoS One*, vol. 9, no. 1, Article ID e87355, 2014.

[53] H. L. Chen, M. J. Chen, S. C. Shih, H. Y. Wang, I. T. Lin, and M. J. Bair, "Socioeconomic status, personal habits, and prevalence of *Helicobacter pylori* infection in the inhabitants of Lanyu," *Journal of the Formosan Medical Association*, vol. 113, no. 5, pp. 278–283, 2014.

[54] T. Uchida, M. Miftahussurur, R. Pittayanon et al., "*Helicobacter pylori* infection in Thailand: a nationwide study of the CagA phenotype," *PLoS One*, vol. 10, no. 9, Article ID e0136775, 2015.

15

Accuracy of Enzyme-Linked Immunosorbent Assays (ELISAs) in Detecting Antibodies against *Mycobacterium leprae* in Leprosy Patients

Omar Ariel Espinosa [ID],[1,2] Silvana Margarida Benevides Ferreira,[3,4] Fabiana Gulin Longhi Palacio,[5] Denise da Costa Boamorte Cortela,[2] and Eliane Ignotti[1,6]

[1]Post Graduation Program in Health Science, Faculty of Medicine, Federal University of Mato Grosso (UFMT), Cuiaba, Mato Grosso, Brazil
[2]Department of Medicine, Faculty of Health Sciences, State University of Mato Grosso (UNEMAT), Caceres, Mato Grosso, Brazil
[3]Cuiabá University (UNIC), Cuiaba, Mato Grosso, Brazil
[4]Post Graduation Program in Nursing, Faculty of Nursing, Federal University of Mato Grosso (UFMT), Cuiaba, Mato Grosso, Brazil
[5]The Brazilian Centre for Evidence-based Healthcare: A Joanna Briggs Institute Centre of Excellence, Sao Paulo, Brazil
[6]Department of Nursing, Faculty of Health Sciences, State University of Mato Grosso (UNEMAT), Caceres, Mato Grosso, Brazil

Correspondence should be addressed to Omar Ariel Espinosa; oespinosa@usp.br

Academic Editor: David Carmena

IgM against *Mycobacterium leprae* may be detected by enzyme-linked immunosorbent assays (ELISAs) based on phenolic glycolipid I (PGL-I) or natural disaccharide octyl bovine serum albumin (ND-O-BSA) as antigens, and the IgG response can be detected by an ELISA based on lipid droplet protein 1 (LID-1). The titers of antibodies against these antigens vary with operational classification. The aim of this study was to compare the accuracy of ELISAs involving PGL-I and ND-O-BSA with that involving LID-1. We included studies that analyze multibacillary and paucibacillary leprosy cases and evaluate the diagnostic accuracy of ELISAs based on LID-1 and/or PGL-I or ND-O-BSA as antigens to measure antibody titers against *M. leprae*. Studies were found via PubMed, the Virtual Health Library Regional Portal, Literatura Latino-Americana e do Caribe em Ciências da Saúde, Índice Bibliográfico Espanhol de Ciências de Saúde, the Brazilian Society of Dermatology, National Institute for Health and Clinical Excellence, Cochrane Library, Embase (the Elsevier database), and Cumulative Index to Nursing and Allied Health Literature. The Quality Assessment of Diagnostic Accuracy Studies served as a methodological validity tool. Quantitative data were extracted using the Standards for Reporting of Diagnostic Accuracy. Sensitivity, specificity, and a diagnostic odds ratio were calculated, and a hierarchical summary receiver-operating characteristic curve and forest plots were constructed. The protocol register code for this meta-analysis is PROSPERO 2017: CRD42017055983. Nineteen studies were included. ND-O-BSA showed better overall performance in terms of sensitivity, specificity, positive and negative likelihood ratios, and diagnostic odds ratio when compared with PGL-I and LID-1. The multibacillary group showed better performance on these parameters (than the paucibacillary group did), at 94%, 99%, 129, 0.05, and 2293, respectively. LID-1 did not provide any advantage regarding the overall estimate of sensitivity in comparison with PGL-I or ND-O-BSA.

1. Introduction

Leprosy is a chronic infectious disease caused by *Mycobacterium leprae* (a microorganism that mainly affects the skin and peripheral nerves) and is considered one of the six most dangerous diseases in developing countries by the World Health Organization (WHO) [1]. Leprosy diagnosis is based on the presence of at least one of the following three cardinal signs: definite loss of sensation in a pale or reddish skin patch, a thickened or enlarged peripheral nerve with loss of sensation and/or weakness of the muscles innervated by that nerve, and the presence of acid-fast bacilli in a slit-skin smear [2].

A continual and slow reduction in the number of new cases has been observed during the last decade, even though more than 200,000 new cases are diagnosed every year. India, Brazil, and Indonesia represent 80% of all cases [3].

A case of leprosy is defined as an individual that has a skin lesion consistent with leprosy, with definite sensory loss, with or without thickened nerves, and/or with positive skin smears [4]. Cases of leprosy are classified operationally as either paucibacillary leprosy (PB) or multibacillary leprosy (MB) depending on the number of skin lesions [5]. Early diagnosis and appropriate treatment of leprosy patients are essential conditions for stopping the transmission and reducing the physical and social consequences of the disease [4].

The discovery of phenolic glycolipid I (PGL-I) in 1980, a specific component of *M. leprae*, and its use in serological assays in patients with leprosy in 1981 are major advances in serological research on the disease [6–8]. Due to the glycolipid nature of PGL-I, the humoral immune response of leprosy patients predominantly involves IgM [9]. The detection of these IgM antibodies represents the best-evaluated and standardized serological test for leprosy [10–15]. In addition to native PGL-I, IgM levels can be measured by means of a synthetic mimotope: a natural disaccharide linked to bovine serum albumin (ND-O-BSA) [15–17]. The IgG response to *M. leprae* can be measured using LID-1 as an antigen: a chimeric protein generated by the fusion of antigens ML0405 and ML2331 [18]. Because it was reported early on that individuals with a high bacillary load have a high IgM titer against PGL-I [19], even in the chronic stage of the disease, the accuracy of the tests based on PGL-I (native or synthetic) and LID-1 has been compared previously in several studies, with the aim of identifying an adequate test for serological diagnosis [15–18, 20–24].

The titers of antibodies against PGL-I, ND-O-BSA, and LID-1 vary, with the clinical presentation being the strongest in MB patients and the weakest or absent in PB patients. The bacterial index may also correlate with antibody titers [20–22].

The Guidelines for the Diagnosis, Treatment and Prevention of Leprosy (WHO) warn that studies of the most commonly used ELISA and lateral flow tests show low sensitivity for PB leprosy, which is often harder to diagnose clinically than MB leprosy. Based on currently available evidence, newer ELISA and other laboratory tests do not represent a clear advantage over current standard diagnostic methods [25].

To date, a number of studies have used ELISAs based on PGL-I, ND-O-BSA, or LID-1 as antigens. The successful implementation of these methods reflects the good performance of these tests. Nonetheless, sensitivity and specificity of these assays vary depending on the geographic origin of the population studied [21]. Therefore, our aims were to conduct a meta-analysis of studies on the accuracy of the available serological tests and to summarize the accuracy of these tests in detecting antibodies against *M. leprae*. The aims were achieved successfully.

2. Methods

The protocol for this meta-analysis was published in the international prospective register of systematic reviews (PROSPERO 2017: CRD42017055983) before its implementation and is described in Supplementary Materials (Text S1). The protocol and final report were developed based on the Cochrane Handbook for Systematic Reviews of Diagnostic Test Accuracy [26].

2.1. The Review Question/Objective. What is the diagnostic accuracy of the commercially available ELISA based on antigen LID-1 as compared to ELISAs based on native antigen PGL-I or synthetic antigen ND-O-BSA for the detection of antibodies against *M. leprae* in patients with leprosy?

More specifically, we performed a meta-analysis of studies on the diagnostic test accuracy of PGL-I, ND-O-BSA, and LID-1 ELISAs to obtain summary points for the accuracy values of the assays for antibodies against *M. leprae*.

2.2. Inclusion Criteria. The mnemonic PIRD (participants, index test, reference test, and diagnosis of interest) was employed for the inclusion criteria as recommended for systematic reviews of diagnostic test accuracy [26]. Studies were included that dealt with MB and PB leprosy cases and evaluated the diagnostic accuracy of ELISAs based on LID-1 and/or PGL-I or ND-O-BSA antigens to measure antibody titers against *M. leprae*.

The gold standard for the diagnosis of leprosy is based on clinical diagnosis. Therefore, only studies that selected and classified patients with leprosy on the basis of clinical diagnosis were included.

2.3. Types of Included Studies. The studies had to have any epidemiological design that afforded a detailed measure of sensitivity, specificity, and receiver-operating characteristic (ROC) curves.

2.4. The Search Strategy. This study was guided by the Preferred Reporting Items for Systematic Reviews and Meta-Analyses (PRISMA) protocol standard proposed by the Cochrane Collaboration® [27]. A three-step search strategy was utilized in this review. First, an initial limited search of Medline was performed by searching for MeSH index terms and related keywords. This search involved an analysis of words contained in the title and abstract and index terms used to describe the article. Second, another search involving all the identified keywords and index terms was performed across all the included databases. Third, a reference list of all dissertations with clearly detailed accurate values was considered. Studies published since 1982—the year when the first ELISA based on the PGL-I antigen was developed to detect antibodies against *M. leprae*—until February 2018 were considered for inclusion in this review. Moreover, only published studies were included because these studies were evaluated by external reviewers. The search strategy can be found in Supplementary Materials (Text S1).

Database searching was carried out in PubMed, which includes Medline and other health databases; in the Virtual Health Library Regional Portal (VHL Regional Portal), which includes Medline, Literatura Latino-Americana e do Caribe em Ciências da Saúde (LILACS), Índice Bibliográfico Espanhol de Ciências de Saúde (IBECS), and other health databases; via the Brazilian Society of Dermatology; at the National Institute for Health and Clinical Excellence (NICE); in the Cochrane Library; in Embase, the Elsevier database; and in the Cumulative Index to Nursing and Allied Health Literature (CINAHL). The databases used to search dissertations as a source of gray literature were Google Scholar and EVIPNet (WHO). The MeSH terms were Leprosy, *Mycobacterium leprae*, Serology, Enzyme-Linked Immunosorbent Assay, Leprosy Multibacillary, and Leprosy Paucibacillary. The keywords were LID-1, PGL-I, ND-O, NDO, IDR1, Specificity, Sensitivity, and Measurement Accuracy. The terms were combined via the boolean operators "AND" and/or "OR" to compose the search strings.

2.5. Assessment of Methodological Quality. The documents selected for retrieval were assessed by two independent reviewers for methodological validity prior to inclusion in this study, by means of standardized critical appraisal instruments from the Quality Assessment of Diagnostic Accuracy Studies (QUADAS 2), which was released in 2011 after revision of the original QUADAS. The QUADAS tool consists of four key domains that evaluate patient selection, an index test, reference standard, and flow and timing (flow of patients through the study and timing of the index tests and reference standard). Each domain is assessed in terms of the risk of bias, and the first three domains are also evaluated in terms of concerns about applicability [28, 29]. Any disagreements between the reviewers were resolved either through discussion or based on the opinion of a third reviewer.

2.6. Data Extraction. Quantitative data were extracted from papers according to the Standards for Reporting of Diagnostic Accuracy (STARD) [30, 31]. A 2 × 2 table was compiled to classify the data as true positive, false positive, true negative, and false negative.

2.7. Data Synthesis. STATA SM/64 (Version 13.1; College Station, TX) with MIDAS and METANDI commands was used for the meta-analysis.

Sensitivity, specificity, positive and negative likelihood ratios (LR+ and LR−), and the diagnostic odds ratio (DOR), with a confidence interval (CI) of 95%, were calculated for each study, and subsequently, the results were combined.

Two forest plots were generated side by side: one for sensitivity and the other for specificity showing the means and 95% CIs of each selected primary study. Through summary receiver-operating characteristic (SROC) curves, the presence or absence of heterogeneity was identified. The meta-analysis was performed based on the hierarchical model of summary receiver-operating characteristic (HSROC) curves [32]. The HSROC curve provides information on the overall performance

(sensitivity, specificity, LR+, LR−, and DOR) of a test via different thresholds.

To evaluate the potential of publication bias, Deeks' funnel plot was constructed, with $p < 0.05$ indicating the presence of publication bias [33]. Fagan's nomogram, conceived to provide posttest probability, was employed to estimate clinical utility of the test values and is based on LR+ and LR− obtained from the meta-analysis [34].

3. Results

Our search yielded 968 citations related to leprosy through the combined application of descriptors in the databases described above. After the eligibility criteria (duplicate texts, articles related to other topics, and text excluded for review criteria or quality methods), 19 baseline studies remained. These studies evaluated the diagnostic accuracy of antigens PGL-I, ND-O-BSA, or LID-1 ELISAs and were included in this meta-analysis after critical appraisal of methodological quality [16–18, 22, 24, 35–48]. The results of our search strategy are shown in a PRISMA flowchart (Figure 1). Excluded studies are summarized in Table S1.

The evaluation of methodological quality revealed that the studies included in this meta-analysis had a "low risk of bias" in patient selection and flow and time domains. Some of the selected studies were "at risk of bias" in the index test (10.5%) and the reference standard domains (15.7%). On the contrary, patient selection and the reference standard showed a "low applicability concern." Only 5.2% of the selected studies yielded "applicability concerns" in the index test (Figure 2). The methodological quality summary bias risk concern and applicability of each domain for each included study are presented in Figure S1. The data extracted from the final selection are given in Table S2.

In the 19 studies included in this meta-analysis, 5512 ELISAs were carried out. These assays were performed on patients classified as MB (33.3%), PB (22.2%), and epidemiological control (44.5%). Concerning the geographic distribution, the samples were collected in Brazil (59%), China (14%), Philippines (11.2%), French Polynesia (8.8%), Spain (2%), Thailand (3%), and Nepal and Australia (2%). The distribution of performed ELISAs by antigen was as follows: PGL-I, 31.5%; ND-O-BSA, 42.1%; and LID-1, 26.4%. The data extracted from the selected studies are given in Table 1.

3.1. Effects of Clinical Manifestations of Leprosy on the Accuracy of Tests. To verify whether leprosy patient groups varied significantly in the performance of the *M. leprae* antigen ELISAs (PGL-I, ND-O-BSA, and LID-1), we carried out a global estimate of the accuracy of each test by group (MB and PB).

A forest plot of sensitivity and specificity of PGL-I in the MB group revealed sensitivity values ranging from 30% to 100% and specificity values from 66% to 100%. The combined sensitivity and specificity were 78% (95% CI 60–90) and 99% (95% CI 91–100), respectively. The sensitivity values for the PB group ranged from 12% to 100%, and the combined sensitivity was 34% (95% CI 11–67; Figure 3(a)).

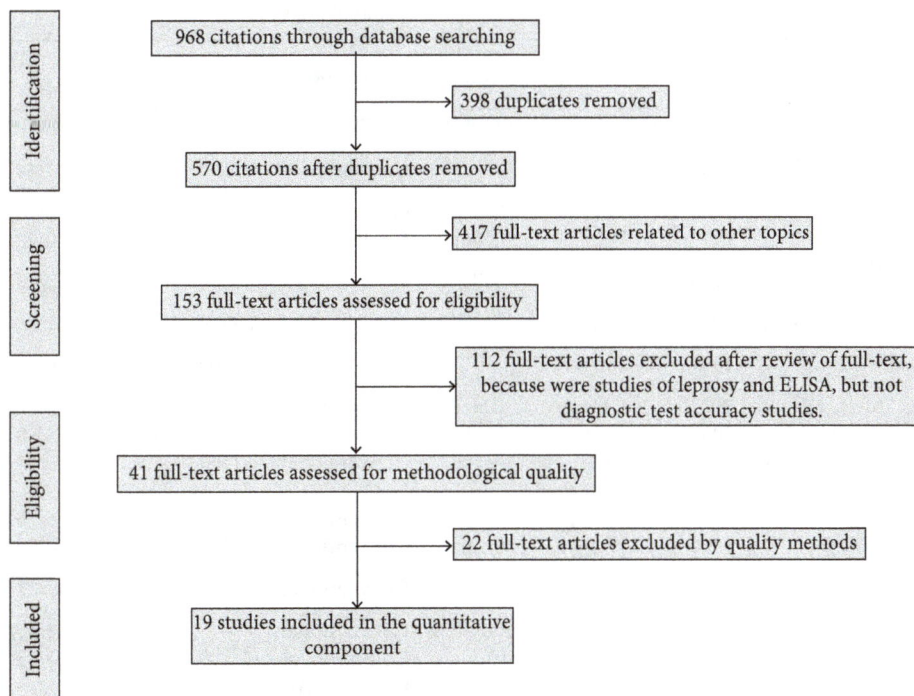

FIGURE 1: A flowchart of the steps performed in the systematic review and meta-analysis.

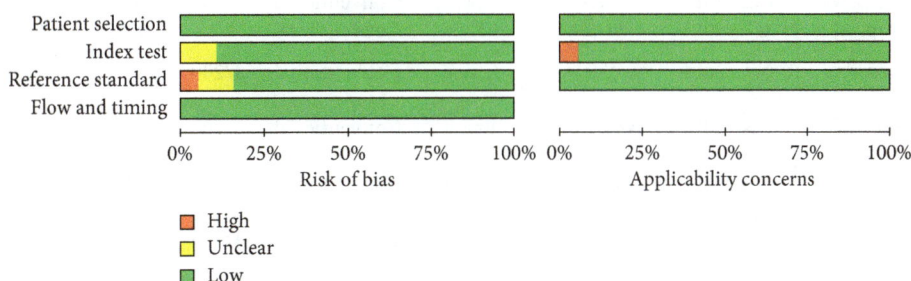

FIGURE 2: Assessment of methodological quality domains in all the studies. Proportions of studies rated as "high," "unclear," and "low" are presented.

In relation to the ND-O-BSA antigen, the MB group sensitivity values ranged from 77% to 100%, and specificity values ranged from 97% to 100%. The combined sensitivity and specificity were 92% (95% CI 81–97) and 99% (95% CI 98–100), respectively. In the PB group, sensitivity values ranged from 15% to 93%, and the combined sensitivity was 56% (95% CI 28–82; Figure 3(b)).

Finally, in terms of the LID-1 antigen, the MB group showed sensitivity values ranging from 35% to 90% and specificity values from 73% to 100%. The combined sensitivity and specificity were 80% (95% CI 66–89) and 97% (95% CI 93–100), respectively. The PB group showed sensitivity values ranging from 3% to 73%, and the combined sensitivity was 20% (95% CI 7–47; Figure 3(c)).

For all ELISA antigens, the combined specificity in the MB group was the same as that in the PB group.

3.2. Publication Bias and Heterogeneity. Deeks' funnel plot was constructed to analyze the potential publication bias for each antigen-specific ELISA in both patient groups. PGL-I Deeks' funnel plots did not reveal any publication bias in the two groups ($p = 0.63$ and 0.69 for groups MB and PB, respectively). For the ND-O-BSA antigen, only Deeks' funnel plot in the MB group did not show publication bias ($p = 580$). On the contrary, studies on the LID-1 antigen showed a publication bias risk in both the MB and PB groups (Figure S2).

The SROC curves for each ELISA antigen revealed a range of 87–100% for the area under the curve (AUC), with a 95% confidence contour and 95% prediction contour for each population studied (Figure S3). The SROC curves did not show heterogeneity among the included studies.

3.3. Accuracy of ELISAs in Detecting M. leprae. By means of the HSROC curves, the accuracy of each type of M. leprae ELISA based on different antigens was evaluated, and a summary point was generated for each population under study (Table 2). When we evaluated the accuracy of PGL-I

TABLE 1: A summary of the included studies.

Antigen	Journal	Year	Author	Country	Method	Dilution	Cut-off OD	TP/total MB	TP/total PB	FN/total EC
PGL-1										
	Aust. NZ J Med	1987	Britton	Australia and Nepal	Conventional	1/100	>0.15	33/44	1/4	0/60
	Int. J. Lepr.	1988	Wu	China	Conventional	1/200	>0.04	76/76	40/40	0/30
	Int. J. Lepr.	1990	Wu	China	Conventional	1/201	>0.2	70/90	11/20	1/30
	Asian Pac J Allergy Immunol.	1990	Praputpittaya	Thailand	Conventional	1/300	>0.056	23/28	5/18	0/33
	Mem. Inst. Oswaldo Cruz	1990	Saad	Brazil	Conventional	1/4000	>0.27	61/74	6/52	4/52
	Lepr. Rev.	1991	Chanteau	French Polynesia	Conventional	1/200	>0.2	20/21	8/23	9/414
	BMC Infect. Dis.	2013	Vaz Cardoso	Brazil	Conventional	1/300	>0.250	90/108	16/104	1/30
	Lepr. Rev.	2003	Torres	Spain	Conventional	1/300	>0.160	15/50	0/10	1/40
	PLoS Neglected Trop. Dis	2017	Frade	Brazil	Conventional	1/400	0.1	15/33	5/7	67/245
ND-O-BSA										
	Int. J. Lepr.	1988	Wu	China	Conventional	1/200	>0.05	76/76	37/40	0/30
	Int. J. Lepr.	1990	Wu	China	Conventional	1/201	>0.2	70/90	11/20	1/30
	Asian Pac. J. Allergy Immunol.	1990	Praputpittaya	Thailand	Conventional	1/300	>0.056	23/28	5/18	0/33
	Int. J. Lepr.	1993	Cellona	Philippines	Conventional	—	0.16	163/193	22/147	7/401
	Int. J. Lepr.	2002	Wu	China	Conventional	1/200	—	53/53	46/50	0/100
	Am. J. Trop. Med. Hyg.	2013	Wen	China	Conventional	—	>0.2	48/49	21/30	1/35
	J. Immunol. Methods	2014	Moura	Brazil	Conventional		>0.2	375/486	88/342	0/69
+LID-1										
	Clin. Vaccine Immunol.	2007	Duthie	Brazil	Conventional	1/1000	0.1	26/30	6/30	1/26
	Mem. Inst. Oswaldo Cruz	2012	Hungria	Brazil	Conventional	1/200	0.3	51/58	6/93	7/282
	Am. J. Trop. Med. Hyg.*	2013	Wen	China	Conventional	—	>0.2	44/49	16/30	0/35
	Biomed Res. Int.	2014	Wen	China	Conventional	1/200	>2 × SD OD EC	7/20	8/11	0/10
	PLoS Neglected Trop. Dis	2016	Amorim	Brazil	Conventional	1/200	>3 × SD OD EC	58/68	5/32	1/98
	Diagn Microbiol. Infect. Dis.	2016	Freitas	Brazil	Conventional	1/200	0.3	42/48	4/60	0/62
	Diagn Microbiol. Infect. Dis.	2017	Hungria	Brazil	Conventional	1/200	0.3	24/30	1/38	2/61
	PLoS Neglected Trop. Dis.	2017	Frade	Brazil	Conventional	1/400	0.1	15/33	5/7	67/245

*Type of sample used: plasma. All other studies used serum. TP/total = true positive/total of cases; FN/total = false negative/total of endemic control; EC = endemic control; +LID-1: Developed by Infectious Disease Research Institute (IDRI).

ELISA assays, acceptable performance was observed only in the MB group. The respective sensitivity, LR+, LR−, and DOR values were as follows: MB group 78% (95% CI 60–90), 90 (95% CI 8–1023), 0.22 (95% CI 0.11–0.44), and 408 (95% CI 23–7041) and PB group 34% (95% CI 11–67), 16 (95% CI 2–121), 0.67 (95% CI 0.42–1), and 22 (95% CI 2.4–247; Figure S4A). ELISAs based on ND-O-BSA showed better performance in both groups: 94% (95% CI 78–98), 129 (95% CI 42–390), 0.05 (95% CI 0.01–0.23), and 2293 (95% CI 279–18844) in group MB and 56% (95% CI 27–81), 76 (95% CI 21–274), 0.43 (95% CI 0.21–0.87), and 174 (95% CI 39–1013) in group PB, respectively (Figure S4B). LID-1 ELISAs showed the worst performance among the three antigens. The respective sensitivity, LR+, LR-, and DOR accuracy data were as follows: in the MB group, 79% (95% CI 66–88), 26 (95% CI 8–90), 0.2 (95% CI 0.11–0.37), and 127 (95% CI 22–721), and in the PB group, 20% (95% CI 7–46), 8.0 (95% CI 3–24), 0.81 (95% CI 0.64–1), and 9.8 (95% CI 2.8–33; Figure S4C).

Specificity values were between 97% and 99% in each type of ELISA and in each group analyzed.

3.4. DOR and Posttest Probability. DORs were considerably higher in the MB group than in the PB group for all the antigens used in the ELISAs.

Fagan's nomogram was built to obtain posttest probability, for which we performed a simulation with a prevalence of 30% for household contacts of leprosy patients from endemic areas in accordance with the included studies. Thus, the probability of someone having the disease and not being detected by the PGL-I ELISA was 9% and 23% in the MB and PB groups, respectively. In contrast, the posttest probability of sick patients with a positive test was 98% and 88% for groups MB and PB (Figure 4(a)). Similarly, the probability of someone having the disease and not being detected by the NO-O-BSA ELISA was 3% and 16% in groups MB and PB, respectively, whereas these values were 98% and 97%,

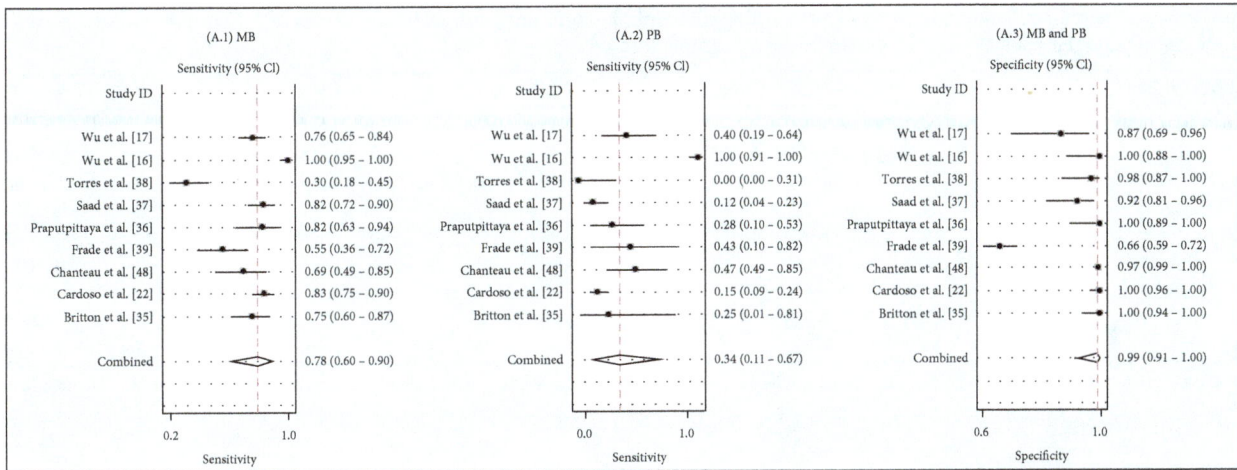

(a)

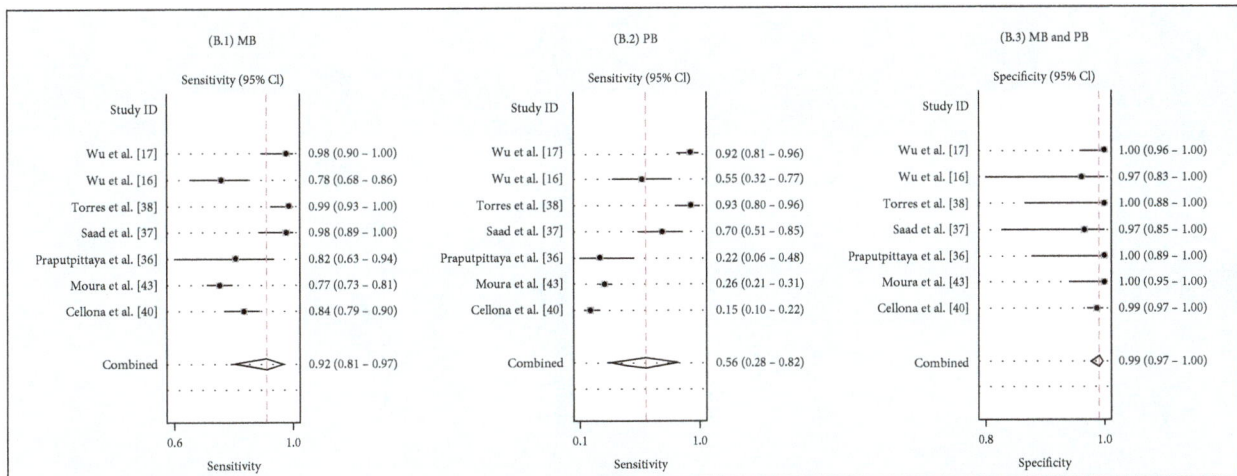

(b)

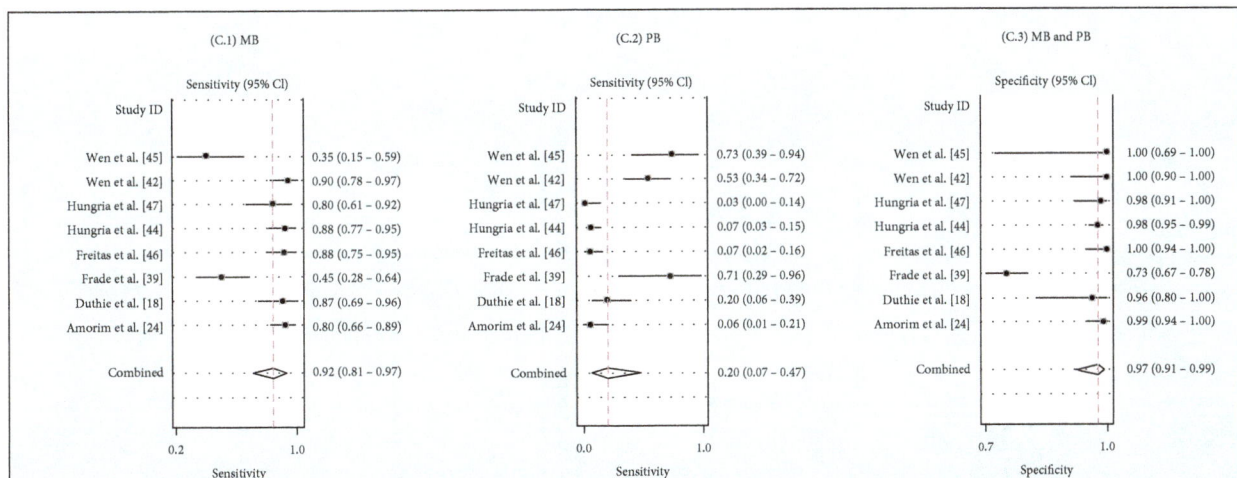

(c)

FIGURE 3: A forest plot of sensitivity of ELISAs by antigen: (a) PGL-I, (b) ND-O-BSA, and (c) LID-1, according to each studied group (MB (A.1, B.1, and C.1) and PB (A.2, B.2, and C.2)). The same specificity was found in both groups for the three ELISAs (A.3, B.3, and C.3). The circle in a square represents sensitivity and specificity, and the horizontal line represents the point estimate (95% CI for each study). Diamonds represent the combined value estimate (95% CI).

TABLE 2: Accuracy of ELISAs for detection of leprosy using different *M. leprae* antigens. Summary points of the HSROC curve accuracy for each *M. leprae* antigen used in the ELISAs for each population studied.

ELISA antigen/Op. class*	Sensitivity %	95% CI	Specificity %	95% CI	LR+	95% CI	LR−	95% CI	DOR	95% CI
PGL-I										
MB	78	60–90	99	91–99	90	8–1023	0.22	0.11–0.44	408	23–7041
PB	34	11–67	97	89–99	16	2–121	0.67	0.42–1	22	2.4–247
ND-O-BSA										
MB	94	78–98	99	97–99	129	42–390	0.05	0.01–0.23	2293	279–18844
PB	56	27–81	99	98–99	76	21–274	0.43	0.21–0.87	174	39–1013
LID-1										
MB	79	66–88	97	91–99	26	8–90	0.2	0.11–0.37	127	22–721
PB	20	7–46	97	92–99	8	3.0–24	0.81	0.64–1	9.8	2.8–33

*Op. class = operational classification; 95% CI = 95% confidence interval; LR− = negative likelihood; LR+ = positive likelihood ratio; DOR = diagnostic odds ratio.

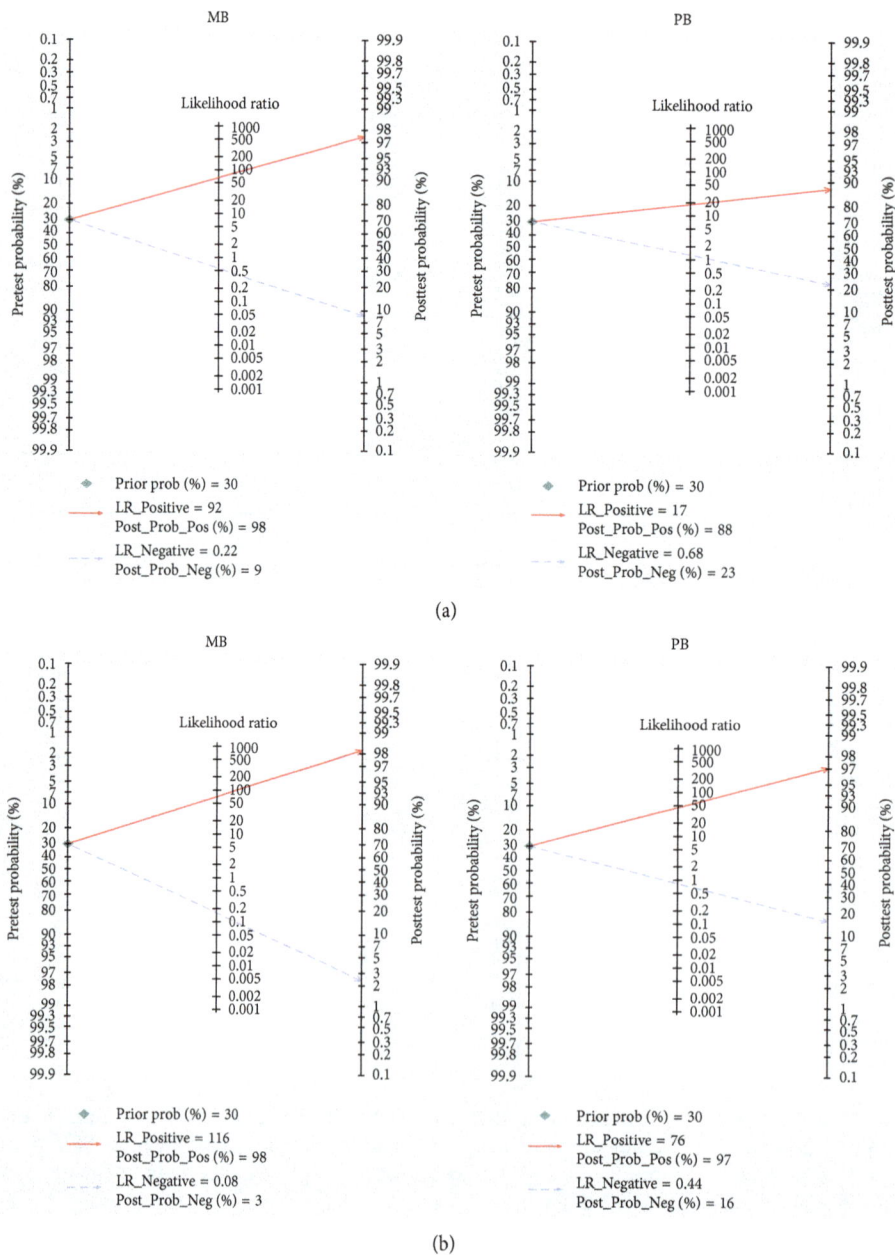

(a)

(b)

FIGURE 4: Continued.

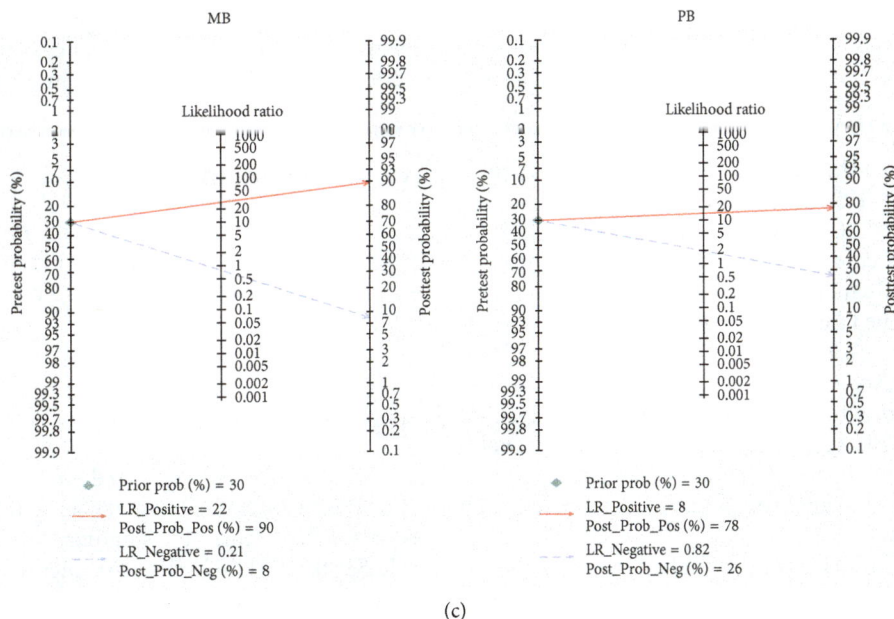

(c)

FIGURE 4: Fagan's nomogram and the posttest probabilities. Fagan's nomogram was built with a prevalence of 30% for household contacts of leprosy patients in an endemic area. If a patient tests positive, the posttest probability that they truly have leprosy would be (a) PGL-I ELISA: 98% for group MB and 88% for group PB; (b) ND-O-BSA ELISA: 98% for group MB and 97% for group PB; and (c) LID-1 ELISA: 90% for group MB and 78% for group PB (solid red line). On the contrary, if this patient tests negative, the posttest probability of having the disease and not being detected would be (a) PGL-I ELISA: 9% for group MB and 23% for group PB; (b) ND-O-BSA ELISA: 3% for group MB and 16% for group PB; and (c) LID-1 ELISA: 8% for group MB and 26% for group PB (dotted blue line).

respectively, for patients with leprosy (Figure 4(b)). For the LID-1 ELISA, the posttest probabilities were 8% and 26% for an individual having the disease and not being diagnosed and 90% and 78% for leprosy patients with a positive test in groups MB and PB, respectively (Figure 4(c)).

4. Discussion

Most of the ELISAs performed in the included studies in this systematic review and meta-analysis were performed in Brazil (59%) and Asia (28.2%, predominantly in China): countries that have different epidemiological profiles [4]. These studies revealed variations in sensitivity and specificity depending on the ELISA antigen and the patient group (MB or PB). These variations may be related to the strains found in each region and immune responses of the patients.

In the present meta-analysis, studies that analyzed ELISA tests involving the ND-O-BSA antigen indicated sensitivity (77–100% for group MB and 15–93% for group PB) and specificity (97–100%) ranges that are more favorable than did studies on PGL-I and LID-1 ELISAs. Sensitivity values among studies from different regions and among studies from the same regions showed great differences, for both the MB and PB groups, as reported previously [21]. Even studies that were designed by the same authors and conducted in the same regions produced different sensitivity values [16, 17]. Specificity values were more similar among the studies analyzed in both groups, MB and PB.

A general diagnostic test accuracy estimate was carried out for each ELISA antigen in both leprosy groups. The

HSROC curves showed better sensitivity (94% (95% CI 78–98) for MB and 56% (95% CI 17–81) for PB) and specificity (99% (95% CI 97–100)) for the ND-O-BSA antigen. In our results, the ELISAs using PGL-I were not subject to conclusive publication bias in either of the groups studied (MB or PB). As for the ELISA involving the ND-O-BSA antigen, only the MB group showed publication bias.

Sensitivity and specificity found for each ELISA matched the accuracy reported by other authors [15, 43, 44, 49]. On the contrary, when we compared the performance reported in these studies with our results, there was no consensus regarding a superior antigen for leprosy ELISAs. This finding may be due to the fact that most of the studies were conducted with conventional ELISAs made in-house and due to other factors like sampling time, sample transport, and sample preservation, which may cause test performance variations. Additionally, there is no standardized cutoff value for any of these ELISA antigens or for either group of patients with leprosy. Nevertheless, we can conclude that all the analyzed antigens have better diagnostic accuracy for MB leprosy, as reported elsewhere in the literature [15, 21, 23, 24, 43, 45, 49, 50]. Very divergent accuracy results in the group of PB patients were found. Based on the estimated median sensitivities found in this patient group, negative tests are not that useful for ruling out PB leprosy patients. Using these serologic tests, PB patients can be diagnosed as negative when they really are not.

The absence of added value for the use of LID-1 was also observed in a recent study, where the researchers detected antibodies against the PGL-I antigen in patients with leprosy by rapid tests [51].

Owing to the presence of anti-BSA antibodies, which may interfere with the test results [52], the ND-O antigen conjugated to human serum albumin (HSA) has been used in ELISAs [15, 43, 49]. Nevertheless, these studies suggest that the BSA or HSA carrier protein of the antigen does not significantly influence the anti-PGL-I seropositivity of the groups under study [15, 43]. The primary literature on ELISAs using the ND-O-HSA antigen was not included because only three studies were found, and at least four are required for a reliable meta-analysis.

The DORs obtained here were higher on average in the MB group than in the PB group. The DOR varies from zero to infinity, with higher values denoting a better discriminatory diagnostic test. Additionally, posttest probability (Fagan's nomogram) was high, specifically within the MB patient group; for each antigen included in our analysis, this result is indicative of good clinical utility of an ELISA as a supplement to clinical diagnosis.

There are some limitations of our study. First of all, there is no standard cutoff value for any ELISA antigen analyzed here and for either group of patients under study (MB or PB). Although this situation did not hamper implementation of our meta-analysis, accuracy variations can occur due to differences in the number of true or false positives or negatives among the studies. Management of outliers varies among authors and affects the measurement of accuracy parameters, resulting in a wide range of sensitivity and specificity estimates across studies, as shown in our study. Second, although the specificity was almost 100%, only a few authors included groups of controls of patients with other diseases such as tuberculosis, and most authors used endemic control samples and a few samples of nonendemic controls. Nevertheless, there was a risk of publication bias in the studies on the ND-O-BSA antigen in the PB group. Few studies indicated whether the samples were from primary or secondary infections, or whether the patients received treatment. Finally, due to different amounts of patient information in the included studies, the data were not divided into additional groups based on other variables, e.g., gender or age.

5. Conclusion

In this meta-analysis, in the MB group, the LID-1 ELISA did not show any advantage with respect to the overall sensitivity estimate (79% (95% CI 66–89)) when compared to native antigen PGL-I (78% (95% CI 60–90)) or to synthetic antigen ND-O-BSA (94% (95% CI 81–97)). Specificity of all the ELISAs in this group was close to 100% for all antigens, whereas in the PB group, all the assays showed lower sensitivity values as compared with the MP group in terms of detection of antibodies against *M. leprae.*

Our results confirm that traditional ELISAs have good accuracy in detecting MB leprosy and poor accuracy in detecting PB leprosy. The WHO research priorities for leprosy include new tools for early detection. To achieve this goal, it is important to have a standardized serological, molecular, or immunological assay that is applicable to different geographic regions with different epidemiological profiles and pathogen strains. In the future, these laboratory tools are expected to become important for the diagnosis of leprosy (MB and PB), for surveillance of household contacts, and for establishing health policy interventions.

Acknowledgments

The authors thank Sumaya McDonald for her contribution to the writing of this manuscript. OAED received a fellowship from Secretaría Nacional de Ciencia, Tecnología e Innovación de Panamá.

Supplementary Materials

Text S1: the protocol registered in Prospero International (PROSPERO 2017: CRD42017055983). Text S2: the literature search strategy. Table S1: a summary of the excluded studies. Table S2: the PRISMA checklist. Figure S1: methodological quality summary of the included studies. Figure S2: analysis of publication bias. Deeks' funnel plot for leprosy ELISAs is based on different antigens. Deeks' funnel plot (asymmetry test for publication bias) did not detect potential publication bias for (A) PGL-I (MB $p = 0.63$ and PB $p = 0.69$). (B) Only ND-O-BSA in the MB group did not show publication bias ($p = 58$). (C) LID-1 showed publication bias in both groups of patients. Figure S3: analysis of heterogeneity. Summary ROC curve plots of sensitivity and specificity for PGL-I (A), ND-O-BSA (B), and LID-1 (C). Each large X represents an individual study in the meta-analysis. The summary operating point is a single sensitivity/specificity point estimated by the results of the studies. AUC = area under the curve. Figure S4: meta-analysis based on the hierarchical method. An HSROC plot displaying diagnostic accuracy results of the included studies by antigen in ELISAs: (A) PGL-I, (B) ND-O-BSA, and (C) LID-1 for different leprosy patient groups (MB and PB). The circle diameter (study estimate) is proportional to the weight given to each study. Summary sensitivity and specificity estimates are marked with a red square. (*Supplementary Materials*)

References

[1] Global leprosy: update on the 2012 situation," *Weekly Epidemiological Record*, vol. 88, no. 35, pp. 365–379, 2013.

[2] World Health Organization, "WHO expert committee on leprosy, 8th report," 2012. World Health Organ Tech Rep Ser 968.

[3] Global leprosy update, 2015: time for action, accountability and inclusion," *Weekly Epidemiological Record*, vol. 91, no. 35, pp. 405–420, 2016.

[4] World Health Organization, "WHO expert committee on leprosy: sixth report," WHO Technical Report Series; 768, World Health Organization, Geneva, Switzerland, 1988.

[5] D. N. Lockwood, E. Sarno, and W. C. Smith, "Classifying leprosy patients—searching for the perfect solution?," *Leprosy Review*, vol. 78, no. 4, pp. 317–320, 2007.

[6] S. W. Hunter and P. J. Brennan, "A novel phenolic glycolipid from *Mycobacterium leprae* possibly involved in

immunogenicity and pathogenicity," *Journal of Bacteriology*, vol. 147, no. 3, pp. 728–735, 1981.

[7] S. N. Payne, P. Draper, and R. J. Rees, "Serological activity of purified glycolipid from *Mycobacterium leprae*," *International Journal of Leprosy and Other Mycobacterial Diseases*, vol. 50, no. 2, pp. 220-221, 1982.

[8] J. S. Spencer, H. J. Kim, W. H. Wheat et al., "Analysis of antibody responses to *Mycobacterium leprae* phenolic glycolipid I, lipoarabinomannan, and recombinant proteins to define disease subtype-specific antigenic profiles in leprosy," *Clinical and Vaccine Immunology*, vol. 18, no. 2, pp. 260–267, 2011.

[9] J. Y. Park, S. N. Cho, J. K. Youn et al., "Detection of antibodies to human nerve antigens in sera from leprosy patients by ELISA," *Clinical and Experimental Immunology*, vol. 87, no. 3, pp. 368–372, 1992.

[10] M. Muñoz, J. C. Beltrán-Alzate, M. S. Duthie, H. Serrano-Coll, and N. Cardona-Castro, "Comparison of enzyme-linked immunosorbent assay using either natural octyl disaccharide-leprosy IDRI diagnostic or phenolic glycolipid-I antigens for the detection of leprosy patients in Colombia," *American Journal of Tropical Medicine and Hygiene*, vol. 98, no. 1, pp. 274–277, 2018.

[11] T. Fujiwara, S. W. Hunter, and S. N. Cho, "Chemical synthesis and serology of disaccharides and trisaccharides of phenolic glycolipid antigens from the leprosy bacillus and preparation of a disaccharide protein conjugate for serodiagnosis of leprosy," *Infection and Immunity*, vol. 43, no. 1, pp. 245–252, 1984.

[12] S. Chanteau, J. L. Cartel, R. Plichart, J. Roux, and M. A. Bach, "PLG I antigen and antibody detection in the control of leprosy in French Polynesia," *Acta Leprologica*, vol. 7, no. 1, pp. 128-129, 1989.

[13] S. Buhrer-Sekula, M. G. Cunha, W. A. Ferreira, and P. R. Klatser, "The use of whole blood in a dipstick assay for detection of antibodies to *Mycobacterium leprae*: a field evaluation," *FEMS Immunology and Medical Microbiology*, vol. 29, no. 3, pp. 197–201, 1998.

[14] S. Buhrer-Sekula, H. L. Smits, G. C. Gussenhoven et al., "Simple and fast lateral flow test for classification of leprosy patients and identification of contacts with high risk of developing leprosy," *Journal of Clinical Microbiology*, vol. 41, no. 5, pp. 1991–1995, 2003.

[15] J. Lobato, M. P. Costa, E. M. Reis et al., "Comparison of three immunological tests for leprosy diagnosis and detection of subclinical infection," *Leprosy Review*, vol. 82, no. 4, pp. 389–401, 2011.

[16] Q. X. Wu, G. Y. Ye, and X. Y. Li, "Serological activity of natural disaccharide octyl bovine serum albumin (ND-O-BSA) in sera from patients with leprosy, tuberculosis, and normal controls," *International Journal of Leprosy and Other Mycobacterial Diseases*, vol. 56, no. 1, pp. 50–55, 1988.

[17] Q. X. Wu, G. Y. Ye, Y. P. Yin, X. Y. Li, Q. Liu, and W. H. Wei, "Rapid serodiagnosis for leprosy—a preliminary study on latex agglutination test," *International Journal of Leprosy and Other Mycobacterial Diseases*, vol. 58, no. 2, pp. 328–333, 1990.

[18] M. S. Duthie, W. Goto, G. C. Ireton et al., "Use of protein antigens for early serological diagnosis of leprosy," *Clinical and Vaccine Immunology*, vol. 14, no. 11, pp. 1400–1408, 2007.

[19] D. B. Young, S. Dissanayake, R. A. Miller, S. R. Khanolkar, and T. M. Buchanan, "Humans respond predominantly with IgM immunoglobulin to the species-specific glycolipid of *Mycobacterium leprae*," *Journal of Infectious Diseases*, vol. 149, pp. 870–873, 1984.

[20] M. S. Duthie, M. N. Hay, E. M. Rada et al., "Specific IgG antibody responses may be used to monitor leprosy treatment efficacy and as recurrence prognostic markers," *European Journal of Clinical Microbiology & Infectious Diseases*, vol. 30, no. 10, pp. 1257–1265, 2011.

[21] M. S. Duthie, R. Raychaudhuri, Y. L. Tutterrow et al., "A rapid ELISA for the diagnosis of MB leprosy based on complementary detection of antibodies against a novel protein-glycolipid conjugate," *Diagnostic Microbiology and Infectious Disease*, vol. 79, no. 2, pp. 233–239, 2014.

[22] L. P. V. Cardoso, R. F. Dias, A. A. Freitas et al., "Development of a quantitative rapid diagnostic test for multibacillary leprosy using smart phone technology," *BMC Infectious Diseases*, vol. 13, p. 497, 2013.

[23] M. L. Penna, G. O. Penna, P. C. Iglesias, S. Natal, and L. C. Rodrigues, "Anti-PGL-I positivity as a risk marker for the development of leprosy among contacts of leprosy cases: systematic review and meta-analysis," *PLoS Neglected Tropical Diseases*, vol. 10, no. 5, article e0004703, 2016.

[24] F. M. Amorim, M. L. Nobre, L. C. Ferreira et al., "Identifying leprosy and those at risk of developing leprosy by detection of antibodies against LID-1 and LID-NDO," *PLoS Neglected Tropical Diseases*, vol. 10, no. 9, article e0004934, 2016.

[25] WHO, *Guidelines for the Diagnosis, Treatment and Prevention of Leprosy*, Licence: CC BY-NC-SA 3.0 IGO, World Health Organization, Geneva, Switzerland, 2017.

[26] J. P. T. Higgins and S. Green, *Cochrane Handbook for Systematic Reviews of Interventions. Version 5.1.0*, The Cochrane Collaboration, London, UK, 2011, http://handbook.cochrane.org.

[27] D. Moher, A. Liberati, J. Tetzlaff, D. G. Altman, and P. Group, "Preferred reporting items for systematic reviews and meta-analyses: the PRISMA statement," *PLoS Medicine*, vol. 6, no. 7, article e1000097, 2009.

[28] P. Whiting, A. W. Rutjes, J. B. Reitsma, P. M. Bossuyt, and J. Kleijnen, "The development of QUADAS: a tool for the quality assessment of studies of diagnostic accuracy included in systematic reviews," *BMC Medical Research Methodology*, vol. 3, p. 25, 2003.

[29] P. F. Whiting, A. W. Rutjes, M. E. Westwood et al., "QUADAS-2: a revised tool for the quality assessment of diagnostic accuracy studies," *Annals of Internal Medicine*, vol. 155, no. 8, pp. 529–536, 2011.

[30] G. J. Meyer, "Guidelines for reporting information in studies of diagnostic test accuracy: the STARD initiative," *Journal of Personality Assessment*, vol. 81, no. 3, pp. 191–193, 2003.

[31] P. M. Bossuyt, J. B. Reitsma, D. E. Bruns et al., "Towards complete and accurate reporting of studies of diagnostic accuracy: the STARD initiative," *Clinical Radiology*, vol. 58, no. 8, pp. 575–580, 2003.

[32] C. M. Rutter and C. A. Gatsonis, "A hierarchical regression approach to meta-analysis of diagnostic test accuracy evaluations," *Statistics in Medicine*, vol. 20, no. 19, pp. 2865–2884, 2001.

[33] J. J. Deeks, P. Macaskill, and L. Irwig, "The performance of tests of publication bias and other sample size effects in systematic reviews of diagnostic test accuracy was assessed," *Journal of Clinical Epidemiology*, vol. 58, no. 9, pp. 882–893, 2005.

[34] T. J. Fagan, "Letter: nomogram for bayes theorem," *New England Journal of Medicine*, vol. 293, no. 5, p. 257, 1975.

[35] W. J. Britton, R. J. Garsia, and A. Basten, "The serological response to the phenolic glycolipid of *Mycobacterium leprae* in Australian and Nepali leprosy patients," *Australian and New Zealand Journal of Medicine*, vol. 17, no. 6, pp. 568–573, 1987.

[36] K. Praputpittaya, V. Suriyanon, C. Hirunpetcharat, K. Rungruengthanakit, and C. Suphawilai, "Comparison of IgM, IgG and IgA responses to *M. leprae* specific antigens in leprosy," *Asian Pacific Journal of Allergy and Immunology*, vol. 8, no. 1, pp. 19–25, 1990.

[37] M. H. Saad, M. A. Medeiros, M. E. Gallo, P. P. Gontijo, and L. S. Fonseca, "IgM immunoglobulins reacting with the phenolic glycolipid-1 antigen from *Mycobacterium leprae* in sera of leprosy patients and their contacts," *Memórias do Instituto Oswaldo Cruz*, vol. 85, no. 2, pp. 191–194, 1990.

[38] P. Torres, J. J. Camarena, J. R. Gomez et al., "Comparison of PCR mediated amplification of DNA and the classical methods for detection of *Mycobacterium leprae* in different types of clinical samples in leprosy patients and contacts," *Leprosy Review*, vol. 74, no. 1, pp. 18–30, 2003.

[39] M. A. C. Frade, N. A. Paula, C. M. Gomes et al., "Unexpectedly high leprosy seroprevalence detected using a random surveillance strategy in midwestern Brazil: a comparison of ELISA and a rapid diagnostic test," *PLoS Neglected Tropical Diseases*, vol. 11, no. 2, article e0005375, 2017.

[40] R. V. Cellona, G. P. Walsh, T. T. Fajardo Jr. et al., "Cross-sectional assessment of ELISA reactivity in leprosy patients, contacts, and normal population using the semisynthetic antigen natural disaccharide octyl bovine serum albumin (ND-O-BSA) in Cebu, the Philippines," *International Journal of Leprosy and Other Mycobacterial Diseases*, vol. 61, no. 2, pp. 192–198, 1993.

[41] Q. Wu, Y. Yin, L. Zhang et al., "A study on a possibility of predicting early relapse in leprosy using a ND-O-BSA based ELISA," *International Journal of Leprosy and Other Mycobacterial Diseases*, vol. 70, no. 1, pp. 1–8, 2002.

[42] Y. Wen, Y. Xing, L. C. Yuan, J. Liu, Y. Zhang, and H. Y. Li, "Whole-blood nested-PCR amplification of *M. leprae*-specific DNA for early diagnosis of leprosy," *American Journal of Tropical Medicine and Hygiene*, vol. 88, no. 5, pp. 918–922, 2013.

[43] R. S. Moura, G. O. Penna, T. Fujiwara et al., "Evaluation of a rapid serological test for leprosy classification using human serum albumin as the antigen Carrier," *Journal of Immunological Methods*, vol. 412, pp. 35–41, 2014.

[44] E. M. Hungria, R. M. Oliveira, A. L. O. M. Souza et al., "Seroreactivity to new *Mycobacterium leprae* protein antigens in different leprosy-endemic regions in Brazil," *Memórias do Instituto Oswaldo Cruz*, vol. 107, no. 1, pp. 104–111, 2012.

[45] Y. Wen, Y. G. You, L. C. Yuan et al., "Evaluation of novel tools to facilitate the detection and characterization of leprosy patients in China," *BioMed Research International*, vol. 2014, Article ID 371828, 7 pages, 2014.

[46] A. A. Freitas, E. M. Hungria, M. B. Costa et al., "Application of *Mycobacterium leprae*-specific cellular and serological tests for the differential diagnosis of leprosy from confounding dermatoses," *Diagnostic Microbiology and Infectious Disease*, vol. 86, no. 2, pp. 163–168, 2016.

[47] E. M. Hungria, A. A. Freitas, M. A. Pontes et al., "Antigen-specific secretion of IFNgamma and CXCL10 in whole blood assay detects *Mycobacterium leprae* infection but does not discriminate asymptomatic infection from symptomatic leprosy," *Diagnostic Microbiology and Infectious Disease*, vol. 87, no. 4, pp. 328–334, 2017.

[48] S. Chanteau, J. L. Cartel, J. P. Boutin, and J. Roux, "Evaluation of gelatin particle agglutination assay for the detection of anti-PGLI antibodies. Comparison with ELISA method and applicability on a large scale study using blood collected on filter paper," *Leprosy Review*, vol. 62, no. 3, pp. 255–261, 1991.

[49] A. C. O. C. Fabri, A. P. Carvalho, S. Araujo et al., "Antigen-specific assessment of the immunological status of various groups in a leprosy endemic region," *BMC Infectious Diseases*, vol. 15, p. 218, 2015.

[50] M. S. Duthie, F. M. Orcullo, J. Abbelana, A. Maghanoy, and M. F. Balagon, "Comparative evaluation of antibody detection tests to facilitate the diagnosis of multibacillary leprosy," *Applied Microbiology and Biotechnology*, vol. 100, no. 7, pp. 3267–3275, 2016.

[51] A. Van Hooij, E. M. Tjon Kon Fat, S. J. F. van den Eeden et al., "Field-friendly serological test for determination of *M. leprae*-specific antibodies," *Scientific Reports*, vol. 7, no. 1, p. 8868, 2017.

[52] C. Sjöwall, A. Kastbom, G. Almroth, J. Wetterö, and T. Skogh, "Beware of antibodies to dietary proteins in "antigen-specific" immunoassays! falsely positive anticytokine antibody tests due to reactivity with bovine serum albumin in rheumatoid arthritis (the Swedish TIRA project)," *Journal of Rheumatology*, vol. 38, no. 2, pp. 215–220, 2011.

16

Comparison of Nasal Colonization of Methicillin-Resistant *Staphylococcus aureus* in HIV-Infected and Non-HIV Patients Attending the National Public Health Laboratory of Central Nepal

Kalash Neupane,[1] Binod Rayamajhee [iD],[2,3] Jyoti Acharya,[4] Nisha Rijal,[4] Dipendra Shrestha,[2] Binod G C [iD],[2,3] Mahesh Raj Pant,[5] and Pradeep Kumar Shah[1]

[1]*Department of Microbiology, Trichandra Multiple Campus, Tribhuvan University, Kathmandu, Nepal*
[2]*National College, Tribhuvan University, Khusibu, Kathmandu, Nepal*
[3]*Department of Infectious Diseases and Immunology, Kathmandu Research Institute for Biological Sciences, Lalitpur, Nepal*
[4]*Department of Bacteriology, National Public Health Laboratory, Teku, Kathmandu, Nepal*
[5]*Department of Microbiology, Kathmandu College of Science and Technology, Kamalpokhari, Kathmandu, Nepal*

Correspondence should be addressed to Binod Rayamajhee; rayamajheebinod@gmail.com

Academic Editor: Lucia Lopalco

Background. *Staphylococcus aureus* is a cardinal source of community- and hospital-acquired infection. HIV infection is a well-recognized risk factor for methicillin-resistant *S. aureus* (MRSA) carriage and infection. Intrinsically developed antibiotic resistance has sharply increased the burden of MRSA which is often associated with morbidity and mortality of the patients. Moreover, nasal carriage of *S. aureus* plays a significant role in spread of community-associated (CA) *S. aureus* infections. *Methods.* This study was conducted from June 2016 to December 2016 at National Public Health Laboratory (NPHL), Kathmandu, with an aim to assess the rate of *S. aureus* nasal carriage and MRSA carriage among HIV-infected and non-HIV patients. A total of 600 nonrepeated nasal swabs were analyzed following standard microbiological procedures, where 300 swabs were from HIV-infected patients while remaining 300 were from non-HIV patients. The isolates were identified on the basis of colony characteristics and a series of biochemical tests. The antibiotic susceptibility test (AST) was performed by the modified Kirby–Bauer disc diffusion method. Inducible clindamycin resistance in isolates was confirmed by the D-test method. *Results.* Overall, out of 600 nasal swabs of patients tested, 125 (20.8%) were *S. aureus* nasal carriers which included 80 out of 300 (26.66%) among HIV-infected patients and 45 (15%) out of 300 among non-HIV patients, and the result was statistically significant ($p = 0.0043$). Among the isolated *S. aureus*, 11 (13.8%) MRSA were confirmed in HIV-infected while 3 (6.7%) MRSA were detected from non-HIV patients. A higher number of *S. aureus* carriers was detected among HIV-infected males 40 (26.49%), whereas MRSA carriage was more prevalent among HIV-infected females 7 (5.1%). Among the HIV-infected, patients of age group 31–40 years were the ones with highest carriage rate 36 (45%), while in non-HIV patients, the highest rate 13 (28.9%) of carriage was detected among the patients of age group 21–30 years. Statistically significant difference was found between *S. aureus* carriage and HIV infection in patients ($p < 0.05$). Higher rate 2/3 (66.7%) of inducible clindamycin resistance in MRSA was detected from non-HIV patients in comparison to HIV-infected patients 7/11 (63.63%) while the result was statistically insignificant ($p > 0.05$). All the MRSA isolates (100%) were resistant against co-trimoxazole while ciprofloxacin showed high rate of sensitivity towards both MSSA and MRSA. None of the isolates were detected as VRSA. The major factors associated with nasal colonization of *S. aureus* were close personal contact, current smoking habit, and working or living in a farm ($p < 0.05$). *Conclusion.* Regular surveillance and monitoring of MRSA nasal carriage and antibiotic susceptibility pattern are of prime importance in controlling *S. aureus* infections especially in high risk groups like HIV-infected patients.

1. Introduction

Staphylococcus aureus is the most prevalent pathogen in community and health care setting and has been a serious threat to human health since its discovery [1]. *S. aureus*, especially methicillin-resistant *S. aureus* (MRSA), is responsible for varieties of maladies ranging from folliculitis to food poisoning. Moreover, it is responsible for causing life-threatening infections such as endocarditis, necrotizing pneumonitis, and osteomyelitis, among others [2]. Community-acquired MRSA (CA-MRSA) strain has emerged as a challenging pathogen which is frequently isolated from military personnel, drug users, athletes, and men who have sex with men [3]. The enduring threat and changing nature of *S. aureus* as a leading infectious pathogen has been well reported [4]. It is a common human skin colonizer, and pathogen armed with various classes of virulence factors including pore-forming toxins, superantigens, phagocytosis inhibitors, and biofilm forming capacity [5].

Some of the most severe infections caused by *S. aureus* include bacteremia, pneumonia, osteomyelitis, toxic shock syndrome, acute endocarditis, myocarditis, meningitis and abscesses in muscles, genitourinary tract infection, infection of central nervous system and various intraabdominal organs [6]. Methicillin-resistant *S. aureus* (MRSA) is a predominant cause of infection both in clinical and community settings which has amplified the disease burden to a major public health problem [7]. Colonizing feature of *S. aureus* is a potential factor for infection, an individual colonized with MRSA strain has a two to twelve fold more risk of subsequent infection [8]. Colonization and infection of MRSA has been recognized more in HIV-infected persons [9]. Moreover, higher prevalence of pathogenic MRSA strains have been documented among HIV-infected pediatric patients [10]. HIV infection and young age are considered as independent risk factors of MRSA infection [1]. High nasal carriage rate of MRSA in HIV infected persons may require early interventions. Hospitalized HIV-infected patients are nearly 17 times more likely to get *S. aureus* infection in comparison to non-HIV patients [11]. Not only this, the increasing prevalence of infections caused by MRSA has been difficult to treat due to the high rate of resistance to commonly prescribed antibiotics [12]. Determination of *S. aureus* nasal carriage rate and antibiotic resistance profiles along with molecular typing of nasal *S. aureus* isolates in healthy populations is necessary to identify risk factors associated with *S. aureus* infection [13–15].

In Nepal, reports on nasal carriage rate in vulnerable groups like HIV sero-positive individuals are very limited. Therefore, this study was carried out to determine the rate of nasal carriage of *S. aureus* in HIV-infected patients which was compared with healthy carriers. Furthermore, the antibiotic resistance patterns of isolates to commonly prescribed antibiotics, was also investigated. This study could be beneficial in management of MRSA infections, particularly in HIV-infected patients, while suggesting appropriate measures for controlling the possible risks of *S. aureus* infections in HIV-infected patients.

2. Methods and Materials

2.1. Study Design. This study was a prospective cross-sectional study. The study was carried out at bacteriology laboratory of National Public Health Laboratory, Teku, Kathmandu. Study population consisted of HIV-infected and non-HIV infected patients from whom nasal swab was collected. A total of 600 nasal swabs were collected for laboratory diagnosis, of which 300 swabs each were from HIV and non-HIV patients. The study duration was 6 months from June 2016 to December 2016. Preformed questionnaire was used to obtain the clinical history and demographic information of each patient. We also collected the information about health conditions and environmental factors of the subjects which were hypothesized to be major factors associated with MRSA colonization in the study population.

2.2. Inclusion and Exclusion Criteria. Patients with known history of HIV infection (seropositive) and noninfection (seronegative) were included in the study. Nasal swabs collected with standard operating procedure were accepted where complete label and strict sterile condition was maintained. Those samples that were improperly labeled and those from the patients who were non-HIV but having other immunodeficiency conditions like renal transplant, cancer, diabetes, liver cirrhosis, malignancy, chronic cardiovascular diseases, or consuming any immunosuppressant medicine were excluded from the study. Additionally, patients who had received any kind of antibiotics within the previous two weeks were also excluded from this study.

2.3. Specimen Collection and Transport. Sampling procedure was done by a well-trained laboratory technician. Nasal swabs were collected by using sterile cotton swabs moistened with sterile normal saline. Each nasal swab was obtained by rotating 2–3 times in the anterior nares of patients' and was transported to bacteriology department quickly for further processing [16]. All the collected swabs were transported in a zip lock bag to the laboratory. No transport medium was used because the bacteriology department and sample collection sites were adjacent to each other and additionally, drying of swab was prevented.

2.4. Laboratory Analysis

2.4.1. Microscopic Observation. The nasal swabs were evenly smeared on clean, dry, and grease-free glass slide. Then smear was heat fixed and stained by Gram stain procedure [17]. The stained smear was observed microscopically using the 100x objective for presence of Gram positive cocci in grape-like clusters.

2.4.2. Culture of Nasal Swabs. Primary culture was done on 5% sheep blood agar, Mac-Conkey agar, and Mannitol salt agar under aseptic conditions. Identification of isolated colonies was done by colony morphology, Gram staining, catalase test, slide coagulase test, and tube coagulase test [18].

2.4.3. Antibiotic Susceptibility Testing. Antibiotic susceptibility test was performed on Mueller Hinton Agar (MHA) by modified Kirby-Bauer disk diffusion method as per the Clinical Laboratory and Standards Institute 2016 guidelines [19] and the obtained results were interpreted accordingly. The antibiotics discs and concentrations used were ciprofloxacin (5 μg), penicillin G (30 μg), gentamicin (30 μg) cotrimoxazole (25 μg), cefoxitin (30 μg), erythromycin (30 μg), tetracycline (30 μg), clindamycin (2 μg), and vancomycin (30 μg). The diameter of zone of inhibition (ZOI) was measured and the results were interpreted. Antimicrobials doses were selected on the basis of prescription frequency by physician. Minimum inhibitory concentration (MIC) values of used antibiotics were unable to determine due to unavailability of all antibiotics powder at the time of study period.

2.4.4. Screening of Methicillin-Resistant S. aureus (MRSA). Screening for methicillin resistance in *S. aureus* was done by using cefoxitin (30 μg) antibiotic disc following modified Kirby-Bauer disc diffusion technique. Those *S. aureus* that showed zone size of $\leq$21 mm around cefoxitin disk were confirmed as MRSA strain.

2.4.5. Screening of Inducible Clindamycin-Resistant S. aureus. The macrolide-inducible clindamycin resistance in *S. aureus* was detected by D test method [20]. 0.5 McFarland standard bacterial suspensions of the test isolate was inoculated on MHA plate and then clindamycin (2 μg) and erythromycin (15 μg) discs were kept 15 mm edge to edge on the same plate. Then the plates were aerobically incubated overnight at 37°C. After the incubation period, flattening of zone (D-shaped) around the clindamycin disc was considered as inducible clindamycin resistance positive in *S. aureus*. Results of erythromycin-resistant *S. aureus* after D-test were interpreted into three phenotypic categories; MS_B (macrolide-streptogramin B), inducible MLS_B ($_iMLS_B$), and constitutive $_cMLS_B$ phenotype.

2.5. Quality Control. Media preparation, inoculation, and culture were performed in strict aseptic conditions. The prepared media were checked for the appearance of pure growth of organisms by using ATCC control strain. Stable strain of *S. aureus* ATCC 25923 was used as the control organism for the laboratory procedures. The thickness of MHA plates was maintained at 4 mm and the pH at 7.2–7.4. Microscope, incubator, centrifuge, refrigerator, water bath, autoclave, and hot air oven were checked regularly to ensure the correct functioning of equipment for the reliability of results. The temperature for all equipment was monitored and recorded.

2.6. Data Analysis. All data were analyzed using SPSS version 21.0. Chi square test was calculated where *p* value of <0.05 was considered statistically significant at 95% of confidence level.

3. Results

Among 600 nasal swabs investigated for determination of *S. aureus* and MRSA nasal carriage, 125 patients were found to be colonized with *S. aureus* among which 80 specimens were from HIV-infected and 45 from non-HIV individuals. The total prevalence of *S. aureus* colonization in HIV was found to be 26.66% while colonization in non-HIV was 15%. The MRSA colonization among the HIV patients was 13.8% (11/80) among 80 *S. aureus* isolates, whereas the MRSA colonization in non-HIV was 6.7% (3/45) among 45 *S. aureus* isolates.

Out of 300 nasal swabs analyzed from HIV-infected individuals, *S. aureus* isolates were 80, of which 26.5% (40/151) were male carriers whereas 23.2% (32/138) were female carriers and among third gender 72.7% (8/11) were *S. aureus* carriers (Table 1). Similarly, out of 45 *S. aureus* isolates from the 300 nasal swabs collected from non-HIV patients; 17.5% (27/154) were isolated from males whereas 12.3% (18/146) were from females. The study reveals that the *S. aureus* carrier percentage was higher among males in HIV-infected as well as in non-HIV patients (Table 2). The nasal carriage rate was not statistically significant with gender of patients ($p > 0.05$).

In HIV-infected patients, a high rate of *S. aureus* nasal carriage was found among the patients of age group 31–40 years with 36 (45%) followed by 21–30 years with 15 (18.8%), 41–50 years with 13 (17.5%), 11–20 years with 8 (10%) whereas *S. aureus* was not detected from the patients of age group 61 year or above (Table 1). Similarly, in non-HIV patients the high rate of *S. aureus* nasal carriage was found among the patients of age group 31–40 years with 12 (26.7%) followed by 11 (24.4%) in age group 41–50 years, 7 (15.6%) in age group 51–60 years, 5 (11.1%) in patients of age group 61 year or above whereas *S. aureus* was not detected from the patients of age group 10 years or less (Table 2). *S. aureus* carrier rate was statistically insignificant in relation to age groups of patients ($p > 0.05$).

Among the 300 HIV-infected patients, the growth of *S. aureus* was found in 80 (26.6%), of which 11 (13.8%) were confirmed as MRSA strains and remaining 69 (86.2%) were methicillin-sensitive *Staphylococcus aureus* (MSSA) (Table 1). On the other hand, from the 300 non-HIV patients 45 (15%) *S. aureus* were isolated where 3 (6.7%) isolates were confirmed as MRSA strain whereas 42 (93.3%) were MSSA strains (Table 2). The results claim higher percentage of MRSA among HIV-infected patients as compared to non-HIV patients. The association between MRSA isolates and HIV-infected patients was found to be statistically significant ($p < 0.05$). More MRSA isolates were isolated from HIV-infected male patients 6(7.5%) than from females 4 (5%) whereas 1 (1.3%) was isolated from third gender patients with known HIV infection. MSSA was found higher 34 (42.5%) in male patients as compared to female patients 28 (35%). Similarly, more MRSA 2 (4.4%) was found among male non-HIV patients whereas one MRSA was reported from female patients. MSSA isolates rate was also higher among male 25 (55.6%) as compared to female 17 (37.8%) patients (Figure 1). MRSA and MSSA carrier rate was statistically insignificant in relation with gender of patients ($p > 0.05$).

TABLE 1: Socio demographic characteristics of the HIV-infected patients and ratio of *S. aureus* carriage.

Demographic features	Type of patients	*S. aureus* (no. (%))	MRSA (no. (%))	No growth	Total (no. (%))
Gender	HIV-infected				
Male	151	40 (50)	6 (7.5)	111 (50.4)	151 (50.3)
Female	138	32 (40)	4 (5)	106 (48.2)	138 (46)
Third gender	11	8 (10)	1 (1.3)	3 (1.4)	11 (3.7)
Total	**300**	**80 (26.7)**	**11 (13.8)**	**220 (73.3)**	**300 (100)**
Age in years					
≤10	18	4 (5)	0	14 (77.8)	18 (6)
11–20	29	8 (10)	2 (2.5)	21 (72.4)	29 (9.7)
21–30	59	15 (18.8)	3 (3.8)	44 (74.6)	59 (19.7)
31–40	93	36 (45)	5 (6.3)	57 (61.3)	93 (31)
41–50	76	13 (17.5)	1 (1.3)	63 (82.9)	76 (25.3)
51–60	21	4 (5)	0	17 (80.9)	21 (7)
≥61	4	0	0	4 (100)	4 (1.3)
Total	**300**	**80 (26.7)**	**11 (13.8)**	**220 (73.3)**	**300 (100)**

TABLE 2: Socio demographic characteristics of the non-HIV patients and ratio of *S. aureus* carriage.

Demographic features	Type of patients	*S. aureus* (no. (%))	MRSA (no. (%))	No growth	Total (no. (%))
Gender	Non-HIV patients				
Male	154	27 (60)	2 (4.4)	127 (49.8)	154 (51.3)
Female	146	18 (40)	1 (2.3)	128 (50.2)	146 (48.7)
Third gender	0	0	0	0	0
Total	**300**	**45 (15)**	**3 (6.7)**	**255 (85)**	**300 (100)**
Age in years					
≤10	16	0	0	16 (100)	16 (5.3)
11–20	33	4 (8.9)	0	29 (87.9)	33 (11)
21–30	45	6 (13.3)	0	39 (86.7)	45 (15)
31–40	101	12 (26.7)	2 (4.4)	89 (88.1)	101 (33.7)
41–50	66	11 (24.4)	1 (2.2)	55 (83.3)	66 (22)
51–60	26	7 (15.6)	0	19 (73.1)	26 (8.7)
≥61	13	5 (11.1)	0	8 (61.5)	13 (4.3)
Total	**300**	**45 (15)**	**3 (6.7)**	**255 (85)**	**300 (100)**

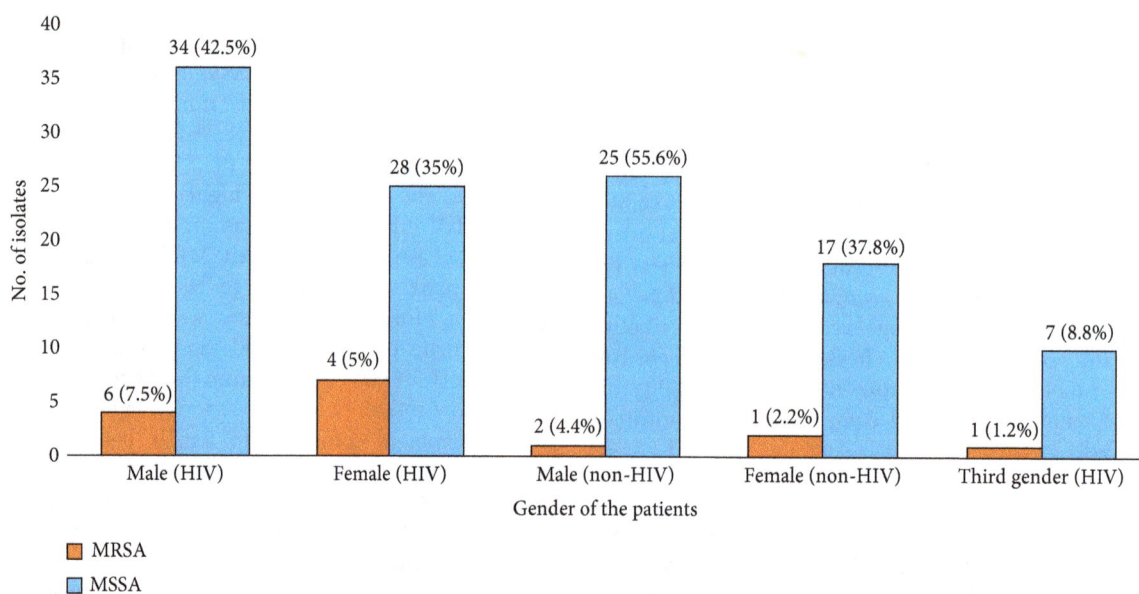

FIGURE 1: Gender-wise distribution of MRSA and MSSA isolates among HIV-infected and non-HIV patients.

Among the *S. aureus* isolates, the highest rate of antibiotic susceptibility was observed against vancomycin (100%) followed by tetracycline (94.4%), cefoxitin (88.8%) and gentamycin (80.8). High rate of resistance was seen towards erythromycin (41.6%) followed by co-trimoxazole (40.8%). Most 10 (71.4%) of the MRSA were resistant towards ciprofloxacin (Table 3).

Among 125 *S. aureus* isolates from HIV-infected and non-HIV patients, percentage of both inducible and constitutive clindamycin resistance was higher in MRSA as compare to MSSA strains. Inducible MLS_B-($iMLS_B$) resistance, constitutive MLS_B resistance, and macrolide-streptogramin B (MS_B) resistance were detected in 30 (24%), 19 (15.2%), and 34 (27.2%) isolates of *S. aureus*, respectively. Higher rate of $iMLS_B$ and $cMLS_B$ was seen among *S. aureus* isolated from HIV-infected patients while the rate of inducible MLS_B resistance was statistically insignificant as to the origin of *S. aureus* isolates i.e. HIV-infected and non-HIV patients ($p > 0.05$) (Table 4).

Nasal colonization rate of *S. aureus* was found significantly higher among the patients who used to work or live on a farm ($p < 0.05$). Similarly, inpatients showed higher rate 69 (55.2%) of *S. aureus* carriage as compared to outpatients 56 (44.8%), which was statistically significant data ($p = 0.005$). Additionally, patients with current smoking habit showed higher rate 76 (60.8%) of *S. aureus* carriage as compare to non-smokers 49 (39.2%) ($p = 0.0051$). Patients who had a job with close human contact were more prone to being a *S. aureus* carrier 89 (71.2%) as compared to those not having close human contact jobs 36 (28.8%) ($p = 0.0076$) (Table 5).

4. Discussion

Colonization of MRSA significantly increases the risk of *S. aureus* infection during hospital stay and even after discharge [21]. Furthermore, nasal carriage of *S. aureus* is a cardinal source of infection and nasopharynx is considered as the main reservoir of *S. aureus* [1]. The outbreaks of MRSA infection especially in group of people like security shelters, health care centers and refugee camps strongly supports the theory that the spread of *S. aureus* requires close personal contact [22]. The rate of nasal carriage depends on various factors like clinical environment, geographical area, occupation of patients, and patient's immune status among others. Previous studies have reported up to 33% nasal colonization of *S. aureus* among HIV-infected population [12].

Total of 600 nasal swabs were analyzed in this study where 300 nasal swabs were from HIV-infected patients and remaining 300 were from non-HIV patients. The prevalence of *S. aureus* in HIV-infected patients was found to be more than the rate in non-HIV patients. This study shows the total prevalence rate of nasal carriage of *S. aureus* to be 20.8% (125/600). HIV-infected patients have higher rate of *S. aureus* nasal carriage than non-HIV infected patients and the result was statistically significant ($p < 0.05$). High rate of *S. aureus* colonization in HIV infected individuals can lead to severe infections in this group of people [23]. Immune status along with an individual behavioral features can play a

positive role in *S. aureus* colonization and subsequent infection [24]. In a similar study carried out by Gonsu et al. (2013) in Cameroon, 40.6% of *S. aureus* nasal carriage was reported, whereas 34.6% of isolated *S. aureus* were MRSA among medical staffs and adult hospitalized patients [25]. Lilian et al. (2013) from Brazil have published a report of 27.2% as the prevalence of nasal colonization with *S. aureus* in patients with HIV/AIDS whereas the rate of MRSA was 21.8% [26]. Furthermore, the study has reported that nasal colonization of *S. aureus* was found to be more among the patients with CD4 cell count <200 cells/mm^3 and who had a high HIV viral load. Hence, HIV-infected patients are more vulnerable group to develop infections due to MRSA. On the other hand, *S. aureus* nasal colonization rate was found 18.4% among the healthy secondary school going students in Iraq whereas only 2.04% isolates were found to be MRSA [27].

The nasal carriage rate of *S. aureus* can be directly linked with underlying diseases, surrounding environment, age of patients and close contact activities [28]. In a study conducted among health care workers of Pakistan, 18.2% were nasal carriers of *S. aureus* where the count was lead my midwives (30%) then maintenance staffs of the hospital (28.6%) where only 1.5% of isolates were MRSA [29]. The real reason behind higher rate of *S. aureus* nasal colonization in midwives is unclear but this could be due to frequent contact with hospitalized patients and longer stay in hospital environment [30]. In a result reported by Khanal et al. (2015) the highest rate of MRSA nasal carriage was noted among hospital nurses which was 7.8% followed by hospital staffs of surgical wards and operating department whereas high number of *S. aureus* isolates (20.8%) were reported from doctors [31].

This study reveals higher rate of *S. aureus* colonization among patients of age group 31–40 years both in HIV-infected and no-HIV patients with prevalence rate 45% and 26.7%, respectively. Similarly, in a study carried out by Reinato et al., they have reported 36.1% of *S. aureus* colonization rate among the HIV/AIDS patients of age group 30–39 years [26]. The risk factors that have been associated with the emergence of MRSA infections among HIV infected individuals are not practically understood well but may be due to some possible risk factors, such as living conditions, prior hospitalization, use of fluoroquinolones and third generation cephalosporin antibiotics, intravenous drug usage, other secondary coinfections and low level of CD4 cells [32]. Some studies have suggested that participation in high risk sexual behaviors, use of public bath, anal intercourse, men who have sex with men (MSM), and sex with multiple partners may flourish the transmission of *S. aureus* and MRSA [33–35].

In this study, more *S. aureus* isolates were reported from males as compared to females both in HIV-infected and non-HIV patients though the result was not statistically significant ($p < 0.05$). The nasal carriage of *S. aureus* is found to be higher among male of active age groups who are mostly involved in outdoor activities, frequently visit to health care centers, and regular exposure to mass of people [31]. In contrast, higher rate of *S. aureus* nasal colonization was reported in female

TABLE 3: Antibiotic susceptibility pattern of MSSA and MRSA bacteria isolated from HIV-infected and non-HIV patients.

Isolates	Type of patients	RXN	Antimicrobial agents (no. (%))							
			CX	CIP	COT	GEN	VA	P	E	TE
MSSA ($n = 69$)	HIV-infected	S	69 (100)	56 (81.2)	45 (65.2)	60 (86.9)	69 (100)	57 (82.6)	41 (59.4)	66 (95.7)
		R	0	13 (18.8)	24 (34.8)	9 (13.1)	0	12 (17.4)	28 (40.6)	3 (4.3)
MSSA ($n = 42$)	Non-HIV	S	42 (100)	33 (78.6)	24 (57.1)	36 (85.7)	42 (100)	39 (92.38)	27 (64.3)	42 (100)
		R	0	9 (21.4)	18 (42.9)	6 (14.3)	0	3 (7.2)	15 (35.7)	0
MRSA ($n = 11$)	HIV-infected	S	0	3 (27.3)	5 (45.5)	3 (27.3)	11 (100)	0	4 (36.4)	8 (72.7)
		R	11 (100)	8 (72.7)	6 (54.5)	8 (72.7)	0	11 (100)	7 (63.6)	3 (27.3)
MRSA ($n = 3$)	Non-HIV	S	0	1 (33.3)	0	2 (66.7)	3 (100)	0	1 (33.3)	2 (66.7)
		R	3 (100)	2 (66.7)	3 (100)	1 (33.3)	0	3 (100)	2 (66.7)	1 (33.3)
Total ($n = 125$)		**S**	**111 (88.8)**	**93 (74.4)**	**74 (59.2)**	**101 (80.8)**	**125 (100)**	**96 (76.8)**	**73 (58.4)**	**118 (94.4)**
		R	**14 (9.2)**	**32 (25.6)**	**51 (40.8)**	**24 (19.2)**	**0**	**29 (23.2)**	**52 (41.6)**	**7 (5.6)**

Key: R = resistant, S = sensitive, RXN = reaction, CX = cefoxitin, CIP = ciprofloxacin, COT = co-trimoxazole, GEN = gentamicin, VA = vancomycin, P = penicillin G, E = erythromycin, TE = tetracycline.

TABLE 4: Clindamycin resistance among MRSA and MSSA strains.

Susceptibility pattern (phenotypes)	E	CD	D-test	MSSA		MRSA		Total S. aureus ($n = 125$) (no. (%))
				HIV-infected ($n = 69$) (no. (%))	Non-HIV ($n = 42$) (no. (%))	HIV-infected ($n = 11$) (no. (%))	Non-HIV ($n = 3$) (no. (%))	
Inducible MLS_B-($iMLS_B$)	R	S	Positive	17 (24.6)	4 (9.5)	7 (63.6)	2 (66.7)	30 (24)
Constitutive MLS_B-($cMLS_B$)	R	R	Negative	11 (15.9)	5 (11.9)	3 (27.3)	0	19 (15.2)
MS_B	R	S	Negative	21 (30.4)	11 (26.2)	1 (9.1)	1 (33.3)	34 (27.2)
Susceptible	S	S	Negative	20 (28.9)	22 (52.4)	0	0	42 (33.6)

Key: R = resistant, S = sensitive, E = erythromycin, CD = clindamycin, MS_B = macrolide–streptogramin B, MLS_B = macrolide–lincosamide–streptogramin B.

TABLE 5: Nasal colonization of S. aureus with respect to risk factors.

Environmental parameters	S. aureus carriers ($n = 125$) (no. (%))	S. aureus non-carriers ($n = 475$) (no. (%))	p value
Farm working/living			
Yes	42 (33.6)	306 (64.4)	**<0.05**
No	83 (66.4)	169 (35.6)	
Job conditions			
With close contact	89 (71.2)	276 (58.1)	**0.0076**
Without close contact	36 (28.8)	199 (41.9)	
Current smoking habit			
Yes	76 (60.8)	222 (46.7)	**0.0051**
No	49 (39.2)	253 (53.3)	
Alcoholic/nonalcoholic (current)			
Alcoholic	69 (55.2)	234 (49.3)	**0.319**
Nonalcoholic	56 (44.5)	241 (50.7)	
Outpatient/inpatient			
Outpatient	56 (44.8)	279 (58.7)	**0.005**
Inpatient	69 (55.2)	196 (41.3)	

(64%) than in male (36%) patients from Iran [36]. Patients with close contact job were more MSSA carriers 71.2% (89/125), as compared to 28.8% (36/125) patients who had no close contact and the result was statistically significant ($p = 0.0076$). Similar result was reported by Oliva et al. where 57% of people who had close contact job were MSSA carriers and 27.1% subjects were MSSA carriers who did not have human contact job [1]. This study shows higher rate of MSSA carriers among patients with current smoking habit ($p = 0.0051$) and patients who used to work or live in farm area ($p < 0.05$). Similarly, there were more MSSA carriers among inpatients (55.2%) in comparison to out-patients (44.8%). The association between type of patients (inpatients/out-patients) and MSSA carriers rate was statistically significant ($p = 0.005$). These results suggest that alcohol consumption, working/living in farm area and job with human contact environment positively contribute towards the spread of MSSA and MRSA. Moreover, hospitalized patients are at greater risk of having CA-MRSA colonization. Individual behavioral factors, environmental, social, HIV-host factors, and all these in united form play a positive role in S. aureus colonization and subsequent series of infection [30].

In this study, 94.4% (118/125) of S. aureus isolates were sensitive to tetracycline followed by cefoxitin 88.8% (111/125), whereas 9.2% (14/125) of isolates were resistant to cefoxitin. High rate of resistance 41.6% was observed against the antibiotic erythromycin followed by co-trimoxazole (40.8%), ciprofloxacin (25.6%) and penicillin G (23.2%), respectively. There was 100% sensitivity to the antibiotic vancomycin. The rate of co-trimoxazole resistance was higher among S. aureus isolated from HIV-infected patients than non-HIV patients. Co-trimoxazole is being used as a major chemoprophylaxis agent for HIV-infected patients for the treatment of various bacterial infections. Increasing rate of antibiotic resistance among MRSA isolates may increase the burden of infections in the community and clinical setting especially in patients with HIV/AIDS [37]. Similar result was reported on antibiotic susceptibility pattern of

S. aureus isolated from health care workers of western Nepal by Khanal et al. (2015) where 93.8% isolates were sensitive to tetracycline and 78.1% were sensitive to cefoxitin whereas 100% MRSA was penicillin resistant [31].

Among 125 *S. aureus* isolates, 24% (30/125) were detected to have inducible clindamycin (iMLS$_B$) resistance whereas high rate of iMLS$_B$ isolates were confirmed from MSSA 70% (21/30) than MRSA 30% (9/30). Additionally, 15.2% (19/125) constitutive MLS$_B$ and 27.2% (34/125) macrolide-streptogramin B (MS$_B$) resistance *S. aureus* were detected where 33.6% (42/125) of *S. aureus* isolates were clindamycin sensitive. None of the MRSA isolates were clindamycin sensitive. The results are not consistent with the findings reported by Prabhu et al. (2011) where 37.52% and 16.66% of *S. aureus* isolates from non-HIV patients were confirmed as iMLS$_B$ and cMLS$_B$ resistance, respectively [38]. The findings of this study show that D-test should be performed in routine antibiotic susceptibility test which could guide the appropriate treatment options during the infection caused by *S. aureus* and MRSA. The rate of iMLS$_B$ resistance of this study is higher as compared to previous reports by Ansari et al. and Adhikari et al. where they have reported 12.4% [39] and 10% [40] of inducible clindamycin-resistant *S. aureus*, respectively. This variation could be due to different clinical settings, type of patients, environment, *S. aureus* with different susceptibility patterns, and behavioral factors of patients [41]. Clindamycin is a drug of choice for the treatment of *S. aureus* infections but constitutive or inducible resistance to this antibiotic has been a major cause of treatment failure. Both MRSA and inducible clindamycin resistance *S. aureus* are serious challenge to health care management of Nepal especially in immunosuppressed groups like patients with HIV/AIDS, tuberculosis, renal transplant, cancer, diabetes, liver cirrhosis, malignancy, and chronic cardiovascular diseases.

High prevalence of nasal colonization along with increased rate of antibiotic resistance in *S. aureus* has posed a great threat to public health of the country and beyond. Compromised immune system and other risk factors including behavioral characters of HIV patients have led to emergence of MRSA which ultimately results in increase burden of community and hospital acquired infections. Increasing treatment failure due to high level of antibiotic resistance of *S. aureus* has expanded the burden of diseases in developing countries. Routine surveillance, proper monitoring of antibiotic resistance pattern and implementation of control strategies to prevent circulation of *S. aureus* strains in both clinical and hospital settings along with early detection of pathogenic MRSA isolates is very crucial for the reduction of morbidity and mortality due to diverse forms of *S. aureus* infections. Hence, routine screening, investigation of *S. aureus* nasal carriage particularly in immune deficient individuals, monitoring of their antibiotic susceptibility and control of *S. aureus* transmission are preventive me2asures for proper management of infections due to *S. aureus*.

5. Conclusion

The findings of this study show high rates of *S. aureus* colonization (mainly MRSA) and subsequent infections among HIV-infected patients. Smoking and alcohol drinking habits pose an individual at higher risk of *S. aureus* infection. Inducible clindamycin resistance (iMLS$_B$) *S. aureus* in HIV patients is increasing. D-test for the detection of iMLS$_B$ can be included as a screening test in routine laboratory investigation. Special attention is urgent to keep transmission and emergence of MRSA strains under control in people living with HIV/AIDS. *S. aureus* isolates showed high frequency of sensitive to tetracycline but we should take in account geographic differences in AST pattern when selecting antibiotic. Control strategies and interventions are very crucial to stop the spread to this "superbug" beyond the border.

6. Limitations

We cannot reveal the exact figure of *S. aureus* colonization without investigating swabs of other probable body sites like groin, pharynx, axillae, and anus. Furthermore, we could not collect the other epidemiological risk factors which could directly affect the MSSA and MRSA colonization and infection pattern. We could not perform/provide the CD4 count data to correlate with the immune status of HIV infected individuals too. Due to limitation of laboratory resources we could not run molecular procedures for confirmation of mecA gene in MRSA isolates. Further investigation in molecular level with collection of broad risk factors of large number of participants from different parts of the nation is required to generalize the result.

Abbreviations

BA: Blood agar
CA: Chocolate agar
CDC: Centers for Disease Control and Prevention
MA: Mac-Conkey agar
MHA: Mueller Hinton agar
MDR: Multidrug resistance
MRSA: Methicillin-resistant *S. aureus*
CLSI: Clinical Laboratory Standards Institute
HIV: Human immunodeficiency virus
AIDS: Acquired immunodeficiency syndrome
ART: Antiretroviral therapy
AST: Antibiotic susceptibility testing
SCCmec: Staphylococcal cassettes chromosome
SOP: Standard operating procedure
PVL: Panton-Valentine Leukocidin
SSTI: Skin-and-soft tissue infection
NPHL: National Public Health Laboratory
WHO: World Health Organization
VRSA: Vancomycin-resistant *S. aureus*.

Authors' Contributions

KN is the primary author, who designed the study methodology, performed laboratory investigations, and prepared the initial manuscript. JA and PKS helped with the designing of the study, analyzing the results, editing and proofreading the article, managing necessary arrangements during laboratory investigations, and supervising the complete study. BR edited, proofread, analyzed the data, and formatted and revised the complete manuscript. NR, DS, BGC, and MRP edited and proofread the article, helped in data analysis, and revised the manuscript for submission. All authors approved the final manuscript before submission to the Canadian Journal of Infectious Diseases and Medical Microbiology.

Acknowledgments

The authors would like to acknowledge all the laboratory staffs of National Public Health Laboratory Teku, Kathmandu, for their valuable support during the study.

References

[1] A. Oliva, M. Lichtner, M. T. Mascellino et al., "Study of methicillin-resistant *Staphylococcus aureus* (MRSA) carriage in a population of HIV-negative migrants and HIV-infected patients attending an outpatient clinic in Rome," *Annali di Igiene, Medicina Preventiva e di Comunità*, vol. 25, no. 2, pp. 99–107, 2013.

[2] S. L. Yousef, S. Y. Mahmoud, and M. T. Eihab, "Prevalence of methicillin-resistant *Staphylococcus aureus* in Saudi Arabia: systemic review and meta-analysis," *African Journal of Clinical and experimental Microbiology*, vol. 14, no. 3, pp. 146–154, 2013.

[3] F. R. DeLeo, M. Otto, B. N. Kreiswirth, and H. F. Chambers, "Community-associated meticillin-resistant *Staphylococcus aureus*," *The Lancet*, vol. 375, no. 9725, pp. 1557–1568, 2010.

[4] J. Sheldon and D. Heinrichs, "The iron-regulated staphylococcal lipoproteins," *Frontiers in Cellular and Infection Microbiology*, vol. 2, p. 41, 2012.

[5] C. Pozzi, E. M. Waters, J. K. Rudkin et al., "Methicillin resistance alters the biofilm phenotype and attenuates virulence in *Staphylococcus aureus* device-associated infections," *PLoS Pathogens*, vol. 8, no. 4, article e1002626, 2012.

[6] V. C. Pereira, D. F. M. Riboli, and M. de Lourdes Ribeiro de Souza, "Characterization of the clonal profile of MRSA isolated in neonatal and pediatric intensive care units of a University Hospital," *Annals of Clinical Microbiology and Antimicrobials*, vol. 13, no. 1, p. 50, 2014.

[7] R. M. Klevens, A. M. Melissa, J. Nadle et al., "Invasive methicillin-resistant *Staphylococcus aureus* infections in the United States," *JAMA*, vol. 298, no. 15, pp. 1763–1771, 2007.

[8] N. Safdar and E. A. Bradley, "The risk of infection after nasal colonization with *Staphylococcus aureus*," *The American Journal of Medicine*, vol. 121, no. 4, pp. 310–315, 2008.

[9] K. J. Popovich, K. Y. Smith, T. Khawcharoenporn et al., "Community-associated methicillin-resistant *Staphylococcus aureus* colonization in high-risk groups of HIV-infected patients," *Clinical Infectious Diseases*, vol. 54, no. 9, pp. 1296–1303, 2012.

[10] A. I. Hidron, E. V. Kourbatova, J. S. Halvosa et al., "Risk factors for colonization with methicillin-resistant *Staphylococcus aureus* (MRSA) in patients admitted to an urban hospital: emergence of community-associated MRSA nasal carriage," *Clinical Infectious Diseases*, vol. 41, no. 2, pp. 159–166, 2005.

[11] A. Senthilkumar, S. Kumar, and J. N. Sheagren, "Increased incidence of *Staphylococcus aureus* bacteremia in hospitalized patients with acquired immunodeficiency syndrome," *Clinical Infectious Diseases*, vol. 33, no. 8, pp. 1412–1416, 2001.

[12] L. S. Parasa, L. C. A. Kumar, P. Sirisha et al., "Epidemiological survey of methicillin resistant *Staphylococcus aureus* in the community and hospital, Gannavaram, Andhra Pradesh, South India," *Reviews in Infection*, vol. 1, no. 2, pp. 117–123, 2010.

[13] W. E. Bischoff, M. L. Wallis, K. B. Tucker, B. A. Reboussin, and R. J. Sherertz, "*Staphylococcus aureus* nasal carriage in a student community prevalence, clonal relationships, and risk factors," *Infection Control and Hospital Epidemiology*, vol. 25, no. 6, pp. 485–491, 2004.

[14] J. Lamaro-Cardoso, H. De Lencastre, Andre Kipnis et al., "Molecular epidemiology and risk factors for nasal carriage of *Staphylococcus aureus* and methicillin-resistant *S. aureus* in infants attending day care centers in Brazil," *Journal of Clinical Microbiology*, vol. 47, no. 12, pp. 3991–3997, 2009.

[15] F. D. Lowy, A. E. Aiello, M. Bhat et al., "*Staphylococcus aureus* colonization and infection in New York State prisons," *Journal of Infectious Diseases*, vol. 196, no. 6, pp. 911–918, 2007.

[16] N. Dhuria, P. Devi, B. Devi, and S. Malhotra, "Prevalence and risk factors for methicillin-resistant *Staphylococcus aureus* colonization in anterior nares of HIV-positive individuals," *udpecker Journal of Medical Sciences*, vol. 2, pp. 26–29, 2013.

[17] A. C. Smith and M. A. Hussey, "Gram stain protocols," in *ACM Microbelibrary-Laboratory Protocols*, American Society for Microbiology, Washington, DC, USA, 2005.

[18] B. A. Forbes, D. E. Sahm, and A. S. Weissfeld, *Bailey and Scott's Diagnostic Microbiology, International Edition*, Mosby, Inc., New York, NY, USA, 12th edition, 2007.

[19] CLSI, *Performance Standards for Antimicrobial Susceptibility Testing*, Clinical and Laboratory Standards Institute, Wayne, PA, USA, 2011.

[20] CLSI, *Performance Standards for Antimicrobial Susceptibility Testing; Twenty-Fifth Informational Supplement, CLSI Document M100-S25*, Clinical and Laboratory Standards Institute, Wayne, PA, USA, 2015.

[21] R. E. Nelson, M. E. Evans, L. Simbartl et al., "Methicillin-resistant *Staphylococcus aureus* colonization and pre-and post-hospital discharge infection risk," *Clinical Infectious Diseases*, 2018.

[22] H. Ringberg, A. C. Petersson, M. Walder, and P. J. H. Johansson, "The throat: an important site for MRSA colonization," *Scandinavian journal of infectious diseases*, vol. 38, no. 10, pp. 888–893, 2006.

[23] W. M. Kyaw, L. K. Lee, W. C. Slong, A. C. L. Plng, B. Ang, and Y. S. Leo, "Prevalence of and risk factors for MRSA colonization in HIV-positive outpatients in Singapore," *AIDS Research and Therapy*, vol. 9, no. 1, p. 33, 2012.

[24] W. C. Mathews, J. C. Caperna, R. E. Barber et al., "Incidence of and risk factors for clinically significant methicillin-resistant *Staphylococcus aureus* infection in a cohort of HIV-infected adults," *Journal of Acquired Immune Deficiency Syndromes*, vol. 40, no. 2, pp. 155–160, 2005.

[25] K. H. Gonsu, S. L. Kouemo, M. Toukam, V. N. Ndze, and S. S. Koulla, "Nasal carriage of methicillin resistant *Staphylococcus aureus* and its antibiotic susceptibility pattern in adult hospitalized patients and medical staff in some hospitals in Cameroon," *Journal of Microbiology and Antimicrobials*, vol. 5, no. 3, pp. 29–33, 2013.

[26] L. A. F. Reinato, D. P. M. Pio, L. P. Lopes, F. M. V. Pereira, A. E. R. Lopes, and E. Gir, "Nasal colonization with *Staphylococcus aureus* in individuals with HIV/AIDS attended in a Brazilian Teaching Hospital," *Revista Latino-Americana de Enfermagem*, vol. 21, no. 6, pp. 1235–1239, 2013.

[27] A. Habeeb, N. R. Hussein, M. S. Assafi, and S. A. Al-Dabbagh, "Methicillin resistant *Staphylococcus aureus* nasal colonization among secondary school students at Duhok City-Iraq," *Journal of Microbiology and Infectious Diseases*, vol. 4, no. 2, pp. 59–63, 2014.

[28] C.-S. Chen, C.-Y. Chen, and Y.-C. Huang, "Nasal carriage rate and molecular epidemiology of methicillin-resistant *Staphylococcus aureus* among medical students at a Taiwanese university," *International Journal of Infectious Diseases*, vol. 16, no. 11, pp. e799–e803, 2012.

[29] N. Akhtar, "Staphylococcal nasal carriage of health care workers," *Journal of College of Physicians and Surgeons Pakistan*, vol. 20, no. 7, pp. 439–443, 2010.

[30] A. I. Hidron, K. Russell, A. Moanna, and D. Rimland, "Methicillin-resistant *Staphylococcus aureus* in HIV-infected patients," *Infection and Drug Resistance*, vol. 3, p. 73, 2010.

[31] R. Khanal, S. Prakash, P. Lamichhane, A. Lamsal, S. Upadhaya, and V. Kumar Pahwa, "Nasal carriage of methicillin resistant *Staphylococcus aureus* among health care workers at a Tertiary Care Hospital in Western Nepal," *Antimicrobial Resistance and Infection Control*, vol. 4, no. 1, p. 39, 2015.

[32] F. R. DeLeo, B. A. Diep, and M. Otto, "Host defense and pathogenesis in *Staphylococcus aureus* infections," *Infectious Disease Clinics of North America*, vol. 23, no. 1, pp. 17–34, 2009.

[33] C. Cianflone, F. Nancy, A. A. Burgi, and B. R. Hale, "Increasing rates of community-acquired methicillin-resistant *Staphylococcus aureus* infections among HIV-infected persons," *International Journal of STD and AIDS*, vol. 18, no. 8, pp. 521–526, 2007.

[34] B. A. Diep, S. R. Gill, R. F. Chang et al., "Complete genome sequence of USA300, an epidemic clone of community-acquired meticillin-resistant *Staphylococcus aureus*," *The Lancet*, vol. 367, no. 9512, pp. 731–739, 2006.

[35] J. D. Szumowski, K. M. Wener, H. S. Gold et al., "Methicillin-resistant *Staphylococcus aureus* colonization, behavioral risk factors, and skin and soft-tissue infection at an ambulatory clinic serving a large population of HIV-infected men who have sex with men," *Clinical Infectious Diseases*, vol. 49, no. 1, pp. 118–121, 2009.

[36] N. Fard-Mousavi, G. Mosayebi, A. Amouzandeh-Nobaveh, A. Japouni-Nejad, and E. Ghaznavi-Rad, "The dynamic of *Staphylococcus aureus* nasal carriage in central Iran," *Jundishapur Journal of Microbiology*, vol. 8, no. 7, 2015.

[37] M. J. A. Reid, A. P. Steenhoff, N. Mannathoko et al., "*Staphylococcus aureus* nasal colonization among HIV-infected adults in Botswana: prevalence and risk factors," *AIDS Care*, vol. 29, no. 8, pp. 961–965, 2017.

[38] K. Prabhu, S. Rao, and V. Rao, "Inducible clindamycin resistance in *Staphylococcus aureus* isolated from clinical samples," *Journal of Laboratory Physicians*, vol. 3, no. 1, p. 25, 2011.

[39] S. Ansari, H. P. Nepal, R. Gautam et al., "Threat of drug resistant *Staphylococcus aureus* to health in Nepal," *BMC infectious diseases*, vol. 14, no. 1, p. 157, 2014.

[40] R. Adhikari, N. D. Pant, S. Neupane et al., "Detection of methicillin resistant *Staphylococcus aureus* and determination of minimum inhibitory concentration of vancomycin for *Staphylococcus aureus* isolated from pus/wound swab samples of the patients attending a tertiary care Hospital in Kathmandu, Nepal," *Canadian Journal of Infectious Diseases and Medical Microbiology*, vol. 2017, Article ID 2191532, 6 pages, 2017.

[41] B. Shrestha, B. M. Pokhrel, and T. M. Mohapatra, "Phenotypic characterization of nosocomial isolates of *Staphylococcus aureus* with reference to MRSA," *Journal of Infection in Developing Countries*, vol. 3, no. 7, pp. 554–560, 2009.

17

In Vitro Activity of Iclaprim against Methicillin-Resistant *Staphylococcus aureus* Nonsusceptible to Daptomycin, Linezolid, or Vancomycin

David B. Huang,[1,2] **Stephen Hawser,**[3] **Curtis G. Gemmell,**[4] **and Daniel F. Sahm**[5]

[1]*Motif BioSciences, New York, NY, USA*
[2]*Rutgers New Jersey Medical School, Trenton, NY, USA*
[3]*IHMA Europe Sàrl, Route de I'Ile-au-Bois 1A, 1870 Monthey, Valais, Switzerland*
[4]*Department of Bacteriology, University of Glasgow Medical School, Glasgow, UK*
[5]*IHMA, Schaumburg, IL, USA*

Correspondence should be addressed to David B. Huang; david.huang@motifbio.com

Academic Editor: Paul-Louis Woerther

Iclaprim is a bacterial dihydrofolate reductase inhibitor in Phase 3 clinical development for the treatment of acute bacterial skin and skin structure infections and hospital-acquired bacterial pneumonia caused by Gram-positive bacteria. Daptomycin, linezolid, and vancomycin are commonly used antibiotics for these indications. With increased selective pressure to these antibiotics, outbreaks of bacterial resistance to these antibiotics have been reported. This *in vitro* pilot study evaluated the activity of iclaprim against methicillin-resistant *Staphylococcus aureus* (MRSA) isolates, which were also not susceptible to daptomycin, linezolid, or vancomycin. Iclaprim had an MIC ≤ 1 µg/ml to the majority of MRSA isolates that were nonsusceptible to daptomycin (5 of 7 (71.4%)), linezolid (26 of 26 (100%)), or vancomycin (19 of 28 (66.7%)). In the analysis of time-kill curves, iclaprim demonstrated $\geq 3 \log_{10}$ reduction in CFU/mL at 4–8 hours for tested strains and isolates nonsusceptible to daptomycin, linezolid, or vancomycin. Together, these data support the use of iclaprim in serious infections caused by MRSA nonsusceptible to daptomycin, linezolid, or vancomycin.

1. Background

Iclaprim represents a diaminopyrimidine that inhibits bacterial dihydrofolate reductase of Gram-positive pathogens [1, 2]. Iclaprim exhibits potent *in vitro* activity against Gram-positive pathogens associated with acute bacterial skin and skin structure infections (ABSSSIs) and nosocomial pneumonia including *Staphylococcus aureus*, *Enterococcus* spp., and *Streptococcus* spp. [1]. Iclaprim demonstrates rapid *in vitro* bactericidal activity in time-kill studies in human plasma [3]. Iclaprim is in Phase 3 clinical development for the treatment of ABSSSI and nosocomial pneumonia. Daptomycin, linezolid, and vancomycin are commonly used antibiotics for these indications (daptomycin is indicated for ABSSSI but not indicated for nosocomial pneumonia); however, increased selective pressure to these antibiotics has resulted in outbreaks of bacterial resistance to these antibiotics. Because of this emerging resistance, this current study was done to evaluate iclaprim's activity against MRSA isolates that were nonsusceptible to daptomycin, linezolid, or vancomycin.

2. Materials and Methods

Antibacterial susceptibility testing was conducted at the Department of Bacteriology, Glasgow Royal Infirmary, Glasgow, Scotland [4], and Eurofins Microbiology Laboratories on a range of MSSA and MRSA strains and isolates with varying susceptibilities to several recognized antistaphylococcal antibiotics. A total of 61 nonduplicative, nonconsecutive isolates of methicillin-resistant *S. aureus* (MRSA), which were nonsusceptible to daptomycin, linezolid, or vancomycin, were obtained from Eurofins repository or from the National

TABLE 1: Iclaprim *in vitro* activity against MRSA isolates nonsusceptible to daptomycin, linezolid, or vancomycin.

MRSA phenotype (number)	Iclaprim MIC ≤ 1, µg/mL (%)	Iclaprim MIC$_{50}$/MIC$_{90}$ (µg/mL)	MIC range (µg/ml)
Daptomycin nonsusceptible ($n = 7$)	5/7 (71.4)	0.25/>8	0.12->8
Linezolid nonsusceptible ($n = 26$)	26/26 (100.0)	0.06/0.25	0.03–1
Vancomycin intermediate ($n = 23$)	16/23 (69.6)	0.25/>8	0.25->8
Vancomycin resistant ($n = 5$)	3/5 (60.0)	0.5/>8	0.25->8

Institutes of Health Network on Antimicrobial Resistance to *Staphylococcus aureus* (NARSA) repository.

Clinical isolates were identified by the submitting laboratories, and identifications were confirmed centrally at Eurofins using the Bruker matrix-assisted laser desorption ionization-time of flight mass spectrometry (MALDI-TOF) biotyper. Susceptibility testing and minimal inhibitory concentration (MIC) interpretations were performed according to broth microdilution protocols. *S. aureus* breakpoints for daptomycin, linezolid, and vancomycin are ≤1, ≤4, and ≤2 µg/mL (4–8 µg/mL were classified as vancomycin-intermediate *S. aureus* and ≥16 were classified as vancomycin-resistant *S. aureus*), respectively. To date, there are no published clinical breakpoints for iclaprim. However, based on a number of factors (e.g., MRSA distribution of MICs, assessment of the pharmacokinetics/pharmacodynamics of iclaprim, and the study of the clinical outcomes of MRSA infections when iclaprim was used in Phase 2 and 3 studies) outlined in the CLSI M23 guideline, an iclaprim MIC ≤ 1 µg/mL for *S. aureus*, including MRSA, has been proposed.

MRSA isolates were tested in cation-adjusted Mueller–Hinton broth (CA-MHB). Quality control and interpretation of results were performed in accordance with CLSI M100-S25 methods [5]. QC ranges for iclaprim were those approved by CLSI and published in M100-S25 [4]. Iclaprim and comparator antibiotic MIC results were within the CLSI published ranges against *S. aureus* ATCC 29213. Isolates were tested with MIC panels (Thermo Fisher Scientific, Cleveland, Ohio, USA) of comparator antibiotics (trimethoprim, trimethoprim-sulfamethoxazole, ceftriaxone, erythromycin, levofloxacin, oxacillin, meropenem, tetracycline, tigecycline, vancomycin, linezolid, and daptomycin).

The analysis of time-kill curves was performed by exposing 10^5–10^6 CFU/mL of each MRSA isolate or strain to iclaprim, daptomycin, linezolid, or vancomycin at 2, 4, and 8x MICs. Bactericidal activity was defined as a ≥ 3 log$_{10}$ reduction in CFU/mL after 24 hours of incubation.

3. Results

The MIC$_{50}$ and MIC$_{90}$ values for the MRSA nonsusceptible to daptomycin, nonsusceptible to linezolid, vancomycin-intermediate, and vancomycin-resistant were >1/>1, 8/>8, 4/8, and >32/>32 µg/mL, respectively. Among the seven MRSA isolates nonsusceptible to daptomycin (all seven had an MIC > 1 to daptomycin), four, two, and one had a vancomycin MIC of 4, 8, and 2 µg/mL, respectively.

Table 1 shows that iclaprim exhibited potent activity against the majority of the 61 MRSA isolates that were nonsusceptible to daptomycin, linezolid, or vancomycin

(MIC$_{50}$ 0.25 µg/mL). In the Glasgow study, all strains and isolates of MRSA and MSSA had an iclaprim MIC ≤ 1 µg/mL. Iclaprim notably exhibited 100% activity against MRSA isolates ($n = 26$) that were nonsusceptible to linezolid. A total of 9 (15.2%) isolates had reduced susceptibility to iclaprim with MICs > 8 µg/mL (Table 1). These isolates were not clustered in time of isolate collection, infection type, and/or geographic region. Figure 1 shows representative time-kill curves of iclaprim (2x, 4x, and 8x MICs for all antibiotics), which exhibited bactericidal activity at 4–8 hours against MRSA strains and isolates nonsusceptible to daptomycin, linezolid, or vancomycin. As expected, representative time-kill curves of daptomycin exhibited no activity against MRSA strains and isolates nonsusceptible to daptomycin, linezolid exhibited no activity against MRSA strains and isolates nonsusceptible to linezolid, and vancomycin exhibited no activity against MRSA strains and isolates nonsusceptible to vancomycin.

4. Discussion

This report shows that iclaprim, without a synergistic combination of a sulfonamide, was highly active and rapidly bactericidal against a collection of 61 MRSA clinical isolates with nonsusceptible phenotypes to daptomycin, linezolid, or vancomycin. The MIC$_{50}$ value of 0.25 µg/mL for MRSA documented in this study was consistent with MIC$_{50}$ values in two previous surveillance reports for 5937 Gram-positive isolates, including MRSA, beta-hemolytic streptococci (most commonly *Streptococcus pyogenes* and *S. agalactiae*), and *S. pneumoniae* [1]. These isolates were collected from patients in the US and EU with skin and soft tissue, blood stream, and respiratory clinical specimens.

Based on MIC distributions of MRSA, assessment of the pharmacokinetics and pharmacodynamics of iclaprim, and the study of the clinical outcomes of MRSA infections when iclaprim was used in Phase 2 and 3 studies, an iclaprim MIC ≤ 1 µg/mL for *S. aureus*, including MRSA, has been proposed as the breakpoint for nonsusceptibility. The 80 mg fixed dose is based on prior animal models of infection studies, which suggest that the pharmacokinetic and pharmacodynamics (PK/PD) drivers, which best correlated with efficacy, were the area under the curve from 0 to 24 hours at steady state (AUC$_{0-24\,h,ss}$), AUC/minimum inhibitory concentration (MIC), and time above the MIC during the dosing interval (T > MIC). In addition, using PK data collected from 470 patients from a Phase 3-complicated skin and skin infection (cSSSI) trials (ASSIST-1 and 2), population PK modeling, and Monte Carlo simulation identified that the fixed iclaprim 80 mg dosage regimen optimally maximized AUC$_{0-24\,h,ss}$, AUC/MIC, and T > MIC while minimizing

(A)

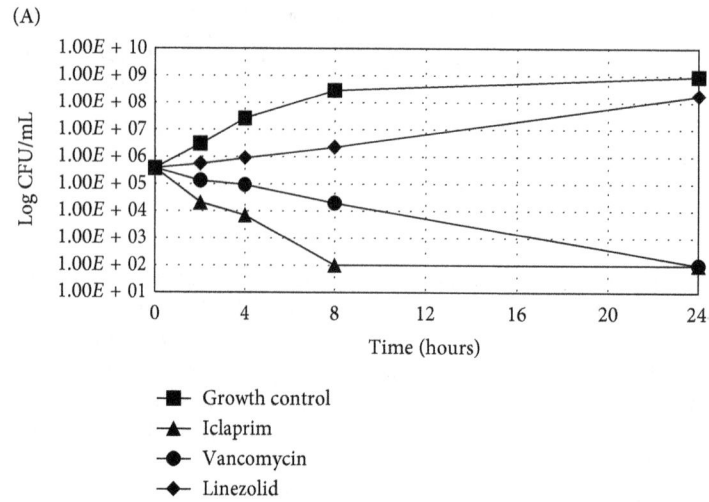

Growth control
Iclaprim
Vancomycin
Linezolid

(B)

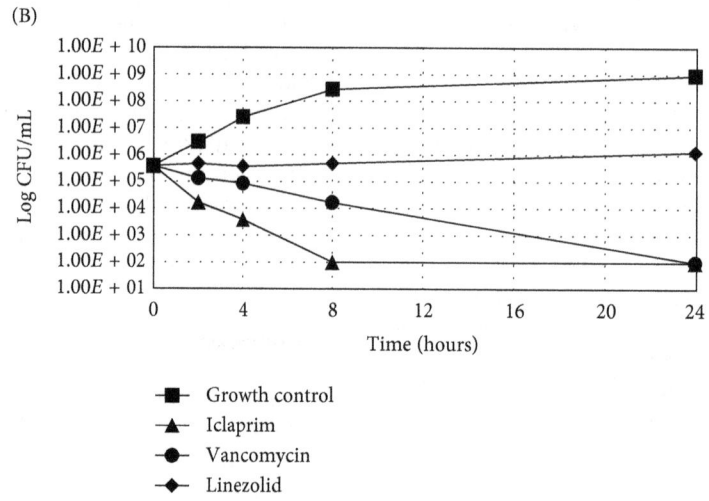

Growth control
Iclaprim
Vancomycin
Linezolid

(C)

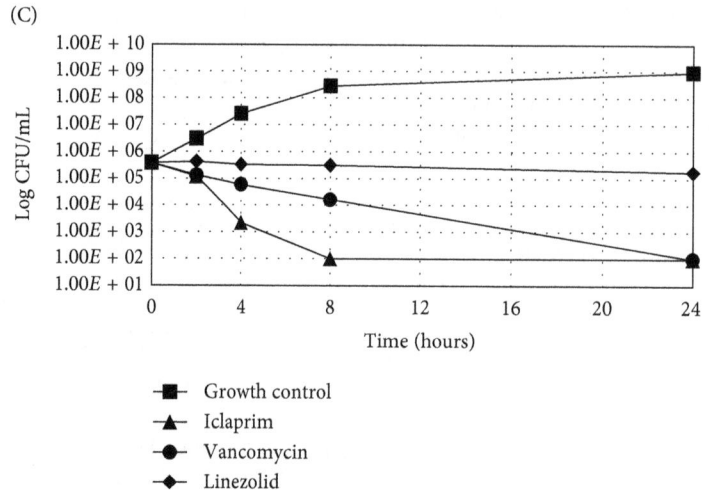

Growth control
Iclaprim
Vancomycin
Linezolid

(a)

(A)

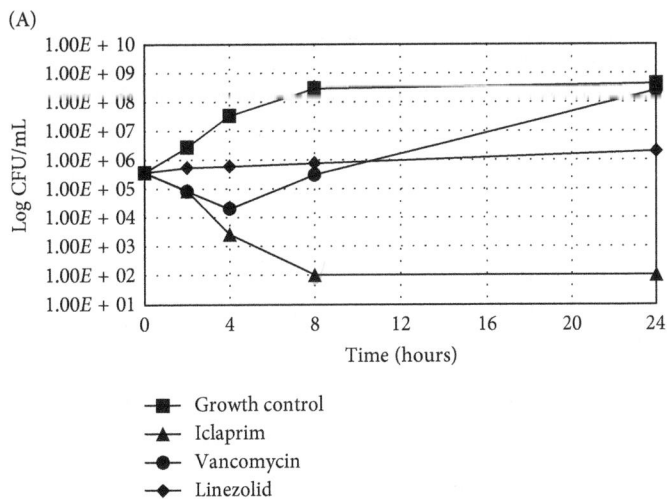

(B)

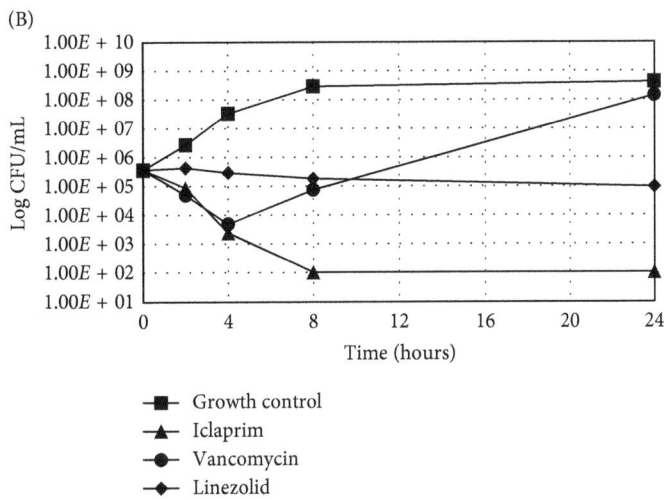

(C)

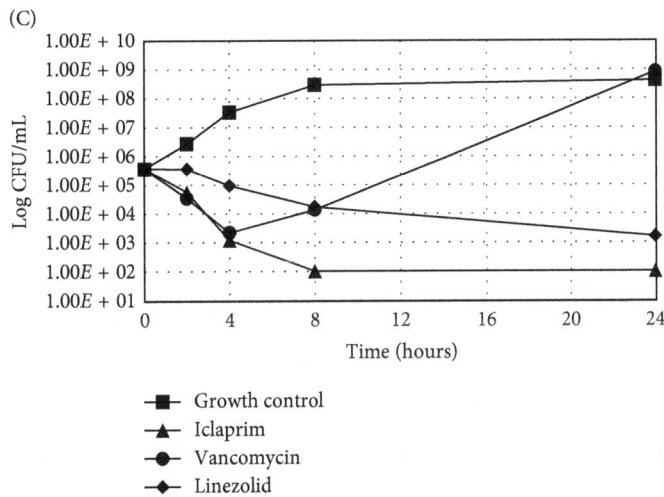

(b)

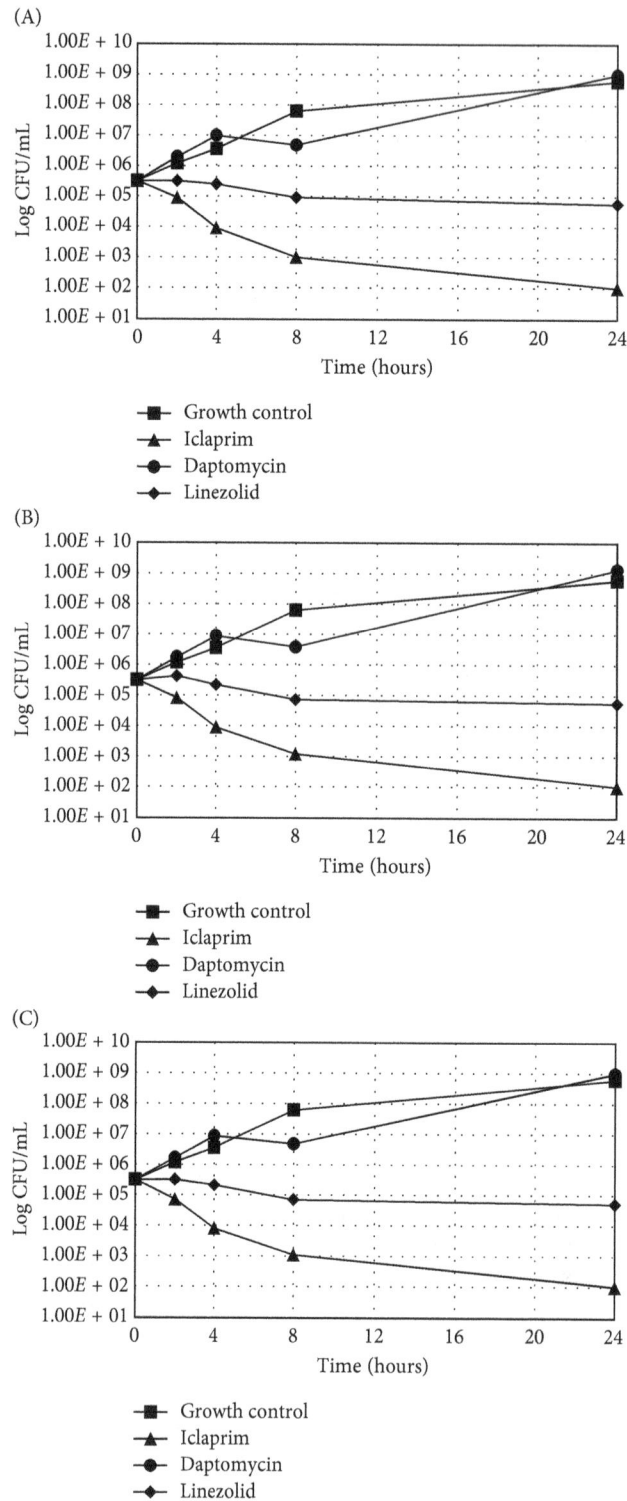

FIGURE 1: Iclaprim time-kill curves against MRSA isolates nonsusceptible to linezolid, resistant to vancomycin, and nonsusceptible to daptomycin, 2x, 4x, and 8x MICs were used for all antibiotics. (a) MRSA, linezolid nonsusceptible strain (MIC ≥ 8 μg/mL), ATCC 986537, NRS271. (A) 2x MIC. (B) 4x MIC. (C) 8x MIC. Iclaprim showed significantly lower CFU at 2 h, 4 h, 8 h, and 24 h compared to control, vancomycin, and linezolid ($P < 0.01$; one-way ANOVA with Tukey's post hoc test). (b) MRSA, vancomycin-resistant strain (MIC ≥ 32 μg/mL), ATCC 1409053, vanA positive. (A) 2x MIC. (B) 4x MIC. (C) 8x MIC. Iclaprim showed significantly lower CFU at 4 h, 8 h, and 24 h compared to control, vancomycin, and linezolid ($P < 0.01$; one-way ANOVA with Tukey's post hoc test). (c) MRSA, daptomycin-resistant strain (MIC ≥ 4 μg/mL) (clinical isolate). (A) 2x MICs. (B) 4x MIC. (C) 8x MIC. Iclaprim showed significantly lower CFU at 4 h, 8 h, and 24 h compared to control, daptomycin, and linezolid ($P < 0.01$; one-way ANOVA with Tukey's post hoc test).

the probability of a $C_{max,ss}$ to $\geq 800\,ng/mL$, a concentration associated with dose-limiting toxicity [6]. Based on PK/PD analyses, iclaprim 80 mg administered over two hours every 12 hours adequately covers *S. aureus* clinical isolates with an iclaprim MIC $\leq 1\,\mu g/mL$; therefore, this dose was selected as the dosing scheme for ongoing Phase 3 clinical trials.

A limitation of this study is the small numbers of daptomycin and linezolid nonsusceptible and vancomycin-resistant MRSA strains to arrive at conclusive activity of iclaprim against these types of strains and dose selection justification for clinical trials, which robust *in vitro* data are necessary. However, these data suggest that larger studies are warranted in examining iclaprim's activity against daptomycin and linezolid nonsusceptible and vancomycin-resistant MRSA. The findings of reduced daptomycin susceptibility and reduced vancomycin susceptibility and resistance have been reported in *S. aureus*. Daptomycin and vancomycin cross-resistance is believed to be related to the physical barrier of a thickened cell wall of MRSA against the penetration of daptomycin and vancomycin molecules [7, 8]. A possible reason as to why iclaprim had reduced activity against such isolates may relate to the mechanism of action of iclaprim, which interferes with folate metabolism in the bacterial cell by competitively blocking the biosynthesis of tetrahydrofolate. This product acts as a carrier of one-carbon fragments and is necessary for the ultimate synthesis of DNA, RNA, and bacterial cell wall proteins. As vancomycin-resistant strains are already altered in terms of cell wall targets, it is likely that some products of folate metabolism are less important [9].

The results of this *in vitro* study suggest that iclaprim may be a useful treatment option for infections caused by MRSA, including those with nonsusceptible phenotypes to daptomycin, linezolid, or vancomycin. Daptomycin, linezolid, and vancomycin are antibiotics that are FDA approved, and the Infectious Diseases Society of America guidelines list these antibiotics as treatment options for skin and skin structure infections (SSSIs) caused by Gram-positive pathogens [10]. New therapeutic options are needed, especially because of reported nonsusceptibility of Gram-positive bacteria to daptomycin, linezolid, and vancomycin and its associated poor outcomes, increased length of stay, healthcare costs, and overall morbidity [11–14].

5. Conclusion

In conclusion, the results from this pilot *in vitro* study show the potent and rapid bactericidal activity of iclaprim against clinical MRSA isolates, including those with nonsusceptible phenotypes to daptomycin, linezolid, or vancomycin. Continued surveillance is warranted to track the continued potency of iclaprim, as well as MRSA isolates nonsusceptible to daptomycin, linezolid, and vancomycin and to detect any potential emergence of resistance.

Acknowledgments

This study was funded by Motif BioSciences.

References

[1] H. S. Sader, T. R. Fritsche, and R. N. Jones, "Potency and bactericidal activity of iclaprim against recent clinical gram-positive isolates," *Antimicrobial Agents and Chemotherapy*, vol. 53, no. 5, pp. 2171–2175, 2009.

[2] P. Schneider, S. Hawser, and K. Islam, "Iclaprim, a novel diaminopyrimidine with potent activity on trimethoprim sensitive and resistant bacteria," *Bioorganic and Medicinal Chemistry Letters*, vol. 13, no. 23, pp. 4217–4221, 2003.

[3] H. Laue, T. Valensise, A. Seguin, S. Lociuro, K. Islam, and S. Hawser, "In vitro bactericidal activity of iclaprim in human plasma," *Antimicrobial Agents and Chemotherapy*, vol. 53, no. 10, pp. 4542–4544, 2009.

[4] C. G. Gemmell and G. Middlemas, "AR-100, a novel diaminopyrimidine: activity against various clinical isolates of gram-positive and gram-negative bacteria," in *Proceedings of 42nd Interscience Conference on Antimicrobial Agents and Chemotherapy (ICAAC)*, San Diego, CA, USA, September 2002.

[5] CLSI M100-S25, *Performance Standards for Antimicrobial Susceptibility Testing: 25th Informational Supplement*, Clinical and Laboratory Standards Institute, Wayne, PA, USA, 2015.

[6] D. B. Huang and T. L. Lodise, "Use of pharmacokinetic/pharmacodynamics (PK/PD) analyses to determine the optimal fixed dosing regimen of iclaprim for Phase III ABSSSI clinical trials," in *Proceedings of IDWeek 2016*, San Diego, CA, USA, October 2016.

[7] L. Z Cui, E. Tominaga, H. Neoh, and K. Hiramatsu, "Correlation between reduced daptomycin susceptibility and vancomycin resistance in vancomycin-intermediate *Staphylococcus aureus*," *Antimicrobial Agents and Chemotherapy*, vol. 50, no. 3, pp. 1079–1082, 2006.

[8] L. Z. Cui, X. Ma, K. Sato et al., "Cell wall thickening is a common feature of vancomycin resistance in *Staphylococcus aureus*," *Journal of Clinical Microbiology*, vol. 41, no. 1, pp. 5–14, 2003.

[9] H. C. Neu and T. D. Gootz, "Antimicrobial chemotherapy," in *Medical Microbiology*, S. Baron, Ed., University of Texas Medical Branch at Galveston, Galveston, TX, USA, 4th edition, 1996.

[10] D. L. Stevens, A. L. Bisno, H. F. Chambers et al., "Practice guidelines for the diagnosis and management of skin and soft tissue infections: 2014 update by the Infectious Diseases Society of America," *Clinical Infectious Diseases*, vol. 59, no. 2, pp. 147–159, 2014.

[11] M. Bassetti, E. Righi, and A. Carnelutti, "New therapeutic options for skin and soft tissue infections," *Current Opinion in Infectious Diseases*, vol. 29, no. 2, pp. 99–108, 2016.

[12] J. Edelsberg, A. Berger, D. J. Weber, R. Mallick, A. Kuznik, and G. Oster, "Clinical and economic consequences of failure of initial antibiotic therapy for hospitalized patients with complicated skin and skin-structure infections," *Infection Control and Hospital Epidemiology*, vol. 29, no. 2, pp. 160–169, 2008.

[13] K. J. Eagye, A. Kim, S. Laohavaleeson, J. L. Kuti, and D. P. Nicolau, "Surgical site infections: does inadequate antibiotic therapy affect patient outcomes?," *Surgical Infections*, vol. 10, no. 4, pp. 323–331, 2009.

[14] E. Nannini, B. E. Murray, and C. A. Arias, "Resistance or decreased susceptibility to glycopeptides, daptomycin, and linezolid in methicillin-resistant *Staphylococcus aureus*," *Current Opinion in Pharmacology*, vol. 10, no. 5, pp. 516–521, 2010.

18

Development of New Tools to Detect Colistin-Resistance among Enterobacteriaceae Strains

Lucie Bardet and **Jean-Marc Rolain**

Aix-Marseille Université, IRD, AP-HM, MEPHI, IHU-Méditerranée Infection, Marseille, France

Correspondence should be addressed to Jean-Marc Rolain; jean-marc.rolain@univ-amu.fr

Academic Editor: Elisabetta Caselli

The recent discovery of the plasmid-mediated *mcr-1* gene conferring resistance to colistin is of clinical concern. The worldwide screening of this resistance mechanism among samples of different origins has highlighted the urgent need to improve the detection of colistin-resistant isolates in clinical microbiology laboratories. Currently, phenotypic methods used to detect colistin resistance are not necessarily suitable as the main characteristic of the *mcr* genes is the low level of resistance that they confer, close to the clinical breakpoint recommended jointly by the CLSI and EUCAST expert systems ($S \leq 2$ mg/L and $R > 2$ mg/L). In this context, susceptibility testing recommendations for polymyxins have evolved and are becoming difficult to implement in routine laboratory work. The large number of mechanisms and genes involved in colistin resistance limits the access to rapid detection by molecular biology. It is therefore necessary to implement well-defined protocols using specific tools to detect all colistin-resistant bacteria. This review aims to summarize the current clinical microbiology diagnosis techniques and their ability to detect all colistin resistance mechanisms and describe new tools specifically developed to assess plasmid-mediated colistin resistance. Phenotyping, susceptibility testing, and genotyping methods are presented, including an update on recent studies related to the development of specific techniques.

1. Introduction

Multidrug-resistant (MDR) bacteria are of a global concern, notably with the description of carbapenemase-producing Enterobacteriaceae [1]. Colistin is an old antibiotic that regained popularity as a last resort treatment to face the worldwide emergence of these pathogens [2]. Colistin is a polycationic and bactericidal drug that targets the lipid A moiety of lipopolysaccharide (LPS), moving its cationic charges, leading to cell wall lysis and bacterial death [3]. The increasing use of colistin has led to emerging resistance, a phenomenon that represents a clinical source of worry [4]. Enterobacteriaceae are Gram-negative bacteria that are often described as the pathogens responsible for human infectious diseases, particularly the *Escherichia coli* and *Klebsiella pneumoniae* species. Until recently, all mechanisms described were of chromosomal origin, mostly mediated by the two-component systems PmrAB and PhoPQ, leading to the addition of positively charged carbohydrates

on the negatively charged lipid A (Figure 1), a phosphoethanolamine by a phosphoethanolamine transferase or a 4-amino-4-arabinose by surexpression of *arnBCADTEF* operon, leading to the loss of polymyxin affinity for the LPS [5]. In November 2015, Liu et al. reported the first plasmid-mediated gene which they named *mcr-1* [6], which encodes for a phosphoethanolamine transferase, and this was followed by the description of variants (*mcr-1.2*, *mcr-1.3*,...) and the genes *mcr-2*, *mcr-3*, *mcr-4*, *mcr-5*, *mcr-6*, *mcr-7*, and *mcr-8* [7–15]. This recent discovery raised concern about the increase and spread of resistance among the Enterobacteriaceae [16] and led to new recommendations for laboratory diagnosis and clinicians [17]. Specifically, the majority of these *mcr-1* strains exhibited a low minimal inhibitory concentration (MIC) of colistin, around 4 μg/ml [6], which is close to the MIC breakpoint according to the EUCAST guidelines (susceptibility ≤ 2 μg/ml and resistance > 2 μg/ml) (http://www.eucast.org). Moreover, several studies have reported the detection of the *mcr-1* gene in carbapenemase-producing

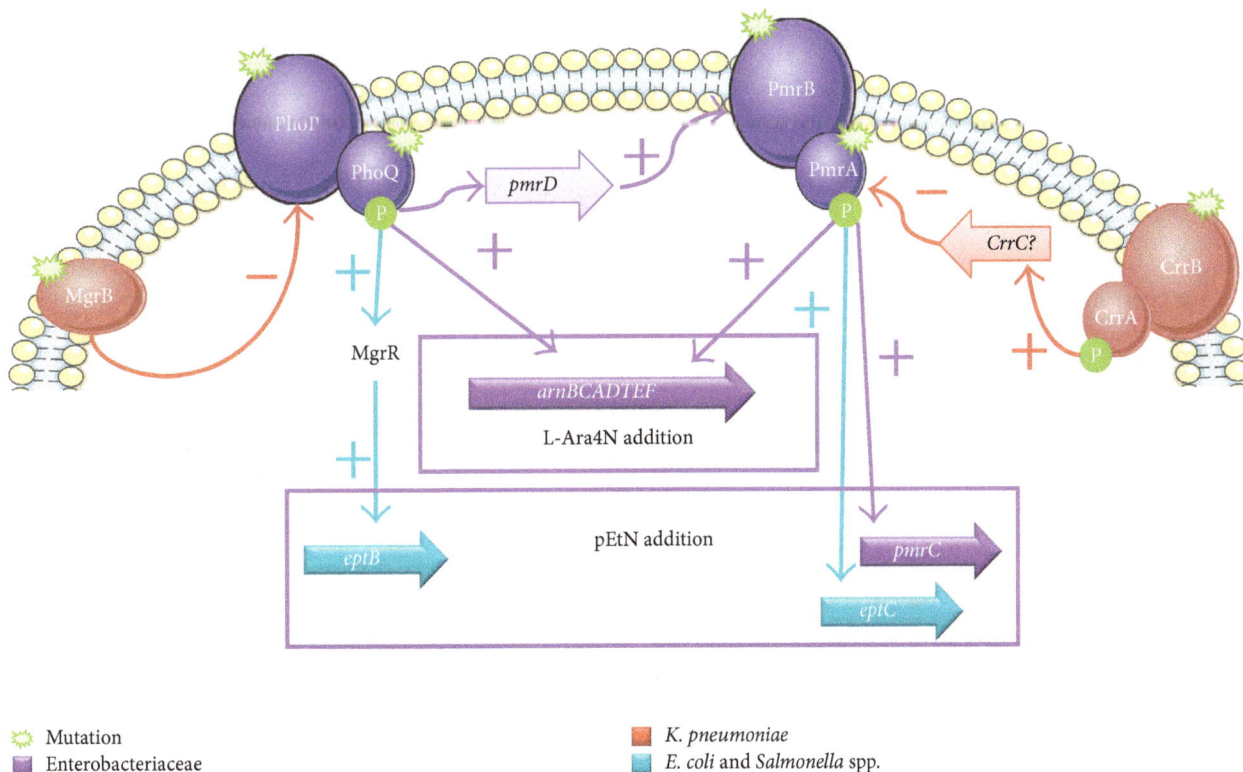

FIGURE 1: Molecular mechanisms of acquired resistance to polymyxins. L-Ara4N: 4-amino-4-arabinose; pEtN: phosphoethanolamine.

Enterobacteriaceae strains, describing coproduction with other plasmid-mediated genes (bla_{NDM-1}, bla_{NDM-5}, bla_{NDM-9}, bla_{KPC-2}, bla_{KPC-3}, bla_{OXA-48}, and $bla_{OXA-181}$) [18–24].

The emergence of antibiotic resistance of clinical interest usually conduces to the development of new tools in clinical microbiology laboratories [25]. Currently, the detection of carbapenemase-producing bacteria is well determined, combining specific culture media, phenotyping testing, antibiotic susceptibility testing, and molecular biology [26–28]. As colistin resistance is a recent global phenomenon, the implementation of rapid and reliable screening tools to detect and analyze colistin-resistant pathogens in such a way as to isolate the patient and adapt the treatment is a necessary approach [29]. Moreover, heteroresistance to colistin is a common phenomenon that is widely underestimated, requiring specific methods [30–32]. Here, we propose an overview of all the screening and analysis methods developed to assess colistin resistance among bacterial pathogens causing infectious diseases in hospitalized patients. This review summarizes the current clinical microbiology diagnosis techniques and their ability to detect all colistin resistance mechanisms, and describes new tools specifically developed to assess plasmid-mediated colistin resistance [33].

Phenotyping, susceptibility testing, and genotyping methods are presented, including an update on recent studies related to the development of specific techniques.

2. Phenotypic Detection Methods

2.1. Selective Culture Media. Culture remains the benchmark method for isolating pathogens within clinical samples, and selective media are continuously developed to isolate specific bacteria [25]. Until recently, there was no specific culture medium for the detection of colistin-resistant strains, and current polymyxin-containing culture media were not able to detect low-level resistant strains because the concentrations of polymyxin in their composition are too high or because they contain other antimicrobial drugs [34–61] (Table 1). Therefore, some in-house media have been developed for colistin-resistant strain screening studies, including strains carrying the *mcr* genes (Supplementary Table S1). These selective culture media were developed by adding low concentrations of colistin (2 or 4 mg/L) to LB nonselective agar or a MacConkey medium, which is selective of Gram-positive contaminants [62, 63]. The chromogenic and nonselective CHROMagar Orientation medium (Biomérieux, Marcy l'Étoile, France) was also used with 4 mg/ml of colistin [64]. They were used in studies to detect the growth of colistin-resistant isolates by directly culturing samples [65–67] or following an enrichment step [68] which could also be selective with the addition of 2 mg/L of colistin to the broth medium [62, 64, 69]. Other anti-infective drugs could be added to avoid contaminants: vancomycin for Gram-positive contaminants [64, 66, 68] and/or amphotericin B for fungal pathogens [67, 68]. For some other studies, such media were developed to screen colistin resistance in bacterial isolates by subculturing them on agar with 2 mg/L of colistin: MH agar [9], COS medium [70], or MacConkey medium [65]. Wong et al. named their medium MHC1 for Mueller–Hinton colistin 1 [71]. Lastly, the selective CNA medium (colistin and nalidixic acid-containing agar), containing 10 mg/L of colistin, could

TABLE 1: Composition of polymyxin-containing agar.

Targeted bacteria	Culture medium	Antibiotics (μg/mL) targeting				References
		Gram-negative strains		Gram-positive strains	Yeast	
		Polymyxins	Others			
Colistin-resistant Gram-negative strains VancoR *Gram-positive strains Gram-negative strains*	LBJMR[a]	4 (C)		Vancomycin 50		
Colistin-resistant	SuperPolymyxin	3.5 (C)		Daptomycin 10 BM 65 Éosine 400	5 (AB)	[75]
Neisseria sp.	Martin–Lewis agar	7.5 (C)	5 (T)	Vancomycin 4	20 (A)	[34]
	Thayer–Martin agar	7.5 (C)		Vancomycin 3	2.57 (N)	[35]
	MTM[b] agar	7.5 (C)	5 (T)	Vancomycin 3	2.57 (N)	[36]
	NYC[c] agar	7.5 (C)	3 (T)	Vancomycin 2	20 (A)	[37]
Burkholderia cepacia	Cepacia medium	30 (B)		Ticarcillin 100		[38]
	OFPBL[d] agar	30 (B)	Bacitracin 3			[39]
	Burkholderia cepacia agar	17.8 (B)	5 (GEN)	Ticarcillin 100		[38]
	Burkholderia cepacia selective agar	71.4 (B)	10 (GEN)	Vancomycin 2.5		[40]
Legionella sp.	BCYE[e] selective agar with GVPC[f]	9.4 (B)	Glycine 3000	Vancomycin 1	80 (CH)	[41]
	CCVC[g]	16 (C)		Vancomycin 0.5 Cefalotin 4	80 (CH)	[42]
	GPVA[h]	11.9 (B)	Glycine 3000	Vancomycin 1	80 (A)	[43]
	PAV[i]	4.76 (B)		Vancomycin 0.5	80 (A)	[44]
	PAC[j]	9.52 (B)		Cefamandole 2	80 (A)	[45]
	DGVP[k]	8 (B)	Glycine 3000	Vancomycin 1		[46]
Campylobacter sp.	*Campylobacter* agar					
	Butzler	0.33 (C)	Bacitracin 338	Novobiocin 5 Cefazolin 15	50 (CH)	[47]
	Skirrow	0.25 (B)	2.5 (T)	Vancomycin 5		[48]
	Blaser–Wang	0.125 (B)	2.5 (T)	Vancomycin 5 Cefalotin 15	2 (AB)	[49]
	Preston	0.125 (B)	5 (T)	Rifampicin 5	50 (CH)	[50]
Brucella spp.	*Brucella* selective medium	1 (B)	Bacitracin 500		100 (CH)	[51]
Vibrio sp.	CPC[l]	66.34 (C) 11.9 (B)				[52]
Gram-positive strains Streptococcus sp. and Gram-positive strains	ANC[m]	10 (C)	Nalidixic acid 10			[53]
Listeria monocytogenes	Oxford medium	20 (C)	Fosfomycin 10	Cefotetan 2 Acriflavine 5	400 (CH)	[54]
	Modified Oxford	10 (C)		Moxalactam 15		[55]
Listeria spp.	PALCAM[n]	10 (B)		Ceftazidime 8 Acriflavine 5		[56]
Bacillus cereus	MYP[o]	10 (B)				[57]
Mycobacteriaceae	Middlebrook 7H11	25 (B)	20 (T)	Carbenicillin 50	10 (AB)	[58]
Clostridium perfringens	SPS[p] agar	10 (B)	Sulfadiazine 120			[59]
	TSN[q] agar	20 (B)	Neomycin 50			[60]
	SFP[r] agar	3.57 (B)	Kanamycin 12			[61]

B: polymyxin B; C: colistin; AB: amphotericin B; A: anisomycin; CH: cycloheximide; MB: methylene blue; N: nystatin; GEN: gentamicin; T: trimethoprim. [a]LBJMR: Lucie Bardet–Jean-Marc Rolain; [b]MTM: modified Thayer–Martin; [c]NYC: New York City; [d]OFPBL: oxidation/fermentation, polymyxin B, bacitracin, and lactose; [e]BCYE: buffered charcoal and yeast extract; [f]GPVC: glycine, polymyxin B, vancomycin, and cycloheximide; [g]CCVC: cefalotin, colistin, vancomycin, and cycloheximide; [h]GPVA: glycine, polymyxin B, vancomycin, and anisomycin; [i]PAV: polymyxin B, anisomycin, and vancomycin; [j]PAC: polymyxin B, anisomycin, and cefamandole; [k]DGVP: dyes, glycine, vancomycin, and polymyxin B; [l]CPC: cellobiose, polymyxin B, and colistin; [m]CNA: colistin and nalidixic acid; [n]PALCAM: polymyxin B, acriflavine, lithium, ceftazidime, esculin, and mannitol; [o]MYP: mannitol, egg yolk, and polymyxin B; [p]SPS: sulfite, polymyxin B, and sulfadiazine, [q]TSN: trypticase, sulfite, and neomycin; [r]SFP: Shahidi-Ferguson perfringens.

detect *mcr-1*-positive isolates, one *E. coli* [72] and one *K. pneumoniae* [73], and was also used with CLED (cysteine lactose electrolyte deficient) medium (BioMérieux, Marcy l'Étoile, France) for screening samples that had or had not been precultured on Trypticase Soy Broth ±2 mg/L of colistin [74].

More specifically, the SuperPolymyxin medium (Elitech Microbio, Signes, France) was developed and intended to specifically detect colistin-resistant strains, including those with a low MIC of colistin and harboring the *mcr-1* gene [75]. The SuperPolymyxin medium has the advantage of facilitating the visualization of *E. coli* strains because it is composed of EMB agar, meaning that they exhibit a metallic green reflect. Its specificity is enabled by 3.5 μg/ml of colistin, 10 μg/ml of daptomycin, and 5 μg/ml of amphotericin B in its composition.

The CHROMagar COL-APSE medium was also developed to detect colistin-resistant strains and was compared to the SuperPolymyxin [76]. Its composition is not precisely described, based on commercial CHROMagar compounds containing colistin sulfate and oxazolidonone antibiotics. The CHROMagar COL-APSE medium presents the advantage to be chromogenic, with the capacity to differentiate colistin-resistant nonfermentative Gram-negative strains as well as Enterobacteriaceae.

The LBJMR medium was also developed to detect all the colistin-resistant bacteria, including those harboring *mcr-1* genes [77]. The LBJMR medium presents the advantage of being versatile, combining colistin-resistant and vancomycin-resistant bacteria screening tools, conferred by 4 μg/ml of colistin sulfate and 50 μg/ml of vancomycin. In particular, the LBJMR medium can be used to detect vancomycin-resistant enterococci (VRE), which represents another emerging field of clinical concern. Both colistin-resistant Enterobacteriaceae and VRE strains are easy to detect on the LBJMR medium with the presence of bromocresol purple and glucose: fermentative strains exhibit yellow colonies on a purple agar. Lastly, it can be used to specifically detect pathogens that are often diagnosed in cystic fibrosis patient samples.

The sensitivities of these three media were excellent to detect colistin-resistant strains.

2.2. Qualitative Detection of Colistin Resistance with Phenotypic Tests

2.2.1. Rapid NP Polymyxin Test for Enterobacteriaceae.
The rapid polymyxin NP test (Elitech, Signes, France) is based on a simple pH test, and detection of colistin resistance is obtained by a color change within 2 hours [78, 79]. The test was evaluated on 200 isolates of Enterobacteriaceae and can be used directly on blood samples [80]. A recent review proposed a diagnosis plan integrating this phenotypic test to confirm colistin resistance of Enterobacteriaceae strains after their growth on a selective medium [29], and its reliability is discussed in several studies [81, 82]. Compared to the broth microdilution (BMD) susceptibility testing method, agreements were excellent to detect *mcr-1* and *mcr-2* strains [83, 84]. The rapid polymyxin test has a good sensitivity to detect *Hafnia* sp. colistin-resistant isolates [79] but failed to detect *Enterobacter* sp. isolates, surely due to their heteroresistance to colistin [85]. This test has to be evaluated with nonfermentative colistin-resistant strains, such as *Acinetobacter baumannii* and *Pseudomonas aeruginosa*.

2.2.2. Micromax Assay for A. baumannii.
The Micromax assay (Halotech DNA SL, Madrid, Spain) is based on the detection of DNA fragmentation and cell wall damage in the presence of colistin [86]. Bacteria are incubated for 60 min with 0.5 μg/ml of colistin, trapped in a microgel, and then incubated with a lysis solution to remove weakened cell walls. The presence of DNA fragments is detected after staining by SYBR Gold fluorochrome and observed by fluorescence microscopy. Resistance corresponds to ≤11% of bacteria with cell wall damage. This method is rapid (3 h 30 min) and showed an excellent sensitivity for the detection of colistin resistance on the 70 *A. baumannii* tested isolates (50 susceptible and 20 resistant), but it is not specific for determining the resistance type.

2.3. Specific Phenotypic Screening Methods for the Detection of MCR-1

2.3.1. Matrix-Assisted Laser Desorption-Ionization Time-of-Flight Mass Spectrometry (MALDI-TOF MS).
The detection of polymyxin-resistant bacteria by MALDI-TOF is a promising and costless approach, as the majority of clinical microbiology laboratories own the required equipment to routinely identify clinical isolates [87]. Currently, the use of MALDI-TOF for detecting the carbapenemase-producing bacteria is described, with the detection of carbapenem hydrolysis [88–90]. As a specific peak was described for lipid A at 1796.2 m/z [91], the MALDI-TOF could be used for the detection of lipid A modifications [92]. Very recently, the MALDIxin test was developed for *E. coli* strains, based on the detection of phosphoethanolamine addition on lipid A, and could specifically detect the *mcr*-positive isolates [93]. Indeed, an additional peak at 1919.2 m/z was observed for all polymyxin-resistant strains, and a second additional peak at 1821.2 m/z was observed for all the *mcr*-positives. The MALDIxin test could detect polymyxin-resistant *E. coli* and also differentiate the chromosome- and plasmid-encoded resistance in 15 minutes, and should be evaluated on other species for which phosphoethanolamine addition is involved in polymyxin resistance.

2.3.2. Inhibition of MCR-1 Activity.
Several studies on the structure of the catalytic domain of the *MCR-1* protein have demonstrated that the phosphoethanolamine transferase is a zinc metalloprotein [94–96], and that zinc deprivation could reduce the colistin MIC in *E. coli* isolates [97]. Screening tests were developed to specifically detect *MCR-1*, based on the difference of colistin susceptibility obtained in the presence or absence of chelators of zinc ion.

The colistin-MAC test consists of the addition of dipicolinic acid (DPA) in the BMD method, leading to a colistin MIC reduction of ≥ 8-fold in case of *MCR-1*-positive strain [98]. 74 colistin-resistant Enterobacteriaceae strains were tested, and 59 of the 61 strains carrying *mcr-1*-like genes were detected by the colistin-MAC test, while the 13 *mcr*-negative strains exhibited discrepancy in results (increase, maintain, or slow decrease) giving a sensitivity of 96.7% and specificity of 100%. Interestingly, the two *mcr-1* strains that were negative with the colistin-MAC test were *K. pneumoniae* strains.

More recently, four assays were tested, based on inhibition by EDTA [99]. The specific detection of *MCR-1* was assessed with the following tests: combined-disk method with diameter differences ≥3 mm, BMD with a reduction of colistin MIC of ≥4-fold, modified rapid polymyxin NP test with the absence of color change, and the alteration of zeta potential $R_{ZP} \geq 2.5$. These assays were performed on 109 Enterobacteriaceae including 59 *mcr-1*-positive *E. coli* and one *mcr-1*-positive *K. pneumoniae*. The modified rapid NP test and zeta potential methods showed excellent sensitivity and specificity and could be inexpensive and simple methods to detect the presence of the *mcr-1* gene.

These tests should be performed on other species harboring the *mcr-1* gene, in particular *K. pneumoniae*, and also on strains harboring other *mcr* genes, to validate their ability.

3. New Recommendations on Polymyxins Susceptibility Testing

Polymyxin susceptibility testing is challenging, as these large and cationic molecules poorly diffuse into the reference cation-enriched Mueller-Hinton (MH2) agar, giving discrepant results, and much more since the description of the *mcr* genes that confer low MICs. Moreover, even in MH2 broth medium, the concentration of cation could largely influence the polymyxin MIC results [64], notably by interacting with the acquired resistance mechanisms of the tested isolates. Defining a reference method for colistin susceptibility testing is a priority, along with the increasing use of polymyxin as last-line therapies.

3.1. Reference Method. Broth microdilution (BMD) is the only approved method for colistin MIC determination by both the European Committee on Antibiotic Susceptibility Testing (EUCAST) and the Clinical and Laboratory Standards Institute (CLSI) [100, 101]. BMD has to be performed with colistin sulfate in untreated polystyrene plates without addition of any surfactant (polysorbate 80) (Table 2). The Mueller–Hinton broth medium has to be cation-adjusted, with a final composition of 20–25 mg/L of calcium and 10–12.5 mg/L of magnesium [102]. EUCAST and CLSI joined their recommendations on the polymyxin breakpoint for MIC of Enterobacteriaceae, *P. aeruginosa* and *Acinetobacter* spp. isolates: susceptible *(S)* if ≤2 μg/ml and resistant *(R)* if >2 μg/ml [100, 103]. In 2017, EUCAST added a new quality control (QC) strain that has to be used to control the performances of a colistin susceptibility method: *E. coli* NCTC 18853 that harbors the *mcr-1* gene, in addition to *E. coli* ATCC 25922 and *P. aeruginosa* ATCC 27853 [104] (Table 2).

Dilution methods consist of adding colistin to the culture medium in such a way as to obtain twofold dilutions and are prepared according to the CLSI guide M07-A10 [101] and ISO 20776-1 standard (International Standard Organization). Broth macrodilution is performed in tubes when reference broth microdilution (BMD) is performed

in 96-well trays. Only colistin sulfate can be used and particular care is required, as the powder is expressed in IU/mg, meaning that the concentrations need to be adjusted according to the CLSI M100 and the manufacturer's instructions [103]. The antibiotic is suspended in sterile water and then diluted in MH2 broth medium before its distribution into 96-well trays. The final bacterial inoculum is 5×10^5 CFU/ml (colony-forming unit) or 5×10^4 CFU/well for the BMD method, prepared using the 0.5 McFarland standard (corresponding to approximately 1 to 2×10^8 CFU/ml) [101]. Trays are then incubated at $35 \pm 1°C$ for 18 ± 2 hours [100, 102]. Results are read visually or with a spectrophotometer.

Broth microdilution is a time-consuming and fastidious way to assess MIC in clinical routines [105, 106]. Many errors can occur, such as an incorrect colistin concentration or dilution. This technique is not well suited to clinical microbiology routines and needs to be automated. Moreover, this method exhibits limitations for assessing heteroresistance. Indeed, the presence of resistant subpopulations can give uninterpretable results due to the presence of skipped wells and has been described for the *Enterobacter* species, as presented in a study of 114 *Enterobacter cloacae* [107]. Population analysis profiling is recommended to confirm heteroresistance [108]. For now, heteroresistance to polymyxins is not correlated with the presence of *mcr* genes.

3.2. Comparative Evaluations of Polymyxin Susceptibility Testing Methods. Evaluating antimicrobial susceptibility testing (AST) methods is performed using a comparison with the reference method, as per the ISO 20776-2 standard [109]: a categorical agreement (CA) is obtained when the strain is in the same clinical category (R, I, S), and an essential agreement (EA) is obtained when the MIC is within plus or minus one doubling dilution from the reference MIC. A very major error (VME) corresponds to a false susceptibility result and is calculated using the resistant strains tested, and a major error (ME), in the case of false resistance, is calculated on the number of susceptible strains. Finally, a minor error (MiE) occurs when a strain is classified as Intermediate *(I)* instead of *S* or *R*, or *S* or *R* instead of *I*. A reliable method will obtain the following scores: CA ≥ 90%, EA ≥ 90%, VME ≤ 3%, and ME ≤ 3% [109]. The results of all the comparative studies performed on colistin susceptibility testing are summarized in Table 3 (in Table S2 for polymyxin B). MIC50 and MIC90 correspond to the MIC that inhibits 50 or 90%, respectively, of the tested strains of the same species.

The surfactant polysorbate 80 was previously added to trays to limit polymyxin adherence to polystyrene and is not yet recommended; however, it could induce VME and *mcr* strains might not be detected [31, 110–112]. Albur et al. demonstrated that the polystyrene trays used also have an influence: using tissue-culture-coated round-bottom trays gave a 5.3-fold increase in MIC values compared to non-coated V-bottom trays [113], for the material used [106] (Table S3). A very recent study compared polystyrene coated trays to glass coated trays and also showed very few differences (Table 3) [114].

TABLE 2: Joint EUCAST-CLSI recommendations on colistin susceptibility testing.

Reference method	Broth microdilution		
Preparation according to ISO 20776-1 standard [102]	(i) Cation-adjusted Mueller-Hinton medium (MH2) (ii) Colistin sulfate (iii) Polystyrene trays without pretreatment (iv) Absence of polysorbate 80 or any surfactant		
MIC breakpoint (μg/ml)	Enterobacteriaceae	*P. aeruginosa*	*Acinetobacter* spp.
EUCAST [100]	$S \leq 2$ and $R > 2$	$S \leq 2$ and $R > 2$	$S \leq 2$ and $R > 2$
CLSI [103]	ECV*: WT ≤ 2 and NWT ≥ 4	$S \leq 2$ and $R \geq 4$	$S \leq 2$ and $R \geq 4$
Quality control [104] (μg/ml)	*E. coli* ATCC 25922	*P. aeruginosa* ATCC 27853	*E. coli* (*mcr-1*) NCTC 18853[#]
Target	0.5–1	1–2	4
Range	0.25–2	0.5–4	2–8

*Epidemiological cutoff values: clinical data and PK/PD are not sufficient to evaluate a clinical breakpoint for the following species: *E. aerogenes*, *E. cloacae*, *E. coli*, *K. pneumoniae*, and *R. ornithinolytica*. WT: wild type; NWT: non-wild type. [#]Recommended by EUCAST; MIC must be 4 μg/ml and only occasionally 2 or 8 μg/ml.

Until 2013, many comparative studies used agar dilution (AD) as the reference method for polymyxins susceptibility testing, a method that differs from the BMD only because the polymyxins are added to a solid MH2 medium [31, 32, 115–126]. Compared to BMD, agar dilution generally gave concordant results for colistin and polymyxin B [31, 110, 127, 128]. VMEs were very uncommon with AD, and this pointed to the AD's potential role in screening, as it presents the advantage to test several strains on the same plates [117, 129]. A recent study compared agar dilution to broth macro- and microdilution on 8 strains and concluded that agar dilution was the most reproducible method, with an excellent distribution of colistin in agar, but that colistin-containing agar plates could be only stored for 7 days [130].

Diffusion methods based on the antibiotic diffusion in agar, whether with the Kirby–Bauer disk diffusion [131] or with the gradient strips, are not reliable for polymyxin testing and should not be used as a large number of studies have obtained high rates of VMEs or poor EA [32, 120, 125, 128, 132–135]. Some studies showed good results but contained only susceptible strains [136–138]. The influence of MH2 agar composition was assessed: agreement was not affected with agar dilution, but important differences were highlighted with Etest (BioMérieux, Marcy l'Étoile, France) [31, 139]. The advantage of the agar diffusion method is the detection of hetero-resistance: colonies present within the inhibition zone correspond to resistant subpopulations [140]. One study compared disc diffusion to Etest method, and a large rate of minor errors occurred [141]. The ColiSpot test consists of replacing the disk of colistin by a drop of a calibrated colistin solution (8 μg/ml). Colistin resistance is revealed in the absence of the inhibition zone. This technique was evaluated with 89 colistin-resistant and 52 colistin-susceptible strains and was developed for veterinarian laboratories [142].

3.3. Commercial Devices Based on Broth Microdilution Reference Method. Several commercial devices based on BMD reference methods were developed to easily assess the reference method by offering ready-to-use systems. Their advantage is the elimination of critical preparation steps of MH2 medium and antibiotic dilutions. These systems were used to detect *mcr-1* strains and were evaluated by EUCAST,

giving correct results, with essential agreement ranging from 82% to 96%, and few MEs or VMEs (http://www.eucast.org/ast_of_bacteria/warnings/) [143].

3.3.1. UMIC Colistine (Biocentric, Bandol, France). UMIC colistine consists of unitary tests composed of 12-well polystyrene strips, one for growth control and 11 containing dehydrated colistin, with concentrations ranging from 0.06 to 64 μg/ml, provided with unitary MH2 tubes. Inoculation is performed simply, after diluting the 0.5 McFarland suspension by 200-fold into the MH2 tubes, by distributing 100 μL of this diluted suspension into the 12 wells of the strip, leading to the rehydration of the antibiotic. The strips are then incubated at $35 \pm 1°$C using the UMIC box to avoid any desiccation. One comparative evaluation on 71 *A. baumannii* isolates and one on 92 Gram-negative isolates including 76 Enterobacteriaceae highlighted the reliability of the UMIC colistine kit [144, 145].

3.3.2. MIC Strip Colistin (MERLIN Diagnostika Bornheim-Hersel, Germany). MIC Strip Colistin also consists in unitary 12-well strips with concentrations of dehydrated colistin ranging from 0.06 to 64 μg/mL, and Micronaut-S is a panel composed of different antibiotics on standard 96-well trays. Those systems can be automated with Micronaut ASTroID that concomitantly performs dilution for antimicrobial susceptibility testing (AST) and deposits on the MALDI-TOF target, simultaneously identifying the same colony being tested.

3.3.3. Sensitest Colistin (Liofilchem, Roseto degli Abruzzi, Italy). It consists of a compact panel of 4 tests containing 7 twofold dilutions of dehydrated colistin (0.25–16 μg/ml). It showed excellent correlation with BMD when tested on 353 isolates, including 259 Enterobacteriaceae, 83 harboring the *mcr-1* gene [146]. Recently, a combined Sensitest colistin/piperacillin-tazobactam was developed, with the same design, providing a unitary test for testing both antibiotics, with colistin concentrations ranging from 0.008 to 128 μg/ml.

TABLE 3: Comparison of different colistin susceptibility testing methods to detect colistin resistance in Gram-negative clinical isolates.

Bacterial species	Reference method	MIC breakpoint	MIC range; % resistant	MIC50 (μg/ml)	MIC90 (μg/ml)	Methods	CA ≥90%	EA ≥90%	ME ≤3%	VME ≤3%	MiE	References
42 A. baumannii isolates	BMD	S≤2 μg/ml; R>2 μg/ml	0.5–4 μg/ml; 0.07%	1 μg/ml	2 μg/ml	BMD in glass-coated plates	92.8	100	0	100		[114]
						AD	78.5	92.8	15.4	100		
						E-test	92.8	16.6	0	100		
						Vitek 2[2] AST-N2812	92.8	61.9	0	100		
353 isolates (83 mcr-1)	BMD	S≤2 μg/ml; R>2 μg/ml	ND; 38.8%	ND	ND	Sensitest	98.9	96	1.46	0.93		[146]
219 isolates		S≤2 μg/ml; R>2 μg/ml	ND; 27.4%	ND	ND	Phoenix 100[3] NMIC-417	96.8	ND	0.6	10		[146]
14 E. coli isolates	BMD	S≤2 μg/ml; R>2 μg/ml	0.25–128 μg/ml; 48%	2	16	Sensititre[1] SEMPA1	94.7	96	10.2	0		[143]
18 K. pneumoniae isolates						Micronaut-S	89.3	96	15.4	5.6		
21 P. aeruginosa isolates						Micronaut-MIC	90.7	99	12.8	5.6		
22 Acinetobacter spp. isolates						Etest, Oxoid MH	81.3	71	5.1	33.3		
						Etest, BBL MH	78.7	43	2.6	41.7		
						Etest, MHE	85.3	47	5.1	25		
						MTS, Oxoid MH	78.7	40	0	44.4		
						MTS, BBL MH	76	49	0	50		
						Sensitest	89.3	88	17.9	2.8		
						UMIC	92	82	7.7	8.3		
117 A. baumannii isolates	BMD	S≤2 μg/ml; R>2 μg/ml	≤0.5–≥16 μg/ml; 24.8%	≤0.5	8	Vitek 2 AST-XN05	89.7	88.9	1.1	37.9		[129]
						Phoenix 100 NMIC/ID-96	88.9	91.5	1.1	41.4		
						AD	87.2	93.2	15.9	3.4		
123 Enterobacteriaceae isolates (14 mcr-1 and 1 mcr-2)	BMD	S≤2 μg/ml; R>2 μg/ml	0.12–128 μg/ml; 67.5%	8	16	Phoenix 100 NMIC-93	91.8	ND	0	12.1		[83]
						Rapid NP	98.3	NA	2.5	1.2		
15 Hafnia alvei isolates 10 Hafnia paralvei isolates	BMD	S≤2 μg/ml; R>2 μg/ml	0.125–32 μg/ml; 96%	8	16	DD	4	NA	0	100		[79]
				8	8	Etest	76	32	0	25		
						Phoenix NMIC-93	100	NA	0	0		
						Rapid NP	100	NA	0	0		
76 Enterobacteriaceae isolates (21 mcr-1)	BMD	S≤2 μg/ml; R>2 μg/ml	0.06–>64 μg/ml; 32.9%	0.25	16	Vitek 2 AST N315	88.2	93.9	0	36		[147]
				2 (4)	8 (8)	Sensititre GNX3F	90.1	89.5	11.8	4		
				0.12	0.5	Etest	92.1	75	5.9	12		
						MicroScan[4] NM44	88.2	NA	15.8	4		

TABLE 3: Continued.

Bacterial species	Reference method	MIC breakpoint	MIC range; % resistant	MIC50 (μg/ml)	MIC90 (μg/ml)	Methods	CA ≥ 90%	EA ≥ 90%	ME ≤ 3%	VME ≤ 3%	MiE	References
246 isolates (absence of mcr genes)	Broth macrodilution	S ≤ 2 μg/ml; R > 2 μg/ml	≤0.5–>8 μg/ml; 12.6%	≤0.5	8	Etest	95.1	92.3	0.4	35.5		[160]
41 K. pneumoniae isolates	BMD	S ≤ 2 μg/ml	2–>128 μg/ml; 95.1%	8	32	BMD-P80	82	95.1	0	18.9	NA	[110]
20 A. baumannii isolates		R > 2 μg/ml		8	32	AD	91.8	55.7	100	3.4		
						Etest	59	50.8	33.3	39.3		
						MTS	67.2	65.6	33.3	41.4		
						Vitek 2 AST EXN8	96.7	70	66.6	0		
290 A. baumannii isolates	BMD	S ≤ 2 μg/ml; R > 2 μg/ml	1–128 μg/ml; 9.3%	2	2	DD 10 μg (9–12 mm)	94.8	NA	0	0	5.2	[136]
						Etest S ≤ 2; R > 4	94.5	2.1	0	55.5	0	
						Etest S ≤ 0.5; R > 2	99.3	≡	0	0	5.5	
						Vitek 2 AST-N136	94.1	44.8	0.38	59.2		
213 Acinetobacter sp. isolates	AD	S ≤ 2 μg/ml; R > 2 μg/ml	≤0.5–≥32 μg/ml; 6.1%	1	2	Vitek 2 AST-N132	99.1	ND	0	15.4		[115]
						Etest	87.3		1	0		
						MicroScan panel type 42	99.1		12.5	15.4		
60 P. aeruginosa isolates	BMD-P80	S ≤ 2 μg/ml; R > 2 μg/ml	≤0.12–≥8 μg/ml; 17.8%			Broth macrodilution	98	83	2.3	0		[128]
20 K. pneumoniae isolates 27 A. baumannii isolates					>8 >8	Etest	91	61	4.5	31.6		
11 A. baumannii isolates	BMD-P80	S ≤ 2 μg/ml	≤0.12–≥8 μg/ml; 20%		>8	BMD	88	34*	12.5	10		[128]
15 K. pneumoniae isolates 24 P. aeruginosa isolates		R > 2 μg/ml			>8	AD Sensititre GNXF	94 96	80 62*	7.5 5	0 0		
11 A. baumannii isolates	BMD-P80	S ≤ 2 μg/ml	≤0.12–≥8 μg/ml; 30%			Etest, BBL MH	78	46	5.7	47		[128]
15 K. pneumoniae isolates 24 P. aeruginosa isolates		R > 2 μg/ml			>8	Etest, Hardy MH Etest, Remel MH	78 84	64 68	2.8 2.8	53 47		
109 P. aeruginosa isolates	BMD	S ≤ 2 μg/ml; R > 2 μg/ml	0%			Phoenix NMIC/ID-76	100	99.1	0	0		[149]
63 E. coli isolates	BMD	S ≤ 2 μg/ml; R > 2 μg/ml	0.12–16 μg/ml; 18.6%	1	1	BMD-P80	99.2	41.3	0	43.5		[112]
61 K. pneumoniae isolates					0.5							
60 Acinetobacter spp. isolates					2							
63 P. aeruginosa isolates					2							

TABLE 3: Continued.

Bacterial species	Reference method	MIC breakpoint	MIC range; % resistant	MIC50 (μg/ml)	MIC90 (μg/ml)	Methods	CA ≥90%	EA ≥90%	ME ≤3%	VME ≤3%	MiE	References
200 Enterobacteriaceae isolates	AD	S≤2 μg/ml; R>2 μg/ml	0.128->128 μg/ml; 28.5%			DD 50 μg; R<15 mm	96.5	NA	0	12.3		[116]
82 K. pneumoniae isolates				0.5	128	DD 10 μg; R≤8; S≥11 mm	93	NA	0	8.8	4.5	
51 E. coli isolates				0.5	0.5	DD 10 μg; R≤11; S≥14 mm	99.5	NA	0	1.7	26.5	
67 E. cloacae isolates				0.5	2	Etest	100	52	0	0	0	
25 P. aeruginosa isolates	AD	S≤2 μg/ml; R>4 μg/ml	0.25->256 μg/ml; 57.1%	2	>256	BMD	81.1	40.5	0	25	5.4	[120]
12 S. maltophilia isolates				>256	>256	Etest	74.3	56.7	0	35	11.4	
						DD 10 μg; R≤10; S≥11 mm	82.8	NA	0	35	2.9	
157 E. coli isolates	AD	S≤2 μg/ml; R>4 μg/ml	0.25-32 μg/ml; 9.6%	0.5	2	DD 150 μg; R<16; S≥20 mm	46.5	NA	1.4	20	49.7	[123]
						DD 10 μg; 2+18H* (10-15)	96.8	NA	0.7	13.3	1.9	
						Etest	96.8	81.5	0.7	0	0.6	
78 P. aeruginosa isolates	BMD	S≤2 μg/ml; R>4 μg/ml	<0.25-2 μg/ml; 0	1	1	Etest	100	79.5	0	0	6.4	[135]
						DD 10 μg	100	NA				
100 A. baumannii isolates	Phoenix	S≤2 μg/ml; R>4 μg/ml		0.5	0.5	DD 10 μg; R≤8; S≥11 mm	100	NA	0	0		[137]
						Etest	100	NA	0	0		
154 Acinetobacter spp. isolates	AD	S≤2 μg/ml; R≥4 μg/ml	≤0.064-≥32; 11.7%	NA	NA	Etest	98.7	88	0.7	5.6		[124]
170 Gram-negative isolates	AD	S≤4 μg/ml; R>4 μg/ml	0.25-128; 31.2%	NA	NA	Etest	100	91.2	0	0		[126]
102 Gram-negative isolates	BMD	S≤2 μg/ml; R>4 μg/ml	<0.5->64 μg/ml; 50%	NA	NA	AD, Oxoid MH	ND	96.8				[31]
						AD, Oxoid Iso-Sensitest		97.9				
						Etest, MH		72.6				
						Etest, ISO		64.2				
						Vitek 2 AST N038		93.1				
						DD 10 μg; R≤10; S≥13 mm		NA				
44 Acinetobacter spp. isolates	AD	S≤2 μg/ml; R>2 μg/ml	1-2 μg/ml; 0	1	2	Vitek 2 AST-N032	100	ND	0	NA	NA	[118]

TABLE 3: Continued.

Bacterial species	Reference method	MIC breakpoint	MIC range; % resistant	MIC50 (µg/ml)	MIC90 (µg/ml)	Methods	CA ≥ 90%	EA ≥ 90%	ME ≤ 3%	VME ≤ 3%	MiE	References
172 Gram-negative isolates	AD	S ≤ 2 µg/ml R > 2 µg/ml	0.5–64; 31.4%			Vitek 22 AST-N032 (n = 32)	82	75.2	0	57.4		[32]
						Etest (n = 137)	86.6	75.0	6.8	27.8		
115 A. baumannii isolates	BMD	S ≤ 2 µg/ml R > 2 µg/ml	≤0.06–512 µg/ml; 19.1%	≤0.06	32	Etest	98.2	16.5	0	1.7		[138]
501 P. aeruginosa isolates (401 CF)	AD	S ≤ 4 µg/ml R > 4 µg/ml	≤0.5–≥16 µg/ml; 17.8%	2	4	BMD 24 h	96		1.2	26.5		[121]
50 A. xylosoxidans isolates				4	≥16	BMD 48 h	93.6		3.9	18.0		
50 S. maltophilia isolates				8	≥16							
70 S. maltophilia	AD	S ≤ 2 µg/ml R > 2 µg/ml	0.12–32 µg/ml; 24.3%	2	4	DD 10 µg; R ≤ 8; S ≥ 11 mm	71.2	NA	0	93.7	5.7	[125]
						Etest	86.4	96.7	5.6	37.5	NA	
200 Gram-negative isolates	BMD	S ≤ 2 µg/ml R > 2 µg/ml	≤1–>128 µg/ml; 15%			DD 10 µg; R ≤ 10; S ≥ 14 mm	94	NA	0	21.8	1.5	[127]
(i) 60 A. baumannii isolates				≤1	2	DD 10 µg; R ≤ 8; S ≥ 11 mm	95		0	31.2	1	
(ii) 80 P. aeruginosa isolates				≤1	≤1							
(iii) 12 S. maltophilia isolates				≤1	32							
35 representatives	BMD	S ≤ 2 µg/ml R > 2 µg/ml	≤1–≥128 µg/ml; 40%			AD	97.1	91.4	47.6	0		[127]

CA: categorical agreement; EA: essential agreement; VME: very major error; MiE: minor error; ME: major error; AD: agar dilution; BMD: broth microdilution; DD: disk diffusion; MH: Mueller–Hinton. Italic values indicate the number of errors and not the percentage when a too few number of strains tested, where R for VME or S for ME. [1]Sensititre panels: ≤0.25–>4 µg/ml except for SEMPA1. [2]Vitek 2 reagent cards: ≤0.5–≥16 µg/ml except for AST-N038 (≤2, 4, and >4 µg/ml) and AST-N032 (1–4 µg/ml). [3]Phoenix 100 cards: ≤1–>4 µg/ml. [4]MicroScan-dried Gram-negative breakpoint combo panel type 42 ≤2 end >4 µg/ml. *Prediffusion test: discs were removed after 2 h of incubation.

3.3.4. The Sensititre System (Thermo Fisher Scientific, Waltham, MA, USA). It presents different antibiotics on 96-well trays with a customizable plate layout. Inoculation, incubation, and reading (based on fluorescence) steps can be automated. Chew et al. [147] recently evaluated a Sensititre GNX3F panel containing both polymyxin B and colistin (0.25–4 mg/L) and presented a sensitivity of 95.2% and 100% in detecting the 21 *mcr-1* isolates tested, respectively.

3.4. Automated Systems. Automated systems were developed to shorten result timeframes by increasing sensitivity, and also to avoid manipulation bias [148], with incubation and real-time reading. However, by combining several antibiotics, the number of concentrations tested is limited, and they cannot give a real MIC (Table 3).

3.4.1. MicroScan WalkAway (Beckman Coulter, San Diego, CA, USA). It uses standard trays that are manually inoculated, and reading is based on fluorometry, with results obtained in 3.5–7H. It is not available on polymyxin B, and essential agreement cannot be evaluated between techniques as the NM44 panel proposes only ≤4 and ≥4 µg/ml for colistin. In the recent study of Chew et al., this panel was able to detect all *mcr-1* tested isolates and presented only one VME on 76 Enterobacteriaceae isolates tested. It also evaluated 213 *Acinetobacter* species and presented 99.1 % categorical agreement against the agar dilution method [115].

3.4.2. Vitek 2 (BioMérieux, Marcy l'Étoile, France). It is a semiautomated system that uses reagent cards containing dehydrated antibiotics and other reagents in a 64-well format. It combines rapid identification and AST using an extrapolated growth algorithm. Various comparative studies performed to evaluate Vitek 2 have returned discrepant results with high rates of VME. In their recent evaluation, Chew et al. [147] demonstrated the efficacy of Vitek 2 in assessing both polymyxin B and colistin MIC with only one VME for each and 96.1% and 93.9% EA, respectively, but it was only able to detect *mcr-1* strains with polymyxin B.

3.4.3. BD Phoenix™ (Becton Dickinson, Le Pont de Claix, France). It performs identification and AST in parallel in 84-well specific plates. Reading is based on an oxidation-reduction indicator in 6–16 hours. One study showed excellent agreement on 109 *P. aeruginosa* strains, but only colistin-susceptible strains were tested [149]. Vourli et al. [129] have shown concerning results testing *Acinetobacter baumannii* strains with very high VME rates (41.4%) despite the study including 24.8% of colistin-resistant strains. This was explained by the majority of errors occurring near the breakpoint (2 instead of 4 µg/ml). Lastly, in the study by Jayol et al. [83], the Phoenix system was able to detect all *mcr*-carrying bacteria, even those with a colistin MIC of 4 µg/ml, but the high rates of VMEs obtained prove its inability to assess heteroresistance.

4. Genotyping and Molecular Screening

4.1. PCR Amplification and Sequencing to Detect Gene Mutations. Molecular biology methods are the most sensitive for determining antibiotic resistance by assessing the presence of resistance genes or mutations conferring resistance. These methods are complementary to the phenotypic techniques and confirm the resistant status of bacterial isolates. The main mutations for Enterobacteriaceae species are located on genes coding the two-component systems PmrA/PmrB and PhoP/PhoQ (Figure 1). Specifically, mutations in the *mgrB* gene—the negative feedback regulator of PhoPQ—notably with the presence of insertional sequences, appeared to be the main resistance mechanism observed in *K. pneumoniae* strains. These colistin resistances are not based on drug-modifying enzymes or the acquisition of a resistance gene which could be easily detected. Screening of potential mutations on these chromosomal genes is done by amplification and sequencing, takes 3 days, and requires that all genes are tested. Sequenced amplicons are then compared by the BLAST tool against the NCBI database to screen possible mutations compared to wild-type genes.

4.2. Real-Time qPCR to Detect the Presence of mcr Genes. The discovery of the acquired gene *mcr-1* justifies the use of molecular detection with RT-PCR, a rapid quantitative technique to detect the presence of the gene. A systematic screening of the gene in colistin-resistant strains was performed [150] (Figure 2). For such purposes, scientists have used the primers of the original study [6], or have designed their own primers for standard PCR [132, 151–160] or RT-PCR, based on SYBR Green assays [64, 151, 161], TaqMan probe [66, 72, 152, 162], or other FAM-labelled probe [9, 71, 163, 164] or HEX-labelled probe [165] (Table 4).

Xavier et al. designed primers to screen *mcr-2* [7], giving a 567 bp product [166]. Some designed their own primers for standard PCR [167–169], and one study developed a TaqMan assay for qPCR [170]. Interestingly, three studies went further by designing a universal primer to detect both *mcr-1* and *mcr-2* genes by standard PCR [166, 171] and a generic primer and a probe to detect them by qPCR [74], but these have not yet been tested on other *mcr* genes. Lastly, primers were designed for detecting *mcr-3* [10], *mcr-4* [11], and *mcr-5* genes [12] by standard PCR (Table 4). A recent study described a multiplex SYBR Green real-time PCR assay for the simultaneous detection of *mcr-1*, *mcr-2*, and *mcr-3* genes [172]. Finally, a multiplex PCR assay for detection of the five *mcr* genes: *mcr-1*, *mcr-2*, *mcr-3*, *mcr-4*, and *mcr-5*, was developed in order to obtain sequential amplicons with a size difference of 200 bp, allowing their fast and simultaneous detection on agarose gels [173].

4.3. PCR to Detect Plasmid Carrying mcr Genes. *mcr-1* is a 1626-base pair-long gene located on a 2607 bp common region flanked on both ends by an IS*Apl1* insertion sequence (IS) in some plasmids [174]. This sequence may form a composite transposon that can potentially move as one complete unit [155, 175, 176]. This insertion sequence appears

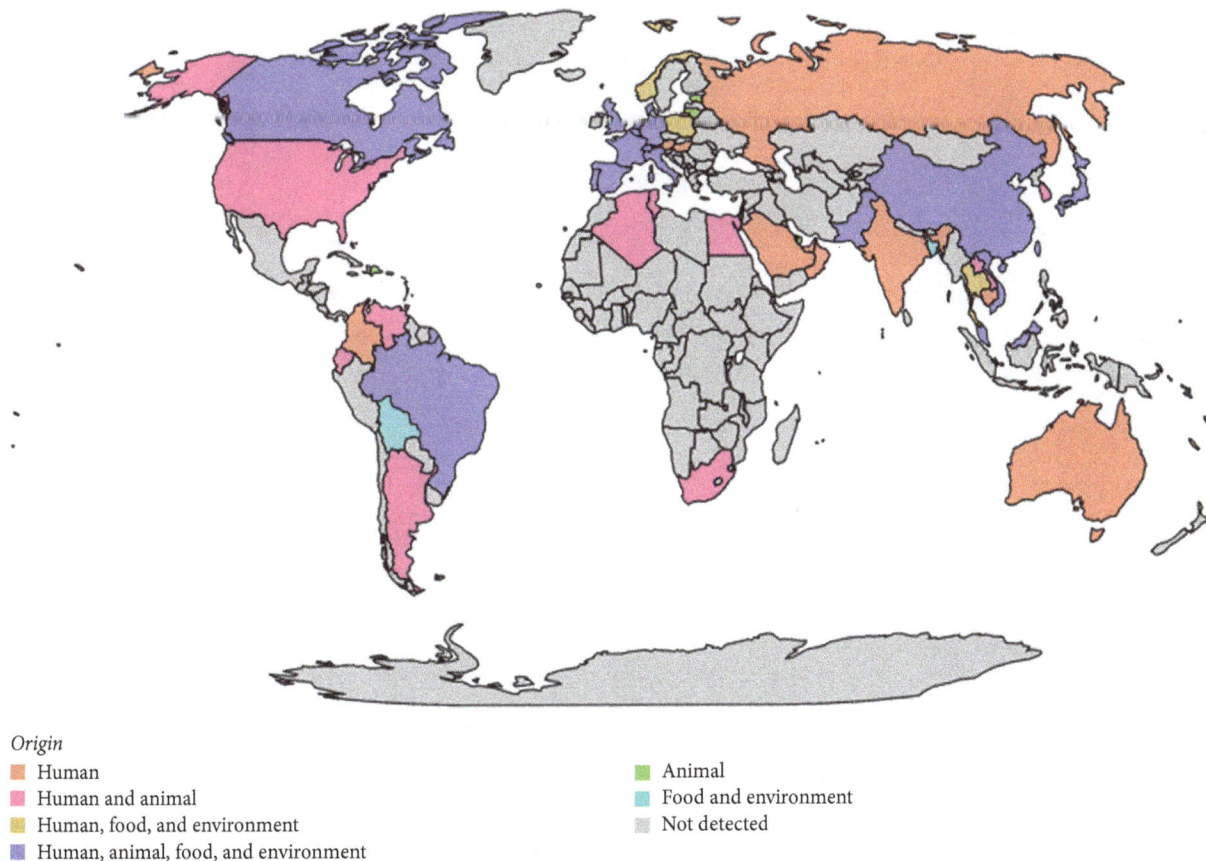

Origin
- ■ Human
- ■ Human and animal
- ■ Human, food, and environment
- ■ Human, animal, food, and environment
- ■ Animal
- ■ Food and environment
- ■ Not detected

FIGURE 2: Worldwide dissemination of the *mcr-1* gene. The map was performed with Magrit mapping application (http://magrit.cnrs.fr).

to be a key component of the mobilome, and its presence is not systematic. Furthermore, only the upstream region can contain IS*Apl1* [165]. Li et al. identified the ability of the Tn6330 transposon (IS*Apl1-mcr-1-orf-*IS*Apl1*) to generate circular IS*Apl1-mcr-1-orf* [177]. Specific primers were developed to screen the upstream presence of this IS transposon by PCR and Sanger sequencing [178–180]. Others have also designed their own system to directly screen on plasmid carrying *mcr*-gene type IncX4 [9, 181], but these methods also exhibit limitations, as a wide distribution has been observed for *mcr-1* among different plasmids (IncI2, IncX4, IncHI2, IncY, IncF, IncP, IncH1, and IncX3), demonstrating the great ability of *mcr* genes to spread.

4.4. Microarray.
Microarray technology allows scientists to analyze dozens of genes at the same time. The Check-MDR CT103 microarray system (Check-Points, Wageningen, the Netherlands) was developed to screen the presence of extended-spectrum beta-lactamase (ESBL) genes (TEM and SHV) and carbapenemase genes (OXA-48, KPC, NDM...) in the same assay and can assay 24 samples at the same time, with an effective detection in 6.5 hours. Recently, a study evaluated this assay for detecting *mcr* genes: sensitivity and specificity were excellent for *mcr-1* and its variants (from *mcr-1.2* to *mcr-1.7* and *mcr-2* genes), but it was not able to detect the new gene *mcr-3* [182]. *mcr-4* has not been assayed yet.

4.5. Loop-Mediated Isothermal Amplification (LAMP).
The Eazyplex SuperBug *mcr-1* kit (Amplex Biosystems Gmbh, Giessen, Germany) was developed to assess the presence of the *mcr-1* gene within 20 minutes [183]. It was effective on 104 microbial strains but needs to be assayed directly on clinical samples. As it was developed before the description of the other *mcr* genes, it can only detect the *mcr-1* gene and the *mcr-1.2* variant.

More recently, another LAMP-based assay was developed to detect *mcr-1* gene and evaluated as a screening tool on 556 multidrug-resistant Enterobacteriaceae [184]. Seven isolates were positive by both standard PCR and LAMP-based assay (6 *E. coli* and 1 *K. pneumoniae*). The results can be assessed by chromogenic visualization. This test constitutes a rapid, specific, and cost-effective tool that exhibits a higher sensitivity than PCR (10-fold). It has to be assayed on clinical samples; as for now, only spiked tools were used.

4.6. Novel Approach with Direct Resistome Analysis.
Genomic screening is an alternative approach for studying resistance and providing a better understanding of the behavior of bacterial isolates [185]. The development of next-generation sequencing has led to lower costs, reduced screening delay, and increased sequencing speeds combined with updated databases providing access to a large amount of information. The *mcr-1* gene was initially discovered by whole

TABLE 4: List of primers designed to detect *mcr* genes by PCR.

Targeted genes	Analyze	Method	Primer sequences	Cycle (nb: steps)	Product (bp)	Study
mcr-1	Original study	Std	CLR F: 5'-CGGTCAGTCCGTTTGTTC-3' CLR R: 5'-CTTGGTCGGTCTGTAGGG-3'	25: 94°C, 30 s; 58°C, 90 s; 72°C, 60 s	309	[6]
	105 colistin-resistant strains	Std	mcr-1_F: 5'-TGTGGTACCGACGCGGTCAG-3' mcr-1_R: 5'-TCAGGGGATGAATGCGGTGC-3'			[152]
	45 colistin-resistant strains in 2 spiked stools	HotStarTaqMasterMix Mcr-1_FAM-BHQ: 5'-CTACAGACGACCAAGCCGA-3' Pr 5 =HEX-C CAAGCCGA-ZEN-GACCAAGGATC-3IABkFQ-3	mcr-1_s: 5'-ATGGCACGGTCTATGATA-3' mcr-1_as: 5'-CGGATAATCCACCTTAACA-3'	45: 95°C, 30 s; 55°C, 30 s; 72°C, 30 s	155	[160]
	In silico study		mcr-1-286F: 5'-ACTTATGGCACGGTCTATGA-3' mcr-1-401R: 5'-ACACCCAAACCAATGATACG-3'	40: 95°C, 10 s; −56°C, 40 s		[162]
	20 strains in 3 spiked stools	SYBR Green	mcr-1-qF1: 5'-ACACTTATGGCACGGTCTATG-3' mcr-1-qR1: 5'-GCACACCCAAACCAATGATAC-3'			[148]
			mcr-1-qF2: 5'-TGGCGTTCAGCAGTCATTAT-3' mcr-1-qR2: 5'-AGCTTACCCACCGAGTAGAT-3'	40: 95°C, 3 s; 60°C, 20 s; 72°C, 7 s	120	[165]
	2046 strains	Std	mcr-1-F: 5'-ATGATGCAGCATACTTCTGTGTG-3' mcr-1-R: 5'-TCAGCGGATGAATGCGGTGC-3'		1646	[148]
	Wastewater samples	SYBR Green	mcr-1-F1: 5'-TGTTCTTGTGGCGAGTGTTG-3' mcr-1-R1: 5'-CGCGCCCATGATTAATAGCA-3'	40: 95°C, 15 s; 60°C, 30 s		[158]
	78 stool	SYBR Green	mcr-1-FW: 5'-AGGCCATCTGCAACACCAA-3' mcr-1-RV: 5'-GCCAACGAGCATACCGACAT-3'	30/40: 95°C, 15 s; −63°C, 10 s; −72°C, 10 s	59	[61]
	100 strains: 18 colistin-resistant strains in 833 faecal samples	TaqMan probe: 6 FAM-GACCGGGACCGGCAATCTTACC-TAMRA	F1: GCAGCATACTTCTGTGTGGTAC R1: ACAAAGCCGAGATTGTCCGCG	35: 95°C, 30 s; −60°C, 1 min	145	[149]
	1495 E. coli strains and 571 KP strains	Std	F1: GCAGCATACTTCTGTGTGGTAC R3: TATGCACGGGAAAGAAACTGGC		554	[150]
	51 strains	Std FastStart Universal Probe Master kit FAM-AACAGGCGGTGGTGATCAGTAGCAT-BHQ	Mcr-1-forward: 5'-GCTCGGTCAGTCCGTTTG-3' Mcr-1-reverse: 5'-GAATGCGGTGCGGTCTTT-3'			[161]
	18 samples		M-F: CATCGCGGACAATCTCGG M-R: AAATCAACACAGGCTTTAGCAC	40: 95°C, 15 s; −60°C, 1 min	116	[161]
	241 isolates	Std	MCR-1-F2: 5'-CTCATGATGCAGCATACTTC-3' MCR-1-R2: 5'-CGAATGGAGTGTGCGGTG-3'		Entire gene	[151]
	Clinical *E. coli* isolates	TaqMan Fast Advanced Master Mix 5'-Cy5-TGCAGACGCACACAATGCCTATGAT-TAO-3'	MCR-1F: 5'-CATCGCTCAAAGTATCCAGTGG-3' MCR-1R: 5'-CCATGTAGATAGACACCGTTCTCAC-3'			[69]
	10,609 *E. coli* isolates (505R)	TaqMan RT-mcr-1_Probe Cy5-AGTTTCTTTCGCGTGCATAAGCCG-BBQ-650	RT-mcr-1_F: TGGCGTTCAGCAGTCATTAT RT-mcr-1_R: AGCTTACCCACCGAGTAGAT	30°C−95°C, 15 s; −60°C, 1 min		[159]
	62 isolates		MCR1_22,697_F1: 5'-CACTTATGGCACGGTCTATGA-3'			[68]

TABLE 4: Continued.

Targeted genes	Analyze	Method	Primer sequences	Cycle (nb: steps)	Product (bp)	Study
	31 colistin-resistant isolates	MCR1_22,763_Pb1 FAM-TGGTCTCGG/ZEN/CTTGGTCGGTCTGTGTAGGGC-3IABkFQ	MCR1_22,810_R1: 5'-CCCAAACCAATGATACGCAT-3'			[157]
	122 faecal samples	Std / TaqMan probe: 5'-TTGACCGGGACGCGCAATCTTA-3' FAM	mcr-1_F: 5'-ATGATGCAGCATACTTCTGTGTGG-3' / mcr-1_R: 5'-GTGCGGTCTTTGACTTTGTCC-3'	45: 15 s, 95°C; −1 min, −60°C	305	[63]
	48 E. coli and 27 KP strains	[6]	mcr-1-F1: 5'-ATGATGCAGCATACTTCTGTG-3' / mcr-1-R1: 5'-TCAGCGGATGAATGCGGGTG-3' / CLR5-F1: 5'-ATGATGCAGCATACTTCTGTGTGG-3' / CLR5-R1: 5'-TCAGCGGATGAATGCGGTGC-3' / CLR5-F: 5'-CGGTCAGTCCGTTTGTTC-3' / Mcr1-Rv2: 5'-CCAGCGTATCCAGCACATTT-3'			[153, 155] [156] [176]
mcr-2	136 colistin-resistant isolates	Std	MCR2-IF: 5'-TGTTGCTTGTGTGCCGATTGGA-3' / MCR2-IR: 5'-AGATGGTAITGTTGGTTGCTG-3'	33: 95°C, 3 min; 65°C, 30 s; 72°C, 1 min	567	[7] [157]
	1200 isolates					[163]
	6 isolates	Std	MCR-2-F(EcoRI): 5'-AACCGAATTCATGACATCACATTCTTG-3' / MCR-2-R (SalI): 5'-CCGGTCGACTTACTGGATAAATGCGCGC-3'	34: 95°C, 1 min; 52°C, 30 s; 72°C, 1 min		[164]
	2396 strains	Std	Mcr-2 full Fw: 5'-ATGACATCACATCACTCTTGG-3' / Mcr-2 full Rv: 5'-TTACTGGATAAATGCGCGC-3'			[165] [65, 166]
	1144 samples					
	436 cultures	TaqMan mcr-2_Probe ROX-ACTGATTATGCGGTGCGGTGACGAG-BHQ-2	Mcr-2_fwd: TTGTCGTGCTGTTATCCTATCG / Mcr-2_rev: CCGTGCCATAAGTATCGGTAAA	30: 95°C, 15 s; −60°C, 1 min		[167]
mcr-1 and mcr-2	1200 isolates	Std	mcr1-2 universal F: ACTTATGGCACGGTCTATGATAC / mcr1-2 universal R: CCGGGGTGACATCAAACA	30: 94°C, 30 s; 58°C, 30 s; 72°C, 2 min	131	[163]
	621 faecal samples	Mcr-generic probe TATCACGCCACAAGATAC	MCR-1/2-Fw: 5'-TAT CGC TAT GTG CTA AAG CC-3' / MCR-1/2-Rv: 5'-TCT TGG TAT TTG GCG GTA TC-3' / Mcr-generic fw: GCCAAATACCAAGAAAATG / Mcr-generic rev: TTATCCATCACGCCTTTT		715bp 98bp	[168] [71]
mcr-3	580 E. coli strains	Std	MCR3-F: 5'-TTGGCACTGTATTTTGCATTT-3' / MCR3-R: 5'-TTAACGAAATTGGCTGGAACA-3'	30: 95°C, 30 s; 50°C, 30 s; 72°C, 45 s	542	[10]

TABLE 4: Continued.

Targeted genes	Analyze	Method	Primer sequences	Cycle (nb: steps)	Product (bp)	Study
mcr-1, mcr-2, and mcr-3	25 isolates; 17 mcr-1 and 8 mcr-3 20 samples	SYBR Green	mcr1-qf: AAAGACGCGGTACAAGCAAC MCR-1 mcr1-qr: GCTGAACATACACGGCACAG mcr2-qf: CGACCAAGCGCGAGTCTAAGG MCR-2 mcr2-qr: CAACTGGCACCAACACACTT mcr3-qf: ACCTCCAGCGTGAGATTGTTCCA MCR-3 mcr3-qr: GCGGTTTCACCAACGACCAGAA	40: 95°C, 30 s; 60°C, 30 s; 72°C, 30 s	213 92 169	[169]
mcr-4	125 isolates	Std	Mcr-4 FW: ATTGGGATAGTCGCCTTTT Mcr-4 RV: TTACAGCCAGAATCATTATCA		487	[11]
mcr-5	12 Salmonella paratyphi B isolates	Std	MCR5_fw: 5′-ATGCGGTTGTCTGCATTTATC-30′ MCR5_rev: 5′-TCATTGTGGTTGTCCTTTTCTG-3′	30: 95°C, 30 s; 50°C, 95 s; 72°C, 95 s	1644	[12]
mcr-1, mcr-2, mcr-3, mcr-4 and mcr-5	49 E. coli and Salmonella isolates	Std	mcr1_fw: AGTCCGTTTGTTCTGTGGC mcr1_rev: AGATCCTTGGTCTCGGCTTG mcr2_fw: CAAGTGTGTTGGTCGCAGTT mcr2_rev: TCTAGCCCGACAAGCATACC mcr3_fw: AAATAAAAATTGTTCCGCTTATG mcr3_rev: AATGGAGATCCCGTTTTT mcr4_fw: TCACTTTCATCACTGCGTTG mcr4_rev: TTGGTCCATGACTACCAATG mcr5_fw: ATGCGGTTGTCTGCATTTATC mcr5_rev: TCATTGTGGTTGTCCTTTTCTG	25: 94°C, 30s; 58°C, 90s; 72°C, 60s	320 715 929 1116 1644	[170]

Std: standard; KP: K. pneumoniae.

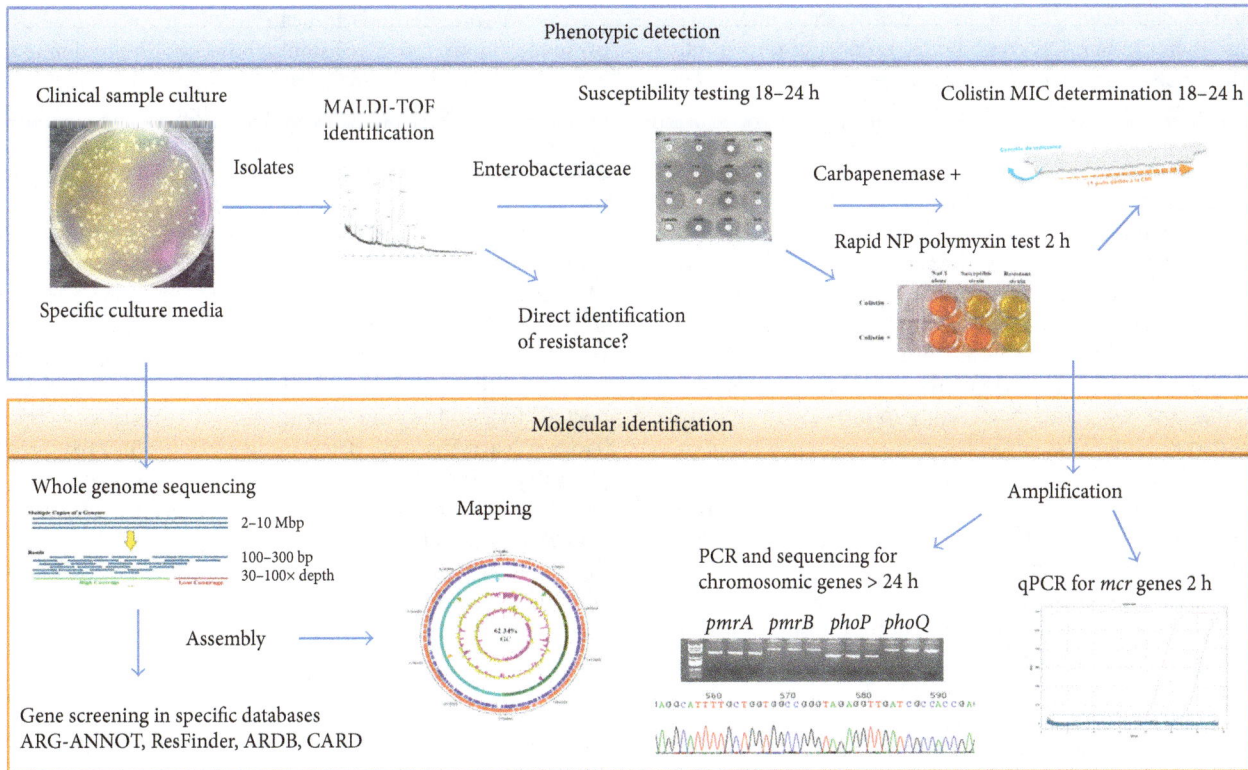

FIGURE 3: Complementarity of phenotypic and genotypic methods in detection and analysis of colistin-resistant bacteria.

TABLE 5: Comparison of detection methods for polymyxin resistance.

Method	Principle	Time	Manual (M); automated (A)	Detection			
				ColR	*mcr*	HR	MIC
Phenotypic							
Selective agar	Selective growth	18 h	M	+	−	+	−
Rapid polymyxin NP	pH change	4 h	M	+	−	−	−
Micromax	Cell wall lysis detection by fluorescence	3 h	M/A	+	−	−	−
MALDI-TOF MS	Specific peak detection	1 h	A	+	+	−	−
MCR-1 inhibition	Chelation with	18 h	M	+	+	±	+
Colistin MAC	Dipicolinic acid						
EDTA assays	EDTA						
AST							
BMD (UMIC, Micronaut-MIC, Sensitest, Micronaut-S, and Sensititre)	Growth inhibition	18 h	M/A	+	−	±	+
Agar diffusion	Measure of growth inhibition zone	18 h	M				
Disk diffusion				−	−	+	−
Gradient strip				−	−	+	+
ColiSpot				+	−	ND	−
Agar dilution	Growth inhibition	18 h	M	−	−	+	+
Automatized system	Growth detection						
MicroScan	Fluorimetry	3.5–7 h	A	+	−	−	−
Vitek 2	Algorithm	4–10 h	A	+	−	−	−
Phoenix	Oxidoreduction	6–16 h	A	+	−	−	−
Genotypic							
Standard PCR	Amplification	3 h	A	+	+	−	−
RT-PCR	Amplification	1 h	A	+	+	−	−
LAMP (Eazyplex, etc.)	Amplification	20 min	A	+	−	−	−
Microarray	DNA hybridization	6.5 h	A	+	−	−	−
NGS	Whole-genome sequencing						
Illumina		4–56 h	A	+	+	−	−
PacBio RS II		0.5–3 h	A	+	+	−	−

ColR: colistin resistance; HR: heteroresistance; +: yes; −: no; ±: sometimes.

genome sequencing during an active livestock monitoring program in China [6]. A considerable number of retrospective studies analyzing previously recorded genomic sequences have since been carried out, showing the global dispersion of the gene [9, 10, 20, 23, 24, 72, 74, 157, 158, 174, 177, 180, 186–204] (Figure 2).

The technologies used to completely sequence the bacterial genome are Illumina (Illumina Inc., San Diego, CA, USA), which produces short sequences (300 bp) and requires several days, and PacBio RS II (Pacific Biosciences, Menlo Park, CA, USA), which produces a single real-time molecule producing long sequences (60kb) in a few hours [205]. The use of Illumina sequencers is not suitable for covering bacterial genomes with multiple repetitive elements because too many sequence pieces are obtained after assembly, whereas PacBio RS II delivers a single sequence without missing regions [174]. Sekizuka et al. performed a hybrid analysis using the two technologies to analyze three Inc2 plasmids and found that they were highly conserved with the exception of the shufflon region, meaning that the combination of the two methods enables to analyze rearragements in highly recombinant regions [174].

The sequences obtained are assembled, the genome is annotated, and then a mapping is carried out against a reference plasmid, in general pHNSHP45 for *mcr-1* [6]. The aligned sequences are then compared to one of the resistance gene databases: Antibiotic Resistance Gene-Annotation [206], ResFinder [207], Comprehensive Antibiotic Resistance Database [208], and Antibiotic Resistance Genes Database [209]. They could also be compared to the plasmid genome, with GenEpid-J [210] or PlasmidFinder, which enabled the discovery of the *mcr-4* gene [11] and presents the advantage of screening multiple genes and detecting the coexistence of several genes including carbapenemases. Lindsey et al. proposed a whole protocol for plasmid sequencing [211]. More specifically, PointFinder was developed to detect chromosomal point mutations associated with antimicrobial resistance [212].

Whole genome sequencing combined with new bioinformatic tools improves our ability to detect several resistance genes at the same time [186, 205] but presents the same limitations than PCR: new genes are not recognized by these techniques, which require the continuous updating of databases [175, 213] that should be merged into a single reference database [213].

5. Conclusion

The recent description of plasmid-mediated colistin-resistant genes has generated concern among the global scientific community about the lack of new antibiotics to treat infections caused by multidrug-resistant pathogens. This concern was raised by the worldwide screening that demonstrated the global spread of bacterial strains harboring the *mcr-1* gene from diverse human and animal origins. Thus, it is necessary to implement an adapted protocol to effectively detect colistin-resistant strains in clinical microbiology laboratories.

Phenotypic methods indicate to the microbiologist the presence of polymyxin-resistant strains but do not define the mechanism involved and the risk of transmission. Molecular methods are rapid and more sensitive but are specific to the resistance genes examined and faced with the large number of molecular mechanisms conferring resistance to polymyxins, should only be used to screen *mcr* genes in clinical microbiology laboratories. Genomic analysis enables the complete screening of resistance genes in genetically identified bacteria from clinical samples but remains an *in silico* study which enables predictions but not resistance observation, as the presence of a resistance gene in a genome does not mean that the corresponding isolate is resistant, supported by studies that identified polymyxin-susceptible bacteria carrying the *mcr-1* gene [92, 165, 213]. Thus, phenotypic and molecular methods are complementary in detecting colistin-resistant pathogens in order to analyze the behavior of the clinical isolate, and it is important to carry them out in parallel [148] (Figure 3). All these techniques and their detection characteristics are summarized in Table 5.

In conclusion, these new techniques need to be combined for a complete understanding of colistin resistance, in particular for strains carrying *mcr* genes, so clinicians can rapidly adapt treatments or isolate the carrier patient in the hospital.

Acknowledgments

This work was supported by the French Government under the "Investissements d'avenir" (Investments for the Future) program managed by the Agence Nationale de la Recherche (ANR, fr: National Agency for Research) (reference: Méditerranée Infection 10-IAHU-03).

References

[1] K. Jeannot, A. Bolard, and P. Plésiat, "Resistance to polymyxins in Gram-negative organisms," *International Journal of Antimicrobial Agents*, vol. 49, no. 5, pp. 526–535, 2017.

[2] S. Biswas, J. M. Brunel, J. C. Dubus, M. Reynaud-Gaubert, and J. M. Rolain, "Colistin: an update on the antibiotic of the 21st century," *Expert Review of Anti-infective Therapy*, vol. 10, no. 8, pp. 917–934, 2012.

[3] R. E. Hancock and D. S. Chapple, "Peptide antibiotics," *Antimicrob Agents Chemother*, vol. 43, no. 6, pp. 1317–1323, 1999.

[4] A. O. Olaitan and J. Li, "Emergence of polymyxin resistance in Gram-negative bacteria," *International Journal of Antimicrobial Agents*, vol. 48, no. 6, pp. 581-582, 2016.

[5] A. O. Olaitan, S. Morand, and J. M. Rolain, "Mechanisms of polymyxin resistance: acquired and intrinsic resistance in bacteria," *Frontiers in Microbiology*, vol. 5, p. 643, 2014.

[6] Y. Y. Liu, Y. Wang, T. R. Walsh et al., "Emergence of plasmid-mediated colistin resistance mechanism *MCR*-1 in animals and human beings in China: a microbiological and molecular biological study," *Lancet Infectious Diseases*, vol. 16, no. 2, pp. 161-168, 2016.

[7] B. B. Xavier, C. Lammens, R. Ruhal et al., "Identification of a novel plasmid-mediated colistin-resistance gene, *mcr*-2, in *Escherichia coli*, Belgium, June 2016," *Eurosurveillance*, vol. 21, no. 27, pp. 6-11, 2016.

[8] V. Di Pilato, F. Arena, C. Tascini et al., "*mcr*-1.2, a new *mcr* variant carried on a transferable plasmid from a colistin-resistant KPC carbapenemase-producing *Klebsiella pneumoniae* strain of sequence type 512," *Antimicrobial Agents and Chemotherapy*, vol. 60, no. 9, pp. 5612-5615, 2016.

[9] Y. Q. Yang, Y. X. Li, T. Song et al., "Colistin resistance gene *mcr*-1 and its variant in *Escherichia coli* isolates from chickens in China," *Antimicrobial Agents and Chemotherapy*, vol. 61, no. 5, pp. e01204-e01216, 2017.

[10] W. Yin, H. Li, Y. Shen et al., "Novel plasmid-mediated colistin resistance gene *mcr*-3 in *Escherichia coli*," *MBio*, vol. 8, no. 3, article e00543-17, 2017.

[11] A. Carattoli, L. Villa, C. Feudi et al., "Novel plasmid-mediated colistin resistance *mcr*-4 gene in *Salmonella* and *Escherichia coli*, Italy 2013, Spain and Belgium, 2015 to 2016," *Eurosurveillance*, vol. 22, no. 31, p. 30589, 2017.

[12] M. Borowiak, J. Fischer, J. A. Hammerl, R. S. Hendriksen, I. Szabo, and B. Malorny, "Identification of a novel transposon-associated phosphoethanolamine transferase gene, *mcr*-5, conferring colistin resistance in d-tartrate fermenting *Salmonella enterica* subsp. enterica serovar Paratyphi B," *Journal of Antimicrobial Chemotherapya*, vol. 72, no. 12, pp. 3317-3324, 2017.

[13] M. AbuOun, E. J. Stubberfield, N. A. Duggett et al., "mcr-1 and mcr-2 (mcr-6.1) variant genes identified in Moraxella species isolated from pigs in Great Britain from 2014 to 2015," *Journal of Antimicrobial Chemotherapy*, vol. 72, no. 10, pp. 2745-2749, 2017.

[14] Y.-Q. Yang, Y.-X. Li, C.-W. Lei, A.-Y. Zhang, and H.-N. Wang, "Novel plasmid-mediated colistin resistance gene mcr-7.1 in Klebsiella pneumoniae," *Journal of Antimicrobial Chemotherapy*, vol. 73, no. 7, pp. 1791-1795, 2018.

[15] X. Wang, Y. Wang, Y. Zhou et al., "Emergence of a novel mobile colistin resistance gene, mcr-8, in NDM-producing Klebsiella pneumoniae," *Emerging Microbes and Infections*, vol. 7, no. 1, 2018.

[16] J. M. Rolain and A. O. Olaitan, "Plasmid-mediated colistin resistance: the final blow to colistin?," *International Journal of Antimicrobial Agents*, vol. 47, no. 1, pp. 4-5, 2016.

[17] Ministère de la santé, *Recommandations pour la prévention de la transmission croisée des bactéries hautement résistantes aux antibiotiques émergentes*, 2014.

[18] J. Sun, R. S. Yang, Q. Zhang et al., "Co-transfer of *bla*NDM-5 and mcr-1 by an IncX3-X4 hybrid plasmid in *Escherichia coli*," *Nature Microbiology*, vol. 1, p. 16176, 2016.

[19] C. C. Lai, Y. C. Chuang, C. C. Chen, and H. J. Tang, "Coexistence of *MCR*-1 and *NDM*-9 in a clinical carbapenem-resistant *Escherichia coli* isolate," *International Journal of Antimicrobial Agents*, vol. 49, no. 4, 2017.

[20] J. F. Delgado-Blas, C. M. Ovejero, L. Abadia-Patino, and B. Gonzalez-Zorn, "Coexistence of *mcr*-1 and bla*NDM*-1 in *Escherichia coli* from Venezuela," *Antimicrobial Agents and Chemotherapy*, vol. 60, no. 10, pp. 6356-6358, 2016.

[21] O. C. Conceição-Neto, C. A. M. Aires, N. F. Pereira et al., "Detection of the plasmid-mediated mcr-1 gene in clinical KPC-2-producing *Escherichia coli* isolates in Brazil," *International Journal of Antimicrobial Agents*, vol. 50, pp. 282-284, 2017.

[22] M. Tacão, S. R. Tavares, P. Teixeira et al., "*mcr*-1 and *bla*KPC-3 in *Escherichia coli* sequence type 744 after meropenem and colistin therapy, Portugal," *Emerging Infectious Diseases*, vol. 23, no. 8, pp. 1419-1421, 2017.

[23] R. Beyrouthy, F. Robin, A. Lessene et al., "*MCR*-1 and OXA-48 in vivo acquisition in KPC-producing *Escherichia coli* after colistin treatment," *Antimicrobial Agents and Chemotherapy*, vol. 61, no. 8, article e02540-16, 2017.

[24] S. Pulss, T. Semmler, E. Prenger-Berninghoff, R. Bauerfeind, and C. Ewers, "First report of an *Escherichia coli* strain from swine carrying an OXA-181 carbapenemase and the colistin resistance determinant *MCR*-1," *International Journal of Antimicrobial Agents*, vol. 50, no. 2, pp. 232-236, 2017.

[25] J. D. Perry, "A decade of development of chromogenic culture media for clinical microbiology in an era of molecular diagnostics," *Clinical Microbiology Reviews*, vol. 30, no. 2, pp. 449-479, 2017.

[26] P. Nordmann and L. Poirel, "Strategies for identification of carbapenemase-producing Enterobacteriaceae," *Journal of Antimicrobial Chemotherapy*, vol. 68, no. 3, pp. 487-489, 2013.

[27] L. Dortet, L. Bréchard, L. Poirel, and P. Nordmann, "Rapid detection of carbapenemase-producing Enterobacteriaceae from blood cultures," *Clinical Microbiology and Infection*, vol. 20, no. 4, pp. 340-344, 2013.

[28] P. Nordmann, L. Poirel, A. Carrër, M. A. Toleman, and T. R. Walsh, "How to detect *NDM*-1 producers," *Journal of Clinical Microbiology*, vol. 49, no. 2, pp. 718-721, 2011.

[29] I. Caniaux, A. van Belkum, G. Zambardi, L. Poirel, and M. F. Gros, "*MCR*: modern colistin resistance," *European Journal of Clinical Microbiology & Infectious Diseases*, vol. 36, no. 3, pp. 415-420, 2017.

[30] M. E. Falagas, G. C. Makris, G. Dimopoulos, and D. K. Matthaiou, "Heteroresistance: a concern of increasing clinical significance?," *Clinical Microbiology and Infection*, vol. 14, no. 2, pp. 101-104, 2008.

[31] J. R. Lo-Ten-Foe, A. M. G. A. de Smet, B. M. W. Diederen, J. A. J. W. Kluytmans, and P. H. J. van Keulen, "Comparative evaluation of the VITEK 2, disk diffusion, etest, broth microdilution, and agar dilution susceptibility testing methods for colistin in clinical isolates, including hetero-resistant *Enterobacter cloacae* and *Acinetobacter baumannii*," *Antimicrobial Agents and Chemotherapy*, vol. 51, no. 10, pp. 3726-3730, 2007.

[32] T. Y. Tan and S. Y. Ng, "Comparison of Etest, Vitek and agar dilution for susceptibility testing of colistin," *Clinical Microbiology and Infection*, vol. 13, no. 5, pp. 541-544, 2007.

[33] L. Bardet, *Development of New Tools for Detection of Colistin-Resistant Gram-Negative Bacteria*, Aix-Marseille Université, Marseille, France, 2017.

[34] J. E. Martin and J. S. Lewis, "Selective culture screening for penicillinase-producing *Neisseria gonorrhoeae*," *The Lancet*, vol. 2, no. 8038, pp. 605-606, 1977.

[35] J. D. Thayer and J. E. Martin, "Improved medium selective for cultivation of *N. gonorrhoeae* and *N. meningitidis*," *Public Heal Reports*, vol. 81, no. 6, pp. 559–562, 1966.

[36] J. E. Martin and A. Lester, "Transgrow, a medium for transport and growth of *Neisseria gonorrhoeae* and *Neisseria meningitidis*," *HSMHA Health Reports*, vol. 86, no. 1, pp. 30–33, 1971.

[37] Y. C. Faur, M. H. Weisburd, M. E. Wilson, and P. S. May, "A new medium for the isolation of pathogenic *Neisseria* (NYC medium). I. Formulation and comparisons with standard media," *Health Laboratory Science*, vol. 10, no. 2, pp. 44–54, 1973.

[38] P. H. Gilligan, P. A. Gage, L. M. Bradshaw, D. V. Schidlow, and B. T. DeCicco, "Isolation medium for the recovery of *Pseudomonas cepacia* from respiratory secretions of patients with cystic fibrosis," *Journal of Clinical Microbiology*, vol. 22, no. 1, pp. 5–8, 1985.

[39] D. F. Welch, M. J. Muszynski, C. H. Pai et al., "Selective and differential medium for recovery of *Pseudomonas cepacia* from the respiratory tracts of patients with cystic fibrosis," *Journal of Clinical Microbiology*, vol. 25, no. 9, pp. 1730–1734, 1987.

[40] D. A. Henry, M. E. Campbell, J. J. LiPuma, and D. P. Speert, "Identification of *Burkholderia cepacia* isolates from patients with cystic fibrosis and use of a simple new selective medium," *Journal of Clinical Microbiology*, vol. 35, no. 3, pp. 614–619, 1997.

[41] P. J. L. Dennis, C. L. R. Bartlett, and A. E. Wright, "Comparison of isolation methods for *Legionella* spp.," in *Proceedings of the 2nd International Symposium*, pp. 294–296, American Society, Washington, DC, USA, 1984.

[42] C. A. Bopp, J. W. Sumner, G. K. Morris, and J. G. Wells, "Isolation of *Legionella* spp. from environmental water samples by low-pH treatment and use of a selective medium," *Journal of Clinical Microbiology*, vol. 13, no. 4, pp. 714–719, 1981.

[43] A. Ta, J. Stout, V. Yu, and M. Wagener, "Comparison of culture methods for monitoring *Legionella* species in hospital potable water systems and recommendations for standardization of such methods," *Journal of Clinical Microbiology*, vol. 33, no. 8, pp. 2118–2123, 1995.

[44] J. Stout, V. L. Yu, R. M. Vickers, and J. Shonnard, "Potable water supply as the hospital reservoir for Pittsburgh pneumonia agent," *The Lancet*, vol. 1, no. 8270, pp. 471–472, 1982.

[45] P. H. Edelstein, "*Legionella*," in *Manual of Clinical Microbiology*, 9th edition, Washington, DC, USA, 2007.

[46] P. R. Murray, E. Baron, J. H. Jorgensen, M. L. Landry, and M. A. Pfaller, *Manual of Clinical Microbiology*, American Society for Microbiology, Washington, DC, USA, 9th edition, 2007.

[47] J. P. Butzler, P. Dekeyser, M. Detrain, and F. Dehaen, "Related *vibrio* in stools," *Journal of Pediatrics*, vol. 82, no. 3, pp. 493–495, 1973.

[48] M. B. Skirrow, "*Campylobacter* enteritis: a "new" disease," *British Medical Journal*, vol. 2, no. 6078, pp. 9–11, 1977.

[49] W. L. Wang, M. Blaser, and J. Cravens, "Isolation of *Campylobacter*," *British Medical Journal*, vol. 2, no. 6129, p. 57, 1978.

[50] F. J. Bolton and L. Robertson, "A selective medium for isolating *Campylobacter jejuni/coli*," *Journal of Clinical Pathology*, vol. 35, no. 4, pp. 462–467, 1982.

[51] L. M. Jones and W. J. B. Morgan, "A preliminary report on a selective medium for the culture of *Brucella*, including fastidious types," *Bulletin of the World Health Organization*, vol. 19, no. 1, pp. 200–203, 1958.

[52] C. Vanderzant and D. F. Splittstoesser, *Compendium of Methods for the Microbiological Examination of Foods*, American Public Health Association, Washington, DC, USA, 1992.

[53] P. D. Ellner, C. J. Stoessel, E. Drakeford, and F. Vasi, "A new culture medium for medical bacteriology," *American Journal of Clinical Pathology*, vol. 45, no. 4, pp. 502–504, 1966.

[54] G. D. W. Curtis, W. W. Nichols, and T. J. Falla, "Selective agents for *Listeria* can inhibit their growth," *Letters in Applied Microbiology*, vol. 8, no. 5, pp. 169–172, 1989.

[55] W. H. Lee and D. McClain, "Improved *Listeria monocytogenes* selective agar," *Applied and Environmental Microbiology*, vol. 52, no. 5, pp. 1215–1217, 1986.

[56] P. van Netten, I. Perales, A. van de Moosdijk, G. D. W. Curtis, and D. A. A. Mossel, "Liquid and solid selective differential media for the detection and enumeration of *L. monocytogenes* and other *Listeria* spp.," *International Journal of Food Microbiology*, vol. 8, no. 4, pp. 299–316, 1989.

[57] D. A. Mossel, M. J. Koopman, and E. Jongerius, "Enumeration of *Bacillus cereus* in foods," *Applied Microbiology*, vol. 15, no. 3, pp. 650–653, 1967.

[58] M. L. Cohn, R. F. Waggoner, and J. K. McClatchy, "The 7H11 medium for the cultivation of mycobacteria," *American Review of Respiratory Disease*, vol. 98, no. 2, pp. 295–296, 1968.

[59] R. Angelotti, H. E. Hall, M. Foter, and K. M. Lewis, "Quantification of *Clostridium perfringens* in foods," *Applied Microbiology*, vol. 10, no. 3, pp. 193–199, 1962.

[60] R. Marshall, "Rapid technique for the enumeration of *Clostridium perfringens*," *Applied Microbiology*, vol. 13, no. 4, pp. 559–563, 1965.

[61] S. A. Shahidi and A. R. Ferguson, "New quantitative, qualitative, and confirmatory media for rapid analysis of food for *Clostridium perfringens*," *Applied Microbiology*, vol. 21, no. 3, pp. 500–506, 1971.

[62] R. J. Meinersmann, S. R. Ladely, J. R. Plumblee et al., "Colistin resistance *mcr*-1-gene-bearing *Escherichia coli* strain from the United States," *Genome Announcements*, vol. 4, no. 5, p. e00898-16, 2016.

[63] M. R. Fernandes, Q. Moura, L. Sartori et al., "Silent dissemination of colistin-resistant *Escherichia coli* in South America could contribute to the global spread of the *mcr*-1 gene," *Eurosurveillance*, vol. 21, no. 17, pp. 1–6, 2016.

[64] V. Donà, O. J. Bernasconi, S. Kasraian, R. Tinguely, and A. Endimiani, "A SYBR® green-based real-time PCR method for improved detection of *mcr*-1-mediated colistin resistance in human stool samples," *Journal of Global Antimicrobial Resistance*, vol. 9, pp. 57–60, 2017.

[65] D. F. Monte, A. Mem, M. R. Fernandes et al., "Chicken meat as a reservoir of colistin-resistant *Escherichia coli* strains carrying *mcr*-1 genes in South America," *Antimicrobial Agents and Chemotherapy*, vol. 61, no. 5, p. e02718-16, 2017.

[66] C. J. H. von Wintersdorff, P. F. G. Wolffs, J. M. van Niekerk et al., "Detection of the plasmid-mediated colistin-resistance gene *mcr*-1 in faecal metagenomes of Dutch travellers," *Journal of Antimicrobial Chemotherapy*, vol. 71, no. 12, pp. 3416–3419, 2016.

[67] S. Buess, M. Nüesch-Inderbinen, R. Stephan, and K. Zurfluh, "Assessment of animals as a reservoir for colistin resistance: no *MCR-1/MCR-2*-producing Enterobacteriaceae detected

in Swiss livestock," *Journal of Global Antimicrobial Resistance*, vol. 8, pp. 33-34, 2017.

[68] K. Zurfluh, R. Stephan, A. Widmer et al., "Screening for fecal carriage of *MCR*-producing Enterobacteriaceae in healthy humans and primary care patients," *Antimicrobial Resistance & Infection Control*, vol. 6, no. 1, p. 28, 2017.

[69] Y. Hu, Y. Wang, Q. Sun et al., "Colistin-resistance gene *mcr-1* in children's gut flora," *International Journal of Antimicrobial Agents*, vol. 50, no. 4, pp. 593–597, 2017.

[70] Y. Wang, G. B. Tian, R. Zhang et al., "Prevalence, risk factors, outcomes, and molecular epidemiology of *mcr*-1-positive Enterobacteriaceae in patients and healthy adults from China: an epidemiological and clinical study," *Lancet Infectious Diseases*, vol. 17, no. 4, pp. 390–399, 2017.

[71] S. C. Y. Wong, H. Tse, J. H. K. Chen, V. C. C. Cheng, P. L. Ho, and K. Y. Yuen, "Colistin-resistant Enterobacteriaceae carrying the *mcr*-1 gene among patients in Hong Kong," *Emerging Infectious Diseases*, vol. 22, no. 9, pp. 1667–1669, 2016.

[72] M. Payne, M. A. Croxen, T. D. Lee et al., "*mcr*-1-positive colistin-resistant *Escherichia coli* in traveler returning to Canada from China," *Emerging Infectious Diseases*, vol. 22, no. 9, pp. 1673–1675, 2016.

[73] Y. Caspar, M. Maillet, P. Pavese et al., "*mcr*-1 colistin resistance in ESBL-producing *Klebsiella pneumoniae*, France," *Emerging Infectious Diseases*, vol. 23, no. 5, pp. 874–876, 2017.

[74] E. M. Terveer, R. H. T. Nijhuis, M. J. T. Crobach et al., "Prevalence of colistin resistance gene (*mcr*-1) containing Enterobacteriaceae in feces of patients attending a tertiary care hospital and detection of a *mcr*-1 containing, colistin susceptible *E. coli*," *PLoS One*, vol. 12, no. 6, Article ID e0178598, 2017.

[75] P. Nordmann, A. Jayol, and L. Poirel, "A universal culture medium for screening polymyxin-resistant Gram-negative isolates," *Journal of Clinical Microbiology*, vol. 54, no. 5, pp. 1395–1399, 2016.

[76] M. H. F. Abdul Momin, D. C. Bean, R. S. Hendriksen, M. Haenni, L. M. Phee, and D. W. Wareham, "CHROMagar COL-APSE: a selective bacterial culture medium for the isolation and differentiation of colistin-resistant Gram-negative pathogens," *Journal of Medical Microbiology*, vol. 66, no. 11, pp. 1554–1561, 2017.

[77] L. Bardet, S. Le Page, T. Leangapichart, and J. M. Rolain, "LBJMR medium: a new polyvalent culture medium for isolating and selecting vancomycin and colistin-resistant bacteria," *BMC Microbiology*, vol. 17, no. 1, pp. 1–10, 2017.

[78] P. Nordmann, A. Jayol, and L. Poirel, "Rapid detection of polymyxin resistance in Enterobacteriaceae," *Emerging Infectious Diseases*, vol. 22, no. 6, pp. 1038–1043, 2016.

[79] A. Jayol, M. Saly, P. Nordmann, A. Ménard, L. Poirel, and V. Dubois, "*Hafnia*, an enterobacterial genus naturally resistant to colistin revealed by three susceptibility testing methods," *Journal of Antimicrobial Chemotherapy*, vol. 72, no. 9, pp. 1–5, 2017.

[80] A. Jayol, V. Dubois, L. Poirel, and P. Nordmann, "Rapid detection of polymyxin-resistant Enterobacteriaceae from blood cultures," *Journal of Clinical Microbiology*, vol. 54, no. 9, pp. 2273–2277, 2016.

[81] Y. D. Bakthavatchalam and B. Veeraraghavan, "Challenges, issues and warnings from CLSI and EUCAST working group on polymyxin susceptibility testing," *Journal of Clinical and Diagnostic Research*, vol. 11, pp. DL03–DL04, 2017.

[82] C. G. Giske and G. Kahlmeter, "Colistin antimicrobial susceptibility testing—can the slow and challenging be replaced by the rapid and convenient?," *Clinical Microbiology and Infection*, vol. 24, no. 2, pp. 93-94, 2017.

[83] A. Jayol, P. Nordmann, P. Lehours et al., "Comparison of methods for detection of plasmid-mediated and chromosomally encoded colistin resistance in Enterobacteriaceae," *Clinical Microbiology and Infection*, vol. 51, no. 2, pp. 3726–3730, 2017.

[84] L. Poirel, Y. Larpin, J. Dobias et al., "Rapid polymyxin NP test for the detection of polymyxin resistance mediated by the *mcr-1/mcr-2* genes," *Diagnostic Microbiology and Infectious Disease*, vol. 90, no. 1, pp. 7–10, 2017.

[85] S. Simar, D. Sibley, D. Ashcraft, and G. Pankey, "Evaluation of the rapid polymyxin NP test for polymyxin B resistance detection using *Enterobacter cloacae* and *Enterobacter aerogenes* isolates," *Journal of Clinical Microbiology*, vol. 55, no. 10, pp. 3016–3020, 2017.

[86] M. Tamayo, R. Santiso, F. Otero et al., "Rapid determination of colistin resistance in clinical strains of *Acinetobacter baumannii* by use of the Micromax assay," *Journal of Clinical Microbiology*, vol. 51, no. 11, pp. 3675–3682, 2013.

[87] J. Osei Sekyere, U. Govinden, and S. Y. Essack, "Review of established and innovative detection methods for carbapenemase-producing Gram-negative bacteria," *Journal of Applied Microbiology*, vol. 119, no. 5, pp. 1219–1233, 2015.

[88] B. Ghebremedhin, A. Halstenbach, M. Smiljanic, M. Kaase, and P. Ahmad-Nejad, "MALDI-TOF MS based carbapenemase detection from culture isolates and from positive blood culture vials," *Annals of Clinical Microbiology and Antimicrobials*, vol. 15, no. 1, p. 5, 2016.

[89] J. Hrabák, E. Chudáčková, and C. C. Papagiannitsis, "Detection of carbapenemases in Enterobacteriaceae: a challenge for diagnostic microbiological laboratories," *Clinical Microbiology and Infection*, vol. 20, no. 9, pp. 839–853, 2014.

[90] P. Seng, M. Drancourt, F. Gouriet et al., "Ongoing revolution in bacteriology: routine identification of bacteria by matrix-assisted laser desorption ionization time-of-flight mass spectrometry," *Clinical Infectious Diseases*, vol. 49, no. 4, pp. 543–551, 2009.

[91] G. Larrouy-Maumus, A. Clements, A. Filloux, R. R. McCarthy, and S. Mostowy, "Direct detection of lipid A on intact Gram-negative bacteria by MALDI-TOF mass spectrometry," *Journal of Microbiological Methods*, vol. 120, pp. 68–71, 2016.

[92] J. O. Sekyere, U. Govinden, L. A. Bester, and S. Y. Essack, "Colistin and tigecycline resistance in carbapenemase-producing Gram-negative bacteria: emerging resistance mechanisms and detection methods," *Journal of Applied Microbiology*, vol. 121, no. 3, pp. 601–617, 2016.

[93] L. Dortet, R. A. Bonnin, I. Pennisi et al., "Rapid detection and discrimination of chromosome- and MCR-plasmid-mediated resistance to polymyxins by MALDI-TOF MS in *Escherichia coli*: the MALDIxin test," *Journal of Antimicrobial Chemotherapy*, pp. 1–9, 2018, In press.

[94] V. Stojanoski, B. Sankaran, B. V. V. Prasad, L. Poirel, P. Nordmann, and T. Palzkill, "Structure of the catalytic domain of the colistin resistance enzyme MCR-1," *BMC Biology*, vol. 14, no. 1, p. 81, 2016.

[95] M. Hu, J. Guo, Q. Cheng et al., "Crystal structure of *Escherichia coli* originated MCR-1, a phosphoethanolamine transferase for colistin resistance," *Scientific Reports*, vol. 6, no. 1, p. 38793, 2016.

[96] G. Ma, Y. Zhu, Z. Yu, A. Ahmad, and H. Zhang, "High resolution crystal structure of the catalytic domain of *MCR*-1," *Scientific Reports*, vol. 6, no. 1, p. 39540, 2016.

[97] P. Hinchliffe, Q. E. Yang, E. Portal et al., "Insights into the mechanistic basis of plasmid-mediated colistin resistance from crystal structures of the catalytic domain of *MCR*-1," *Scientific Reports*, vol. 7, p. 39392, 2017.

[98] M. Coppi, A. Cannatelli, A. Antonelli et al., "A simple phenotypic method for screening of *MCR*-1-mediated colistin resistance," *Clinical Microbiology and Infection*, vol. 24, no. 2, pp. 201.e1–201.e3, 2017.

[99] F. Esposito, M. R. Fernandes, R. Lopes et al., "Detection of colistin-resistant *mcr*-1-positive *Escherichia coli* by use of assays based on inhibition by EDTA and zeta potential," *Journal of Clinical Microbiology*, vol. 55, no. 12, pp. 3454–3465, 2017.

[100] European Committee on Antimicrobial Susceptibility Testing (EUCAST), *Breakpoint Tables for Interpretation of MICs and Zone Diameters,* Vol. 8, EUCAST, Växjö, Sweden, 2018.

[101] CLSI, Clinical and Laboratory Standards Institute, *M07-A10: Methods for Dilution Antimicrobial Susceptibility Tests for Bacteria That Grow Aerobically; Approved Standard,* Vol. 35, CLSI, Wayne, PA, USA, 10th edition, 2015.

[102] ISO 20776-1:2006, *Clinical Laboratory Testing and In Vitro Diagnostic Test Systems–Susceptibility Testing of Infectious Agents and Evaluation of Performance of Antimicrobial Susceptibility Test Devices–Part 1: Reference Method for Testing the In Vitro Activity of Antimicrobial Agents against Rapidly Growing Aerobic Bacteria Involved in Infectious Diseases n.d*, https://www.iso.org/standard/41630.html.

[103] Clinical and Laboratory Standards, *M100–S27: Performance Standards for Antimicrobial Susceptibility Testing*, Clinical and Laboratory Standards, Wayne, PA, USA, 2017.

[104] European Committee on Antimicrobial Susceptibility Testing (EUCAST), *Routine and Extended Internal QualityControl for Mic Determination and Disk Diffusion as Recommendedby EUCAST,* Vol. 8, EUCAST, Växjö, Sweden, 2018.

[105] K. H. Jerke, M. J. Lee, and R. M. Humphries, "Polymyxin susceptibility testing: a cold case reopened," *Clinical Microbiology Newsletter*, vol. 38, no. 9, pp. 69–77, 2016.

[106] R. M. Humphries, "Susceptibility testing of the polymyxins: where are we now?," *Pharmacotherapy*, vol. 35, no. 1, pp. 22–27, 2015.

[107] D. Landman, J. Salamera, and J. Quale, "Irreproducible and uninterpretable polymyxin B MICs for *Enterobacter cloacae* and *Enterobacter aerogenes*," *Journal of Clinical Microbiology*, vol. 51, no. 12, pp. 4106–4111, 2013.

[108] A. Poudyal, B. P. Howden, J. M. Bell et al., "In vitro pharmacodynamics of colistin against multidrug-resistant *Klebsiella pneumoniae*," *Journal of Antimicrobial Chemotherapy*, vol. 62, no. 6, pp. 1311–1318, 2008.

[109] ISO 20776-2:2007, *Clinical Laboratory Testing and In Vitro Diagnostic Test Systems–Susceptibility Testing of Infectious Agents and Evaluation of Performance of Antimicrobial Susceptibility Test Devices–Part 2: Evaluation of Performance of Antimicrobial Susceptibility Test Devices n.d*, 2018, https://www.iso.org/standard/41631.html.

[110] K. Dafopoulou, O. Zarkotou, E. Dimitroulia et al., "Comparative evaluation of colistin susceptibility testing methods among carbapenem-nonsusceptible *Klebsiella pneumoniae* and *Acinetobacter baumannii* clinical isolates," *Antimicrobial Agents and Chemotherapy*, vol. 59, no. 8, pp. 4625–4630, 2015.

[111] C. A. Sutherland and D. P. Nicolau, "To add or not to add polysorbate 80: impact on colistin MICs for clinical strains of Enterobacteriaceae and *Pseudomonas aeruginosa* and quality controls," *Journal of Clinical Microbiology*, vol. 52, no. 10, p. 3810, 2014.

[112] H. S. Sader, P. R. Rhomberg, R. K. Flamm, and R. N. Jones, "Use of a surfactant (polysorbate 80) to improve MIC susceptibility testing results for polymyxin B and colistin," *Diagnostic Microbiology and Infectious Disease*, vol. 74, no. 4, pp. 412–414, 2012.

[113] M. Albur, A. Noel, K. Bowker, and A. MacGowan, "Colistin susceptibility testing: time for a review," *Journal of Antimicrobial Chemotherapy*, vol. 69, no. 5, pp. 1432–1434, 2014.

[114] L. Singhal, M. Sharma, S. Verma et al., "Comparative Evaluation of Broth Microdilution with Polystyrene and Glass-Coated Plates, Agar Dilution, E-Test, Vitek, and Disk Diffusion for Susceptibility Testing of Colistin and Polymyxin B on Carbapenem-Resistant Clinical Isolates of Acinetobacter baum," *Microbial Drug Resistance*, 2018.

[115] S. Y. Lee, J. H. Shin, K. Lee et al., "Comparison of the Vitek 2, MicroScan, and Etest methods with the agar dilution method in assessing colistin susceptibility of bloodstream isolates of *Acinetobacter* species from a Korean University Hospital," *Journal of Clinical Microbiology*, vol. 51, no. 6, pp. 1924–1926, 2013.

[116] S. M. Maalej, M. R. Meziou, F. M. Rhimi, and A. Hammami, "Comparison of disc diffusion, Etest and agar dilution for susceptibility testing of colistin against Enterobacteriaceae," *Letters in Applied Microbiology*, vol. 53, no. 5, pp. 546–551, 2011.

[117] B. Behera, P. Mathur, A. Das et al., "Evaluation of susceptibility testing methods for polymyxin," *International Journal of Infectious Diseases*, vol. 14, no. 7, pp. e596–e601, 2010.

[118] T. Y. Tan, L. S. Y. Ng, and K. Poh, "Susceptibility testing of unconventional antibiotics against multiresistant *Acinetobacter* spp. by agar dilution and Vitek 2," *Diagnostic Microbiology and Infectious Disease*, vol. 58, no. 3, pp. 357–361, 2007.

[119] T. Y. Tan, "Comparison of three standardized disc susceptibility testing methods for colistin," *Journal of Antimicrobial Chemotherapy*, vol. 58, no. 4, pp. 864–867, 2006.

[120] S. M. Moskowitz, E. Garber, Y. Chen et al., "Colistin susceptibility testing: evaluation of reliability for cystic fibrosis isolates of *Pseudomonas aeruginosa* and *Stenotrophomonas maltophilia*," *Journal of Antimicrobial Chemotherapy*, vol. 65, no. 7, pp. 1416–1423, 2010.

[121] M. Hogardt, S. Schmoldt, M. Götzfried, K. Adler, and J. Heesemann, "Pitfalls of polymyxin antimicrobial susceptibility testing of *Pseudomonas aeruginosa* isolated from cystic fibrosis patients," *Journal of Antimicrobial Chemotherapy*, vol. 54, no. 6, pp. 1057–1061, 2004.

[122] M. Richter and R. Rosselló-Móra, "Shifting the genomic gold standard for the prokaryotic species definition," *Proceedings of the National Academy of Sciences of the United States of America*, vol. 106, no. 45, pp. 19126–19131, 2009.

[123] F. Boyen, F. Vangroenweghe, P. Butaye et al., "Disk prediffusion is a reliable method for testing colistin susceptibility in porcine *E. coli* strains," *Veterinary Microbiology*, vol. 144, no. 3-4, pp. 359–362, 2010.

[124] A. Nemec and L. Dijkshoorn, "Variations in colistin susceptibility among different species of the genus

Acinetobacter," *Journal of Antimicrobial Chemotherapy,* vol. 65, no. 2, pp. 367–369, 2010.

[125] A. C. Nicodemo, M. R. E. Araujo, A. S. Ruiz, and A. C. Gales, "In vitro susceptibility of *Stenotrophomonas maltophilia* isolates: comparison of disc diffusion, Etest and agar dilution methods," *Journal of Antimicrobial Chemotherapy,* vol. 53, no. 4, pp. 604–608, 2004.

[126] F. W. Goldstein, A. Ly, and M. D. Kitzis, "Comparison of Etest with agar dilution for testing the susceptibility of *Pseudomonas aeruginosa* and other multidrug-resistant bacteria to colistin," *Journal of Antimicrobial Chemotherapy,* vol. 59, no. 5, pp. 1039-1040, 2007.

[127] A. C. Gales, A. O. Reis, and R. N. Jones, "Contemporary assessment of antimicrobial susceptibility testing methods for polymyxin B and colistin: review of available interpretative criteria and quality control guidelines," *Journal of Clinical Microbiology,* vol. 39, no. 1, pp. 183–190, 2001.

[128] J. A. Hindler and R. M. Humphries, "Colistin MIC variability by method for contemporary clinical isolates of multidrug-resistant Gram-negative bacilli," *Journal of Clinical Microbiology,* vol. 51, no. 6, pp. 1678–1684, 2013.

[129] S. Vourli, K. Dafopoulou, G. Vrioni, A. Tsakris, and S. Pournaras, "Evaluation of two automated systems for colistin susceptibility testing of carbapenem-resistant *Acinetobacter baumannii* clinical isolates," *Journal of Antimicrobial Chemotherapy,* vol. 72, no. 9, pp. 2528–2530, 2017.

[130] A. Turlej-Rogacka, B. B. Xavier, L. Janssens et al., "Evaluation of colistin stability in agar and comparison of four methods for MIC testing of colistin," *European Journal of Clinical Microbiology & Infectious Diseases,* vol. 37, no. 2, pp. 345–353, 2017.

[131] A. W. Bauer, W. M. Kirby, J. C. Sherris, and M. Turck, "Antibiotic susceptibility testing by a standardized single disk method," *American Journal of Clinical Pathology,* vol. 45, no. 4, pp. 493–496, 1966.

[132] L. J. Rojas, M. Salim, E. Cober et al., "Colistin resistance in carbapenem-resistant *Klebsiella pneumoniae*: laboratory detection and impact on mortality," *Clinical Infectious Diseases,* vol. 314, p. ciw805, 2016.

[133] L. R. R. Perez, "Evaluation of polymyxin susceptibility profile among KPC-producing *Klebsiella pneumoniae* using Etest and MicroScan WalkAway automated system," *APMIS,* vol. 123, no. 11, pp. 951–954, 2015.

[134] A. Lat, S. A. Clock, F. Wu et al., "Comparison of polymyxin B, tigecycline, cefepime, and meropenem MICs for KPC-producing *Klebsiella pneumoniae* by broth microdilution, Vitek 2, and Etest," *Journal of Clinical Microbiology,* vol. 49, no. 5, pp. 1795–1798, 2011.

[135] I. M. van der Heijden, A. S. Levin, E. H. De Pedri et al., "Comparison of disc diffusion, Etest and broth microdilution for testing susceptibility of carbapenem-resistant *P. aeruginosa* to polymyxins," *Annals of Clinical Microbiology and Antimicrobials,* vol. 6, no. 1, p. 8, 2007.

[136] P. Piewngam and P. Kiratisin, "Comparative assessment of antimicrobial susceptibility testing for tigecycline and colistin against *Acinetobacter baumannii* clinical isolates, including multidrug-resistant isolates," *International Journal of Antimicrobial Agents,* vol. 44, no. 5, pp. 396–401, 2014.

[137] M. Sinirtaş, H. Akalin, and S. Gedikoğlu, "Investigation of colistin sensitivity via three different methods in *Acinetobacter baumannii* isolates with multiple antibiotic

resistance," *International Journal of Infectious Diseases,* vol. 13, no. 5, pp. e217–e220, 2009.

[138] L. A. Arroyo, A. Garcia-Curiel, M. E. Pachón-Ibáñez et al., "Reliability of the E-test method for detection of colistin resistance in clinical isolates of *Acinetobacter baumannii,*" *Journal of Clinical Microbiology,* vol. 43, no. 2, pp. 903–905, 2005.

[139] R. Girardello, P. J. M. Bispo, T. M. Yamanaka, and A. C. Gales, "Cation concentration variability of four distinct Mueller-Hinton agar brands influences polymyxin B susceptibility results," *Journal of Clinical Microbiology,* vol. 50, no. 7, pp. 2414–2418, 2012.

[140] L. Bardet, S. Baron, T. Leangapichart, L. Okdah, S. M. Diene, and J. M. Rolain, "Deciphering heteroresistance to colistin in a *Klebsiella pneumoniae* isolate from Marseille, France," *Antimicrobial Agents and Chemotherapy,* vol. 61, no. 6, p. e00356-17, 2017.

[141] I. Galani, F. Kontopidou, M. Souli et al., "Colistin susceptibility testing by Etest and disk diffusion methods," *International Journal of Antimicrobial Agents,* vol. 31, no. 5, pp. 434–439, 2008.

[142] E. Jouy, M. Haenni, L. Le Devendec et al., "Improvement in routine detection of colistin resistance in *E. coli* isolated in veterinary diagnostic laboratories," *Journal of Microbiological Methods,* vol. 132, pp. 125–127, 2017.

[143] E. Matuschek, J. Åhman, C. Webster, and G. Kahlmeter, "Antimicrobial susceptibility testing of colistin–evaluation of seven commercial MIC products against standard broth microdilution for *Escherichia coli, Klebsiella pneumoniae, Pseudomonas aeruginosa,* and *Acinetobacter* spp.," *Clinical Microbiology and Infection,* 2017.

[144] P. Plésiat, K. Jeannot, and P. Triponney, "Évaluation comparative de la détermination du test de sensibilité à la colistine UMIC (Biocentric) chez Pseudomonas aeruginosa," in *Proceedings of the 36ème Réunion Interdiscip. Chim. Anti-Infectieuse,* Paris, France, December 2016.

[145] L. Bardet, L. Okdah, S. Baron, S. Le Page, and J. Rolain, "Évaluation du test UMIC Colistine de détermination de la CMI," in *Proceedings of the 37ème Réunion Interdiscip. Chim. Anti-Infectieuse,* Paris, France, December 2017.

[146] E. Carretto, F. Brovarone, G. Russello et al., "Clinical validation of the Sensitest Colistin, a broth microdilution based method to evaluate colistin MICs," *Journal of Clinical Microbiology,* vol. 56, no. 4, 2018.

[147] K. L. Chew, M. V. La, R. T. P. Lin, and J. W. P. Teo, "Colistin and polymyxin B susceptibility testing for carbapenem-resistant and *mcr*-positive Enterobacteriaceae: comparison of Sensititre, MicroScan, Vitek 2, and Etest with broth microdilution," *Journal of Clinical Microbiology,* vol. 55, no. 9, pp. 2609–2616, 2017.

[148] T. Cimmino, S. Le Page, D. Raoult, and J. M. Rolain, "Contemporary challenges and opportunities in the diagnosis and outbreak detection of multidrug-resistant infectious disease," *Expert Review of Molecular Diagnostics,* vol. 16, no. 11, pp. 1163–1175, 2016.

[149] T. Giani, M. I. Morosini, M. M. D'Andrea, M. García-Castillo, G. M. Rossolini, and R. Cantón, "Assessment of the Phoenix[TM] automated system and EUCAST breakpoints for antimicrobial susceptibility testing against isolates expressing clinically relevant resistance mechanisms," *Clinical Microbiology and Infection,* vol. 18, no. 11, pp. E452–E458, 2012.

[150] R. L. Skov and D. L. Monnet, "Plasmid-mediated colistin resistance (*mcr*-1 gene): three months later, the story unfolds," *Eurosurveillance*, vol. 21, no. 9, p. 30155, 2016.

[151] S. Bontron, L. Poirel, and P. Nordmann, "Real-time PCR for detection of plasmid-mediated polymyxin resistance (*mcr*-1) from cultured bacteria and stools," *Journal of Antimicrobial Chemotherapy*, vol. 71, no. 8, pp. 2318–2320, 2016.

[152] S. Chabou, T. Leangapichart, L. Okdah, S. Le Page, L. Hadjadj, and J. M. M. Rolain, "Real-time quantitative PCR assay with Taqman® probe for rapid detection of *MCR*-1 plasmid-mediated colistin resistance," *New Microbes and New Infections*, vol. 13, pp. 71–74, 2016.

[153] J. Quan, X. Li, and Y. Chen, "Prevalence of *mcr*-1 in *Escherichia coli* and *Klebsiella pneumoniae* recovered from bloodstream infections in China: a multicentre longitudinal study," *The Lancet Infectious Diseases*, vol. 17, no. 4, pp. 400–410, 2017.

[154] S. S. Elnahriry, H. O. Khalifa, A. M. Soliman et al., "Emergence of plasmid-mediated colistin resistance gene *mcr*-1 in a clinical *Escherichia coli* isolate from Egypt," *Antimicrobial Agents and Chemotherapy*, vol. 60, no. 5, pp. 3249-3250, 2016.

[155] L. Falgenhauer, S. E. Waezsada, Y. Yao et al., "Colistin resistance gene *mcr*-1 in extended-spectrum beta-lactamase-producing and carbapenemase-producing Gram-negative bacteria in Germany," *Lancet Infectious Diseases*, vol. 16, no. 3, pp. 282-283, 2016.

[156] H. Ye, Y. Li, Z. Li et al., "Diversified *mcr*-1-harbouring plasmid reservoirs confer resistance to colistin in human gut microbiota," *mBio*, vol. 7, no. 2, p. e00177-16, 2016.

[157] A. Walkty, J. A. Karlowsky, H. J. Adam et al., "Frequency of *MCR*-1-mediated colistin resistance among *Escherichia coli* clinical isolates obtained from patients in Canadian hospitals (CANWARD 2008–2015)," *CMAJ Open*, vol. 4, no. 4, pp. E641–E645, 2016.

[158] R. Gao, Y. Hu, Z. Li et al., "Dissemination and mechanism for the *MCR*-1 colistin resistance," *PLoS Pathogens*, vol. 12, no. 11, p. e1005957, 2016.

[159] A. Cannatelli, T. Giani, A. Antonelli, L. Principe, F. Luzzaro, and G. M. Rossolini, "First detection of the *mcr*-1 colistin resistance gene in *Escherichia coli* in Italy," *Antimicrobial Agents and Chemotherapy*, vol. 60, no. 5, pp. 3257-3258, 2016.

[160] G. D. Wright, "Antibiotic resistance in the environment: a link to the clinic?," *Current Opinion in Microbiology*, vol. 13, no. 5, pp. 589–594, 2010.

[161] I. Lekunberri, J. L. Balcázar, and C. M. Borrego, "Detection and quantification of the plasmid-mediated *mcr*-1 gene conferring colistin resistance in wastewater," *International Journal of Antimicrobial Agents*, vol. 50, no. 6, pp. 734–736, 2017.

[162] A. Irrgang, N. Roschanski, B. A. Tenhagen et al., "Prevalence of *mcr*-1 in *E. coli* from livestock and food in Germany, 2010–2015," *PLoS One*, vol. 11, no. 7, Article ID e0159863, 2016.

[163] R. H. T. Nijhuis, K. T. Veldman, J. Schelfaut et al., "Detection of the plasmid-mediated colistin-resistance gene *mcr*-1 in clinical isolates and stool specimens obtained from hospitalized patients using a newly developed real-time PCR assay," *Journal of Antimicrobial Chemotherapy*, vol. 71, no. 8, pp. 2344–2346, 2016.

[164] D. Yang, Z. Qiu, Z. Shen et al., "The occurrence of the colistin resistance gene *mcr*-1 in the Haihe River (China)," *International Journal of Environmental Research and Public Health*, vol. 14, no. 6, p. 576, 2017.

[165] E. Snesrud, A. C. Ong, and B. Corey, "Analysis of serial isolates of *mcr*-1-positive *Escherichia coli* reveals a highly active IS *Apl*1 transposon," *Antimicrobial Agents and Chemotherapy*, vol. 61, no. 5, p. e00056-17, 2017.

[166] N. Lima Barbieri, D. W. Nielsen, Y. Wannemuehler et al., "*mcr*-1 identified in avian pathogenic *Escherichia coli* (APEC)," *PLoS One*, vol. 12, no. 3, Article ID e0172997, 2017.

[167] J. Sun, Y. Xu, R. Gao et al., "Deciphering *MCR*-2 colistin resistance," *mBio*, vol. 8, no. 3, p. e00625-17, 2017.

[168] N. Liassine, L. Assouvie, M. C. Descombes et al., "Very low prevalence of *MCR*-1/*MCR*-2 plasmid-mediated colistin resistance in urinary tract Enterobacteriaceae in Switzerland," *International Journal of Infectious Diseases*, vol. 51, pp. 4-5, 2016.

[169] S. Simmen, K. Zurfluh, M. Nüesch-Inderbinen, and S. Schmitt, "Investigation for the colistin resistance genes *mcr*-1 and *mcr*-2 in clinical Enterobacteriaceae isolates from cats and dogs in Switzerland," *ARC Journal of Animal and Veterinary Sciences*, vol. 2, no. 4, pp. 26–29, 2016.

[170] N. Roschanski, L. Falgenhauer, M. Grobbel et al., "Retrospective survey of *mcr*-1 and *mcr*-2 in German pig-fattening farms, 2011-2012," *International Journal of Antimicrobial Agents*, vol. 50, no. 2, pp. 266–271, 2017.

[171] L. Poirel, A. Jayol, and P. Nordmann, "Polymyxins: antibacterial activity, susceptibility testing, and resistance mechanisms encoded by plasmids or chromosomes," *Clinical Microbiology Reviews*, vol. 30, no. 2, pp. 557–596, 2017.

[172] J. Li, X. Shi, W. Yin et al., "A multiplex SYBR Green real-time PCR assay for the detection of three colistin resistance genes from cultured bacteria, feces, and environment samples," *Frontiers in Microbiology*, vol. 8, pp. 1–5, 2017.

[173] A. Rita Rebelo, V. Bortolaia, J. S. Kjeldgaard et al., "Multiplex PCR for detection of plasmid-mediated colistin resistance determinants, mcr-1, mcr-2, mcr-3, mcr-4 and mcr-5 for surveillance purposes," *Eurosurveillance*, vol. 23, no. 6, 2018.

[174] T. Sekizuka, M. Kawanishi, M. Ohnishi et al., "Elucidation of quantitative structural diversity of remarkable rearrangement regions, shufflons, in IncI2 plasmids," *Scientific Reports*, vol. 7, no. 1, p. 928, 2017.

[175] M. Doumith, G. Godbole, P. Ashton et al., "Detection of the plasmid-mediated *mcr*-1 gene conferring colistin resistance in human and food isolates of *Salmonella enterica* and *Escherichia coli* in England and Wales," *Journal of Antimicrobial Chemotherapy*, vol. 71, no. 8, pp. 2300–2305, 2016.

[176] N. Stoesser, A. J. Mathers, C. E. Moore, N. P. J. Day, and D. W. Crook, "Colistin resistance gene *mcr*-1 and pHNSHP45 plasmid in human isolates of *Escherichia coli* and *Klebsiella pneumoniae*," *Lancet Infectious Diseases*, vol. 16, no. 3, pp. 285-286, 2016.

[177] R. Li, M. Xie, J. Lv, E. Wai-Chi Chan, and S. Chen, "Complete genetic analysis of plasmids carrying *mcr*-1 and other resistance genes in an *Escherichia coli* isolate of animal origin," *Journal of Antimicrobial Chemotherapy*, vol. 72, no. 3, pp. 696–699, 2017.

[178] K. Veldman, A. van Essen-Zandbergen, M. Rapallini et al., "Location of colistin resistance gene *mcr*-1 in Enterobacteriaceae from livestock and meat," *Journal of Antimicrobial Chemotherapy*, vol. 71, no. 8, pp. 2340–2342, 2016.

[179] J. Campos, L. Cristino, L. Peixe, and P. Antunes, "*MCR*-1 in multidrug-resistant and copper-tolerant clinically relevant Salmonella 1,4,[5],12:i:- and S. Rissen clones in Portugal, 2011 to 2015," *Eurosurveillance*, vol. 21, no. 26, p. 30270, 2016.

[180] M. F. Anjum, N. A. Duggett, M. AbuOun et al., "Colistin resistance in *Salmonella* and *Escherichia coli* isolates from a pig farm in Great Britain," *Journal of Antimicrobial Chemotherapy*, vol. 71, no. 8, pp. 2306–2313, 2016.

[181] L. Poirel, N. Kieffer, A. Brink, J. Coetze, A. Jayol, and P. Nordmann, "Genetic features of *MCR*-1-producing colistin-resistant *Escherichia coli* isolates in South Africa," *Antimicrobial Agents and Chemotherapy*, vol. 60, no. 7, pp. 4394–4397, 2016.

[182] O. J. Bernasconi, L. Principe, R. Tinguely et al., "Evaluation of a new commercial microarray platform for the simultaneous detection of β-lactamase and *Mcr*-1/-2 genes in Enterobacteriaceae," *Journal of Clinical Microbiology*, vol. 55, no. 10, pp. 3138–3141, 2017.

[183] C. Imirzalioglu, L. Falgenhauer, J. Schmiedel et al., "Evaluation of a LAMP-based assay for the rapid detection of plasmid-encoded colistin resistance gene *mcr*-1 in Enterobacteriaceae isolates," *Antimicrobial Agents and Chemotherapy*, vol. 61, no. 4, p. e02326-16, 2017.

[184] D. Zou, S. Huang, H. Lei et al., "Sensitive and rapid detection of the plasmid-encoded colistin-resistance Gene *mcr*-1 in Enterobacteriaceae isolates by loop-mediated isothermal amplification," *Frontiers in Microbiology*, vol. 8, pp. 1–7, 2017.

[185] J. L. Martinez, T. M. Coque, and F. Baquero, "What is a resistance gene? Ranking risk in resistomes," *Nature Reviews Microbiology*, vol. 13, no. 2, pp. 116–123, 2015.

[186] Y. Wang, R. Zhang, J. Li et al., "Comprehensive resistome analysis reveals the prevalence of *NDM* and *MCR*-1 in Chinese poultry production," *Nature Microbiology*, vol. 2, p. 16260, 2017.

[187] A. Gundogdu and O. U. Nalbantoglu, "Humans as a source of colistin resistance: in silico analysis of public metagenomes for the *mcr*-1 gene in the gut microbiome," *Erciyes Medical Journal*, vol. 38, no. 2, pp. 59–61, 2016.

[188] D. P. Thanh, H. T. Tuyen, T. N. T. Nguyen et al., "Inducible colistin resistance via a disrupted plasmid-borne *mcr*-1 gene in a 2008 Vietnamese *Shigella sonnei* isolate," *Journal of Antimicrobial Chemotherapy*, vol. 71, no. 8, pp. 2314–2317, 2016.

[189] R. J. Meinersmann, S. R. Ladely, J. L. Bono et al., "Complete genome sequence of a colistin resistance gene (*mcr*-1)-bearing isolate of *Escherichia coli* from the United States," *Genome Announcements*, vol. 4, no. 6, p. e01283-16, 2016.

[190] M. F. Kluytmans-van den Bergh, P. Huizinga, M. J. Bonten et al., "Presence of *mcr*-1-positive Enterobacteriaceae in retail chicken meat but not in humans in the Netherlands since 2009," *Eurosurveillance*, vol. 21, no. 9, p. 30149, 2016.

[191] S. Malhotra-Kumar, B. B. Xavier, A. J. Das et al., "Colistin-resistant *Escherichia coli* harbouring *mcr*-1 isolated from food animals in Hanoi, Vietnam," *Lancet Infectious Diseases*, vol. 16, no. 3, pp. 286-287, 2016.

[192] P. McGann, E. Snesrud, R. Maybank et al., "*Escherichia coli* harboring *mcr*-1 and *bla*CTX-M on a novel IncF plasmid: first report of *mcr*-1 in the USA," *Antimicrobial Agents and Chemotherapy*, vol. 60, no. 7, pp. 4420-4421, 2016.

[193] O. J. Bernasconi, E. Kuenzli, J. Pires et al., "Travelers can import colistin-resistant Enterobacteriaceae, including those possessing the plasmid-mediated *mcr*-1 gene," *Antimicrobial Agents and Chemotherapy*, vol. 60, no. 8, pp. 5080–5084, 2016.

[194] M. R. Fernandes, J. A. McCulloch, M. A. Vianello et al., "First report of the globally disseminated IncX4 plasmid carrying the *mcr*-1 gene in a colistin-resistant *Escherichia coli* sequence type 101 isolate from a human infection in Brazil," *Antimicrobial Agents and Chemotherapy*, vol. 60, no. 10, pp. 6415–6417, 2016.

[195] M. Corbella, B. Mariani, C. Ferrari et al., "Three cases of *mcr*-1-positive colistin-resistant *Escherichia coli* bloodstream infections in Italy, August 2016 to January 2017," *Eurosurveillance*, vol. 22, no. 16, p. 30517, 2017.

[196] S. Guenther, L. Falgenhauer, T. Semmler et al., "Environmental emission of multiresistant *Escherichia coli* carrying the colistin resistance gene *mcr*-1 from German swine farms," *Journal of Antimicrobial Chemotherapy*, vol. 72, pp. 1289–1292, 2017.

[197] M. Fritzenwanker, C. Imirzalioglu, K. Gentil, L. Falgenhauer, F. M. Wagenlehner, and T. Chakraborty, "Incidental detection of a urinary *Escherichia coli* isolate harbouring *mcr*-1 of a patient with no history of colistin treatment," *Clinical Microbiology and Infection*, vol. 22, no. 11, pp. 954-955, 2016.

[198] J. A. Ellem, A. N. Ginn, S. C. A. Chen, J. Ferguson, S. R. Partridge, and J. R. Iredell, "Locally acquired *mcr*-1 in *Escherichia coli*, Australia, 2011 and 2013," *Emerging Infectious Diseases*, vol. 23, no. 7, pp. 1160–1163, 2017.

[199] Y. Qian, J. B. Bulitta, C. A. Peloquin, and P. N. Holden, *Crossm Polymyxin Combinations Combat Era*, 2017.

[200] S. B. Jørgensen, A. Søraas, L. S. Arnesen, T. Leegaard, A. Sundsfjord, and P. A. Jenum, "First environmental sample containing plasmid-mediated colistin-resistant ESBL-producing *Escherichia coli* detected in Norway," *APMIS*, vol. 125, no. 9, pp. 10–12, 2017.

[201] T. He, R. Wei, L. Zhang et al., "Characterization of *NDM*-5-positive extensively resistant *Escherichia coli* isolates from dairy cows," *Veterinary Microbiology*, vol. 207, pp. 153–158, 2017.

[202] K. Rutherford, J. Parkhill, J. Crook et al., "Artemis: sequence visualization and annotation," vol. 16, no. 10, pp. 944-945, 2000.

[203] A. O. Olaitan, S. Chabou, L. Okdah, S. Morand, and J. M. Rolain, "Dissemination of the *mcr*-1 colistin resistance gene," *Lancet Infectious Diseases*, vol. 16, no. 2, p. 147, 2016.

[204] Y. Zhang, K. Liao, H. Gao et al., "Decreased fitness and virulence in ST10 *Escherichia coli* harboring *bla*NDM-5 and *mcr*-1 against a ST4981 strain with *bla*NDM-5," *Frontiers in Cellular and Infection Microbiology*, vol. 7, p. 242, 2017.

[205] A. C. Schürch and W. van Schaik, "Challenges and opportunities for whole-genome sequencing-based surveillance of antibiotic resistance," *Annals of the New York Academy of Sciences*, vol. 1388, no. 1, pp. 108–120, 2017.

[206] S. K. Gupta, B. R. Padmanabhan, S. M. Diene et al., "ARG-ANNOT, a new bioinformatic tool to discover antibiotic resistance genes in bacterial genomes," *Antimicrobial Agents and Chemotherapy*, vol. 58, no. 1, pp. 212–220, 2014.

[207] E. Zankari, H. Hasman, S. Cosentino et al., "Identification of acquired antimicrobial resistance genes," *Journal of Antimicrobial Chemotherapy*, vol. 67, no. 11, pp. 2640–2644, 2012.

[208] A. G. McArthur, N. Waglechner, F. Nizam et al., "The comprehensive antibiotic resistance database," *Antimicrobial Agents and Chemotherapy*, vol. 57, no. 7, pp. 3348–3357, 2013.

[209] B. Liu and M. Pop, "ARDB-antibiotic resistance genes da-tabase," *Nucleic Acids Research*, vol. 37, pp. 443–447, 2009.

[210] S. Suzuki, M. Ohnishi, M. Kawanishi, M. Akiba, and M. Kuroda, "Investigation of a plasmid genome database for colistin-resistance gene *mcr-1*," *Lancet Infectious Diseases*, vol. 16, no. 3, pp. 284-285, 2016.

[211] R. L. Lindsey, D. Batra, L. Rowe et al., "High-quality genome sequence of an *Escherichia coli* o157 strain carrying an *mcr-1* resistance gene isolated from a patient in the United States," *Genome Announcements*, vol. 5, no. 11, p. e01725-16, 2017.

[212] E. Zankari, R. Allesøe, K. G. Joensen, L. M. Cavaco, O. Lund, and F. M. Aarestrup, "PointFinder: a novel web tool for WGS-based detection of antimicrobial resistance associated with chromosomal point mutations in bacterial pathogens," *Journal of Antimicrobial Chemotherapy*, vol. 72, no. 10, pp. 2764–2768, 2017.

[213] M. J. Ellington, O. Ekelund, F. M. Aarestrup et al., "The role of whole genome sequencing in antimicrobial susceptibility testing of bacteria: report from the EUCAST Subcommittee," *Clinical Microbiology and Infection*, vol. 23, no. 1, pp. 2–22, 2017.

19

Herpes Zoster Burden in Canadian Provinces: A Narrative Review and Comparison with Quebec Provincial Data

Marie-Claude Letellier,[1] **Rachid Amini** ⓘ**,**[2] **Vladimir Gilca** ⓘ**,**[1,2,3] **Gisele Trudeau,**[2] **and Chantal Sauvageau**[1,2,3]

[1]*Université Laval, Quebec City, Canada*
[2]*Institut National de Santé Publique du Québec, Quebec City, Canada*
[3]*Centre Hospitalier Universitaire de Québec—Université Laval, Quebec City, Canada*

Correspondence should be addressed to Rachid Amini; rachid.amini@inspq.qc.ca

Academic Editor: Aim Hoepelman

Background. The main aim of this review was to assess incidence rates and trends of medically attended and death cases of herpes zoster in Canada. *Methods.* The search was conducted in five databases (PubMed, Cochrane, Embase, PsycNET, and Web of Science). Data on herpes zoster-related consultations and hospitalisations and deaths were also extracted from three Quebec provincial administrative databases (RAMQ, MED-ECHO, and ISQ). *Results.* The electronic search yielded 587 publications. Seventeen publications satisfied inclusion criteria. These publications reported data from eleven studies. Ten studies used provincial databases, and one study used the Canadian Primary Care Sentinel Surveillance Network electronic database. Seven studies evaluated overall rates of medically attended cases (consultations and hospitalisations). Four of these studies reported an increase in rates of medically attended cases during the study period; one study reported stable rates, and two studies reported only an average rate. The rates varied from 316 to 450/100,000 p.y. The Quebec analysis shows similar rates with a slight decreasing trend (from 369 to 350/100,000 p.y.). Incidence rates of consultations were reported separately in three studies. Two studies reported an increase in rates (from 258 to 348/100,000 p.y. and from 324 to 366/100,000 p.y.), and the third study reported a decrease (from 525 to 479/100,000 p.y.). Hospitalization rates were reported separately in two studies, both reporting a decrease (from 12 to 8 cases/100,000 p.y. and from 9 to 4 cases/100,000 p.y.). Quebec data also showed a decrease, from 9 to 6 cases/100,000 p.y. One study reported herpes zoster-related deaths. In this study, the reported death rate was 0.7/1,000,000 p.y. in the overall population and 5.5/1,000,000 p.y. in those aged ≥65 years. Quebec analysis showed a death rate of 1.2/1,000,000 p.y. in the overall population and 8.6/1,000,000 p.y. in those aged ≥65 years. *Conclusions.* The results of the reviewed studies and our analysis of Quebec provincial data indicate important variations in the reported overall incidence rates of medically attended herpes zoster cases in Canada. The trends in time are heterogeneous in studies in which hospitalisations and medical consultations were pooled together. We observed a decrease in hospitalization rates and a slight increase in consultation rates in studies reporting hospitalisations and consultations separately. These results consolidate the understanding of the herpes zoster burden in Canada and might be used as a tool in decision-making regarding future preventive interventions.

1. Background

Varicella zoster virus results in varicella (chickenpox) as primary infection. The virus remains latent in the sensory ganglia and can reactivate later in life, causing herpes zoster, also known as shingles. While children are the main contributors to varicella burden, the elderly are particularly affected by herpes zoster. The implementation of the varicella vaccine in childhood vaccination programs has substantially decreased disease incidence and related complications, including hospitalizations and deaths [1]. The potential impact of this decrease on the herpes zoster burden is not well understood. Some authors have raised the concern that high varicella vaccine coverage is followed by a decrease of virus circulation, and as a result, a decrease of natural boosting could lead to an increase in herpes zoster incidence [2, 3]. Uncertainties regarding this hypothesis led to an increase in the number of studies on the herpes zoster epidemiology [4, 5].

Varicella vaccine has been available in Canada since 1999 and has been largely used in provincial publicly funded childhood vaccination programs since the early 2000s. In the province of Quebec, such a program was implemented in 2006. A few years after program implementation, a decrease in consultations, hospitalizations, and deaths associated with varicella was reported [6]. The first live attenuated herpes zoster vaccine was approved for use in Canada in 2009. This vaccine is recommended for adults aged 60 years and over and is authorized for use in some subpopulations at risk for herpes zoster aged 50 years and over. The use of the live attenuated vaccine is limited because of several reasons including relatively low short- and midterm efficacy [7], its relatively high price, the recommendation to an age group in which vaccines' uptake is relatively low, the cost-effectiveness of a publicly funded programs remains questionable, and it is not publicly funded in most Canadian provinces. By 2018, only one out of ten Canadian provinces implemented a publicly funded herpes zoster immunization program [8]. The recent approval of a new promising recombinant herpes zoster vaccine [9] raises the question about its optimal use and potential impact on herpes zoster burden.

We conducted a review of Canadian studies examining herpes zoster burden. The main aim of this review was to assess incidence rates and trends of medically attended and death cases related to herpes zoster in Canadian jurisdictions with no or very low herpes zoster vaccination coverage at the time of study conduction. Moreover, we extracted and analysed data on the same issue from the Quebec provincial administrative databases. It was thought that such a review and analysis will provide useful information for (i) a better understanding of the impact of varicella vaccination on the epidemiology of herpes zoster, (ii) an estimation of herpes zoster burden, (iii) future cost-effective estimations of different potential immunisation programs, and (iv) decision-making regarding herpes zoster prevention.

2. Methods

2.1. Literature Search, Selection, and Eligibility Criteria. The main search for this systematic review was conducted on May 24, 2018. Five databases (PubMed, Cochrane, Embase, PsycNET, and Web of Science) were searched, using the keywords "shingles or herpes zoster or zona" and "epidemiology or incidence or burden" and "Canada." We also conducted several additional searches based on a review of citations from relevant publications. No language, publication year, or age group restrictions were applied. After conducting the first search, all titles were reviewed for relevance. After excluding nonpertinent titles (e.g., limited to diagnosis, clinical manifestation, treatment, or clinical trial reports), we read all abstracts, and for those meeting the outcomes of interest, full articles were read to determine

their eligibility for inclusion. To be eligible, the articles should have presented Canadian data on herpes zoster-related consultations, hospitalizations, and/or deaths. Two authors (MCL and VG) reviewed selected articles for eligibility and resolved discordances by discussion.

2.2. Quebec Data. We extracted data on herpes zoster-related consultations and hospitalisations, hospitalisations separately, and deaths from three provincial administrative databases: RAMQ (Régie de l'Assurance Maladie du Québec), MED-ECHO (Maintenance et Exploitation des Données pour l'Étude de la Clientèle Hospitalière), and ISQ (Institut de la statistique du Québec). The data received from RAMQ were aggregated and did not allow us to separate consultations from hospitalisations. Data on consultations and hospitalisations (RAMQ database) and hospitalisations separately (MED-ECHO database) were available for the period from 1996 to 2015 and on death causes for the period from 1996 to 2013 (ISQ database). Herpes zoster diagnoses with the code 053.x in the ninth edition and B02.x in the tenth edition of the International Classification of Diseases (ICD) were extracted. For hospitalisations, only cases with herpes zoster as the principal or first secondary diagnosis were retained for this analysis. An incident case was defined as the first herpes zoster diagnosis during a calendar year. To verify for a potential double counting, a second analysis was performed by defining as incident only the first-time herpes zoster diagnosis during the entire study period (1996–2015). A death was included in the analysis if herpes zoster was the underlying cause of death.

Incidence rates of consultations and hospitalisations and deaths were calculated for the overall provincial population and for people aged 65 years and over. Overall incidence rates were standardized for age with the 2007 Quebec population as reference (data obtained from ISQ). Both Quebec analysis and reviewed studies were restricted exclusively to anonymous data. Thus, no research ethics board approval was required.

3. Results

The electronic database search yielded 587 hits; 130 were duplicates in two or more databases and were excluded. The remaining 457 citations were screened by title and abstract, and 390 were excluded because of lack of any preestablished outcome or population of interest. The 67 articles potentially containing outcomes of interest were read fully. Seventeen of them satisfied inclusion criteria and were included in the review (Figure 1). These seventeen articles reported data from ten original studies that were conducted in 4 Canadian provinces (British Columbia [4, 10], Manitoba [11–13], Alberta [14–16], and Ontario [17, 18]), and one study was conducted based on the Canadian Primary Care Sentinel Surveillance Network electronic database (CPCSSN) [19]. The main features of the included studies are presented in Table 1.

There was wide variation between studies' periods (Figure 2). Some studies considered one unique period

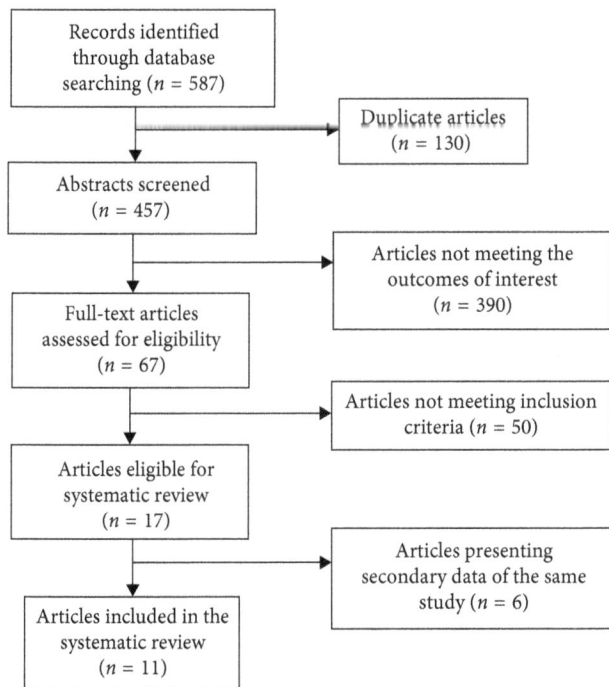

FIGURE 1: Flow chart of study selection for systematic review.

[4, 11–13, 15, 16, 18, 19], while others subdivided study periods into pre- and postvaricella vaccination program implementation [10, 14, 17]. Ten studies used provincial administrative databases and ICD classification (Table 1). However, there were some differences in the definition of an incident case in included studies. Some studies reported only the first episode [10, 11, 15, 17, 18], and others counted a subsequent episode if separated from the first one by at least 6 months [14], one year [4], or two years [13]. Studies reported crude and/or standardized incidence rates for overall population or rates by age groups. Incidence rates standardized for age were generally lower than crude ones. Finally, three different age criteria were used when assessing herpes zoster incidence rates among the elderly: 60 years and over [17], 65 years and over [4, 11, 12, 19], and 66 years and over [18].

Seven studies evaluated incidence rates of medically attended cases (consultations and hospitalisations) [10, 13–18]. Four of these studies reported an increase in incidence rates of medically attended cases during the study period; one study reported relatively stable rates (Figure 3(a)), and two studies reported only the average incidence rate for the analysed period. In the five studies reporting the rates trend, the incidence rates of medically attended cases varied from 316 to 570 cases per 100,000 person-years (p.y.). One of these studies [13] limited eligibility criteria to cases aged 20 years and over. This study reported the highest incidence rates. When excluding this study, the incidence rates of medically attended cases varied from 316 to 450 cases per 100,000 p.y. The analysis of Quebec data shows similar incidence rates of medically attended cases with a slight decreasing trend (from 369 to 350 cases per 100,000 p.y.; rate ratio: 0.95 (95% CI: 0.94–0.96)). This trend is due to a slight decrease in incidence rates in

individuals under the age of 60. The most pronounced decrease was observed in children aged 0–9 years in the postvaricella vaccination period (2006–2015) when compared to the prevaccination period (from 83 to 65 cases per 100,000 p.y.; rate ratio: 0.79 (95% CI: 0.76–0.82)).

Incidence rates of consultations were reported separately in three studies (Figure 3(b)). Two studies reported an increase in consultations rates (from 258 to 348 cases [11] and from 324 to 366 cases [4] per 100,000 p.y.), and the third study reported a decrease (from 525 to 479 cases per 100,000 p.y. [17]).

Hospitalization rates were reported separately in two studies, both reporting a decrease (from 12 to 8 cases per 100,000 p.y. [4] and from 9 to 4 cases per 100,000 p.y. [17]; Figure 3(c)). Quebec data also showed a decrease, from 9 to 6 cases per 100,000 p.y. Three other studies reported a decrease of the percentage of hospitalized cases from 4-5% to 2-3% [10, 14, 15] without presenting hospitalisation rates.

All studies reported higher incidence rates for consultations, hospitalisations, and overall consultations and hospitalisations in the older population (60–66 years and over) when compared to younger population (Table 1).

Only one study reported herpes zoster-related deaths. In this study, the reported death rate was 0.7 per 1,000,000 p.y. in the overall population and 5.5 per 1,000,000 p.y. in those aged 65 years and over [4]. Quebec analysis shows a death rate of 1.2 per 1,000,000 p.y. in the overall population and 8.6 per 1,000,000 p.y. in those aged 65 years and over.

The second analysis of Quebec data with a restrictive definition of an incident case as the first-time consultations and hospitalizations for herpes zoster during the entire study period brought relatively little change to the results of the primary analysis; the overall number of cases decreased by less than 9% (from 543,290 to 495,111 cases), without a change in the general trend.

One study evaluated the prevalence of herpes zoster in patients with and without common chronic diseases. The age- and sex-adjusted herpes zoster prevalence in patients with chronic diseases was statistically significantly higher when compared to those observed in individuals without chronic diseases. Namely, the prevalence ratio was 1.57 for patients with diabetes, 1.83 for those with chronic obstructive pulmonary disease, 2.58 in case of neoplasm, and 6.46 for those with HIV/AIDS [19].

A recent Canadian study evaluated the effectiveness of the live attenuated herpes zoster vaccine in individuals aged 50 years and older. In this study, the vaccine effectiveness decreased from year to year, and by the fifth year, the vaccine offered no protection against the incident disease. The adjusted vaccine effectiveness in years one to five following vaccination, respectively, was 50.0% (95% CI: 44.7, 54.8), 34.5% (95% CI: 27.3, 41.0), 31.5% (95% CI: 21.8, 39.9), 30.5% (95% CI: 13.9, 44.3), and 14.0% (95% CI: −21.0, 39.0) [16].

4. Discussion

We searched publications in peer-reviewed scientific papers available in the five most comprehensive databases. This search found 11 original Canadian studies conducted in four

TABLE 1: Canadian studies presenting herpes zoster incidence rates of outpatient visits and hospitalizations.

Author and year of publication	Periods; province; number of incident herpes zoster cases (N)	Cases identification	Incidence rates (per 100,000 person-years) (standardized unless stated otherwise)		
			Consultations (outpatient visits)	Hospitalizations	Outpatient visits + hospitalizations
Brisson et al. 2001 [11]	1979–1997; Manitoba; N: not documented	(i) Annual billing claims database; first claim with a herpes zoster ICD-9 code (ii) Hospital length of stay ≥ 1 day; hospitalisations with herpes zoster (HZ) ICD-9 code in one of the first three positions	*Crude rates* (i) All ages: increase from 258 to 348 during the study period (ii) ≥ 65 years: average rate of 812	*Crude rates* (i) ≥ 65 years: average rate of 86	Not documented
Russell et al. 2007 [15]	1986–2002; Alberta; N: not documented	(i) Provincial registration database (ii) Physician claims data system (iii) Hospital morbidity inpatient database (iv) First-time healthcare service utilisation for an HZ ICD-9/10 code in any position	Not documented	(i) All ages: decrease of hospitalized cases from 5% in 1993 to 3% in 2002	*Crude rates* (i) All ages: increasing rate from 1986 to 2002 (roughly from 280 to 440 according to the presented figure)
Edgar et al. 2007 [4]	1994–2003; British Columbia; (i) N of outpatient visits = 114,596 (ii) N of hospitalizations = 3,887	(i) Physician billing data; physician visit for an HZ ICD-9 code (ii) Hospitalisations for an HZ ICD-9/10 code regardless of its position (iii) Physician visits and hospitalizations ≥ 365 days apart were included	(i) All ages: increase from 324 to 366 (ii) ≥ 65 years: average crude rate of 703	(i) All ages: decrease from 12 to 8 (ii) ≥ 65 years: average crude rate of 51	Not documented
Brisson et al. 2008 [12]	2000–2003; Manitoba; N: not documented	(i) Hospitalisations for an HZ ICD code in the first position vs. any position	Not documented	*Crude rates among ≥ 65-year-olds* (i) HZ code in any position: average rate of 3 for 65–69 years and 30 for ≥80 years (ii) HZ code in the first position: average rate of 1 and 9 for 65–69 years and ≥ 80 years, respectively	Not documented
Tanuseputro et al. 2011 [17]	1992–2010; Ontario; (i) N of outpatient visits = 686,763 (ii) N of hospitalizations = 14,240	(i) First outpatient visit for an HZ ICD-9 code (ii) First hospitalization for an HZ ICD-9/10 code in any position (in a sensitivity analysis: hospitalization with HZ as primary diagnosis only)	(i) All ages: decrease from 525 to 479 (ii) ≥ 60 years: average crude rate of 740 during 2005–2009	(i) All ages: decrease from 9 to 4 (and from 5 to 2 in a sensitivity analysis with HZ as primary diagnosis)	(i) All ages: steady mean annual rate between 309 during 1992–1998 (prevaricella vaccine availability) and 303 during 2005–2009 (publicly available vaccine) Rate ratio (2005–2009 vs. 1992–1998) = 0.98 (0.82–1.14)

TABLE 1: Continued.

Author and year of publication	Periods; province; number of incident herpes zoster cases (N)	Cases identification	Incidence rates (per 100,000 person-years) (standardized unless stated otherwise)		
			Consultations (outpatient visits)	Hospitalizations	Outpatient visits + hospitalizations
Russell et al. 2014 [14]	1994–2010; Alberta; N of outpatients and inpatients = 174,711	(i) Supplemental enhanced service event system (physician claims records) (ii) Alberta communicable disease reporting system (iii) Morbidity and ambulatory care reporting databases (hospital inpatients and hospital emergency department visits) (iv) First health service utilisation for an HZ ICD-9/10 code in any position (v) HZ codes ≥ 180 days after the first diagnosis classified as recurrent episodes	Not documented	(i) All ages: decrease of hospitalized cases from 5% during prelicensure of the varicella vaccine period (1994–1998) to 3% during the publicly available varicella vaccination period (2002–2010)	*Crude rates (recurrent episodes included)* (i) All ages: increase from 350 to 450
Antoniou et al. 2014 [18]	1997–2009; Ontario; N = 19,143	(i) Prescription drugs database (ii) Physician claims records database (iii) Hospitalisation admissions database (iv) Emergency department visits database (v) New diagnosis of HZ: first HZ ICD-9/10 code or first antiviral treatment for HZ	Not documented	Not documented	*Crude rates* (i) ≥ 66 years: average rate of 1,232 (1,171 for patients not receiving statin and 1,325 for statin users)
Marra et al. 2016 [10]	1997–2012; British Columbia; N = 238,295	(i) Medical services plan and hospital discharge database (ii) PharmaNet (outpatient prescription database) (iii) HZ ICD-9/10 code in any position without any evidence of HZ or postherpetic neuralgia in the previous 12 months (iv) Sensitivity analysis: HZ diagnosis with antiviral treatment received within 7 days	Not documented	(i) All ages: decrease of hospitalized cases from 4% during prelicensure of the varicella vaccine period (1997–1999) to 2% during the publicly funded vaccination period (2005–2012)	(i) All ages: increase from 316 to 449 (and from 162 to 300 in a sensitivity analysis with case definition as an HZ diagnosis with an antiviral treatment) Rate ratio (publicly funded varicella vaccination vs. prelicensure period) = 1.22 (1.20–1.24)

TABLE 1: Continued.

Author and year of publication	Periods; province; number of incident herpes zoster cases (N)	Cases identification	Incidence rates (per 100,000 person-years) (standardized unless stated otherwise)		
			Consultations (outpatient visits)	Hospitalizations	Outpatient visits + hospitalizations
Friesen et al. 2016 [13]	1997–2013; Manitoba; N: not documented	(i) Physician claims database (ii) Hospital discharge database (iii) First HZ ICD-9/10 code in any position (iv) Multiple episodes included if a minimum of 2 years had elapsed since the first-time HZ and ≥ 180 days had elapsed since the last HZ diagnosis	Not documented	Not documented	(i) ≥ 20 years: steady rate at 470 from 1997-1998 to 2008-2009 and increase since 2009-2010 to reach 570 in 2013-2014
McDonald et al. 2017 [16]	2009–2015; Alberta; N of outpatients and inpatients = 49,243	(i) Physician claims database (ii) Morbidity and ambulatory care reporting database (iii) First HZ ICD-9/10 code in any position	Not documented	Not documented	*Crude rates* (i) ≥ 50 years: average rate of 903 (ii) Incidence rates increased from 581 in 50–54 years to 130 in ≥ 75 years
Queenan et al. 2017 [19]	2013–2015; Canadian Primary Care Sentinel Surveillance Network; N of outpatients = 3,281	(i) Surveillance system electronic database (ii) HZ ICD-9 code in any position	*Prevalence in ≥ 18 years* (i) One year: 0.32% (ii) By age: (1) 18–39 years: 0.12% (2) 40–64 years: 0.35% (3) ≥ 64 years: 0.67% (iii) By status: (1) No chronic disease: 0.21% (2) Diabetes: 0.69% (3) COPD: 0.69% (4) Any neoplasm: 1.07% (5) HIV/AIDS: 1.00%	Not documented	Not documented
Quebec analysis	1996–2015; Quebec; N of outpatients and inpatients = 543,290	(i) Physician claims records; first HZ ICD-9/10 code during a calendar year or during the entire study period (ii) Hospital discharge database; first HZ ICD-9/10 code as the main diagnosis or the first secondary diagnosis	Not documented	(i) All ages: decrease from 9 to 6 (ii) ≥ 65 years: decrease from 50 to 31	(i) All ages: decrease from 369 during 1996–2000 (prelicensure of varicella vaccine) to 350 during 2006–2015 (publicly funded varicella vaccination period) Rate ratio (2006–2015 vs. 1996–2000) = 0.95 (0.94–0.95) (ii) ≥ 65 years: average rate of 949 (steady over the study period)

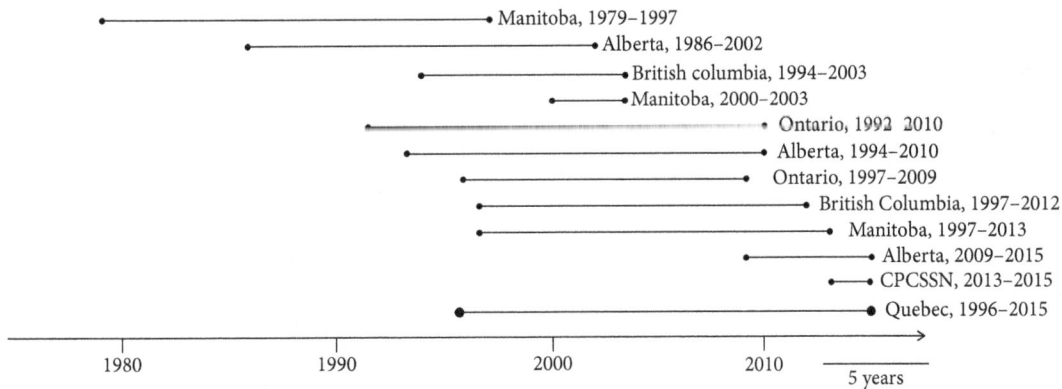

FIGURE 2: Studies' periods and duration.

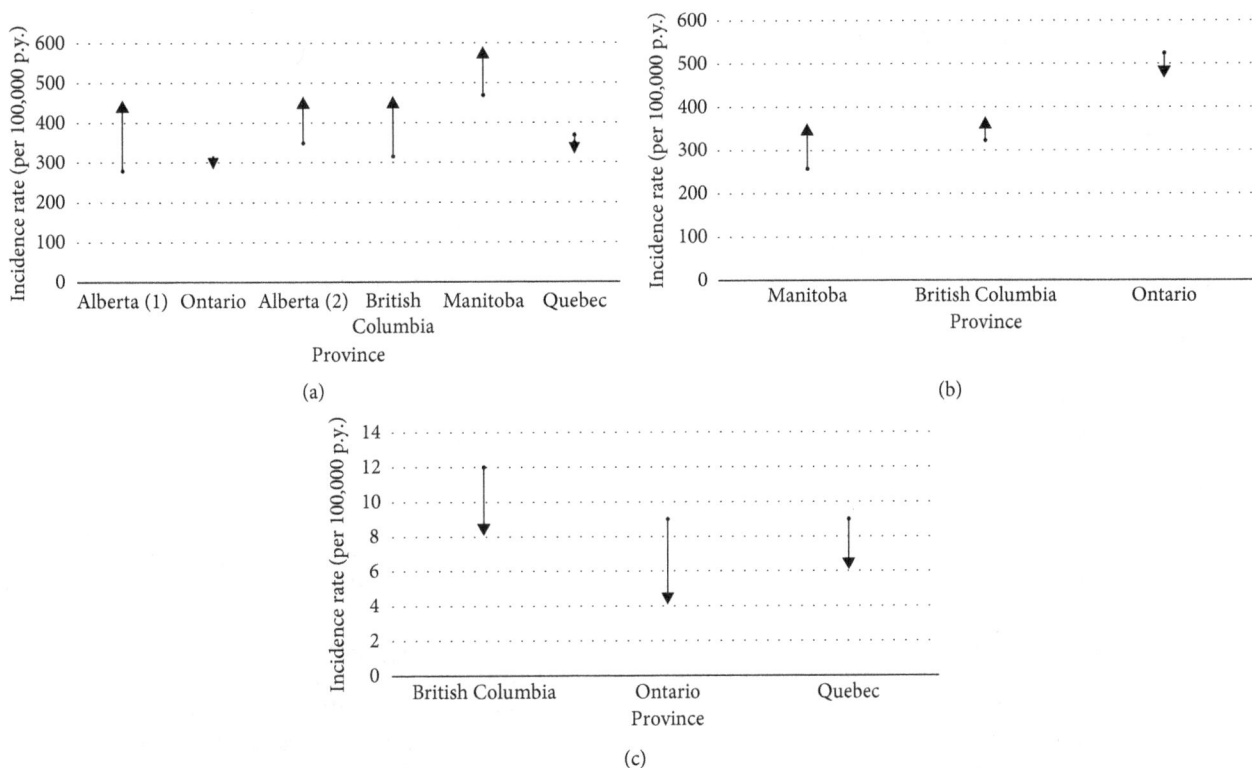

FIGURE 3: Incidence rates of hospitalisations and consultations (a), consultations (b), and hospitalisation (c) for herpes zoster by Canadian Province.

different provinces (British Columbia: 2 studies; Alberta: 3 studies; Manitoba: 3 studies; and Ontario: 2 studies), and one study used the Canadian Primary Care Sentinel Surveillance Network database. These studies include data from 1979 to 2015. Over time, in Canada, a trend of a decrease in hospitalization rates and a slight increase in consultation rates was observed. The shift toward ambulatory care during the last decades and the availability of antiviral treatments can explain the decrease in hospitalizations. Higher chances of survival of immunosuppressed patients and an aging population can explain at least partially the reported increase in herpes zoster consultations in some but not all studies. When medically attended cases were analysed and presented

in an aggregated manner (consultations and hospitalisations), some discrepancies were observed among studies' results. Four studies reported an increase, one study reported no change, while Quebec analysis showed a slight decrease of the incidence of all medically attended cases. These discrepancies might be explained by different time periods analysed, by different definitions used for an incident case, and by the methodology used when analysing and presenting data (i.e., crude and/or standardized incidence for age).

The Canadian publications available suggest there has been no important, if any, impact of varicella vaccination on overall medically attended herpes zoster rates. More in-depth analysis of Quebec data suggests some positive impact of varicella vaccination on incidence rates of medically attended herpes zoster cases in children (a decrease of 21% in children aged 0–9 years). Because the period of time since varicella vaccination programs implementation in Canadian provinces is relatively short (11–16 years), the longer term impact of these programs on herpes zoster burden at this point is unknown.

The large populations included in provincial databases used in eleven published Canadian studies and in our analysis (overall >30 millions) and their wide geographical distribution allow us to presume that the observed results are representative for Canada. Overall, this review shows relatively small variations in the burden of herpes zoster during the last 3-4 decades. In our opinion, the main factors influencing these variations and trends are the aging population, healthcare systems organization changes, and new available treatments. With an aging population and no efficient prevention in place, the burden of herpes zoster is expected to increase.

Herpes zoster incidence does not seem to follow geographic trends [20, 21], and the results of this systematic review support this observation. A recent systematic review of studies conducted worldwide shows that herpes zoster incidence varies but stays in a certain range. The lowest incidence rate (131 cases per 100,000 p.y.) was reported in an older study conducted in the United States between 1945 and 1959, and the highest was reported in a South Korean study (997 cases per 100,000 p.y.) between 2003 and 2007 [20]. An European review showed incidence rates between 200 and 457 cases per 100,000 p.y. [21]. The lowest and the highest of these incidence rates were reported in Iceland (1990–1995) and Belgium (1994–2003), respectively. Overall, Canadian incidence rates were in the same range with those reported in many other countries, including those reported in the United States [22]. The consistency of our results with those from other countries and geographical regions suggests our estimate of the burden of herpes zoster from the healthcare system perspective is valid and might be helpful when deciding about future preventive interventions.

Consistently with previous published data [23, 24], a Canadian study shows increased risk for herpes zoster in patients with common chronic diseases including diabetes and chronic obstructive pulmonary disease [19]. Furthermore, one recent study confirms the relatively low short-term-only effectiveness of the live attenuated vaccine. With such low effectiveness and an estimated vaccine uptake of 8% among persons aged 60 years and over [7], little impact on herpes zoster burden might be expected. The latter is at least partially supported by little variation in herpes zoster burden in the last 3-4 decades.

This review and analysis has some limitations. First, we limited our search to the peer-reviewed literature. As such, some data reported in the grey literature could have been missed. Second, the studies included and the Quebec analysis were based on data retrieved from existing administrative databases. This approach is subject to potential information biases, which may have impacted the results. In the Quebec study, as well as in the ten studies included in this systematic review, the herpes zoster diagnosis codes have not been validated. However, in the recent Canadian study using the CPCSSN data, the ICD-9 code 053 has been shown to have a sensitivity of 100% and a positive predictive value of 84% [19]. Some studies conducted in the United States found similar results for the ICD-9 code 053 with a sensitivity of 98% and a positive predictive value varying between 84% and 94% [5, 25–27]. These figures suggest that specific ICD codes may be reliable to estimate herpes zoster incidence. Third, a given proportion of herpes zoster cases without medical care seeking are not reported to databases. Thus, the obtained results reflect herpes zoster burden from the healthcare perspective only and do not allow to estimate the societal burden. Fourth, in order to verify for a potential double counting, we used two definitions for an incident case (i.e., first-time reported case during a calendar year and first-time reported case during the entire study period). Both definitions are arbitrary, and the second one does not include recurrent cases. However, the difference of 8.9% in cases captured with the first definition and the second definition is congruent with recently published results from a large study, which reported a recurrence of the disease in 6.4% of patients [28]. This suggests that our main analysis with the definition of an incident case as the first diagnosis during a calendar year estimates reasonably well both first-time and recurrent medically attended cases of herpes zoster.

5. Conclusion

The results of the reviewed studies and our analysis of Quebec provincial data indicate important variations in the reported overall incidence rates of medically attended herpes zoster cases in Canada. The trends in time are heterogeneous in studies in which hospitalisations and medical consultations were pooled together. The results are more consistent in studies which analysed the hospitalisations and medical consultations separately. The latter studies' results suggest a decrease in hospitalization rates and a slight increase in consultation rates. In our opinion, these trends are mainly explained by changes in the management of consulting cases, improved access to ambulatory medical services, and availability of antiviral medication. The results of this review and Quebec analysis consolidate the understanding of the herpes zoster burden in Canada and might be used as a tool in decision-making regarding preventive interventions including future cost-effective evaluations of potential immunization programs.

Abbreviations

RAMQ: Régie de l'Assurance Maladie du Québec
MED-   Maintenance et Exploitation des Données pour
ECHO: l'Étude de la Clientèle Hospitalière
ISQ: Institut de la statistique du Québec
p.y.:   Person-years.

Authors' Contributions

All authors have read and approved the final manuscript. M.-C.L., C.S., and G.T. conducted the methodology. M.-C.L. and R.A. collected the data. C.S. and M.-C.L. designed the study. M.-C.L., V.G., R.A., and G.T. conducted the research, analyzed the data, performed the validation of the results, and wrote the paper. R.A. extracted the data. C.S. had primary responsibility for the final content.

Acknowledgments

We thank Dr. Rodica Gilca for critically reading the manuscript and for her helpful scientific advice. We also thank Isabelle Petillot and Marie-France Richard for technical assistance with manuscript preparation. This review and analysis was financially supported by the Quebec Ministry of Health and Social Services.

References

[1] J. I. Cohen, "Clinical practice: herpes zoster," *New England Journal of Medicine*, vol. 369, no. 3, pp. 255–263, 2013.

[2] M. Brisson, N. J. Gay, W. J. Edmunds, and N. J. Andrews, "Exposure to varicella boosts immunity to herpes-zoster: implications for mass vaccination against chickenpox," *Vaccine*, vol. 20, no. 19-20, pp. 2500–2507, 2002.

[3] M. Brisson, G. Melkonyan, M. Drolet, G. De Serres, R. Thibeault, and P. De Wals, "Modeling the impact of one- and two-dose varicella vaccination on the epidemiology of varicella and zoster," *Vaccine*, vol. 28, no. 19, pp. 3385–3397, 2010.

[4] B. L. Edgar, E. Galanis, C. Kay, D. Skowronski, M. Naus, and D. Patrick, "The burden of varicella and zoster in British Columbia 1994–2003: baseline assessment prior to universal vaccination," *Canada Communicable Disease Report*, vol. 33, no. 11, pp. 1–15, 2007.

[5] A. O. Jumaan, O. Yu, L. A. Jackson, K. Bohlke, K. Galil, and J. F. Seward, "Incidence of herpes zoster, before and after varicella-vaccination-associated decreases in the incidence of varicella, 1992-2002," *Journal of Infectious Diseases*, vol. 191, no. 12, pp. 2002–2007, 2005.

[6] N. Ouhoummane, N. Boulianne, G. De Serres, P. De Wals, and M. Brisson, *Fardeau de la varicelle et du zona au Québec, 1990–2008: Impact du Programme Universel de Vaccination*, Rapport no. 978-2-550-63185-9, Institut National de Santé Publique du Québec, Québec, Canada, 2011.

[7] X. C. Liu, K. A. Simmonds, M. L. Russell, and L. W. Svenson, "Herpes zoster vaccine (HZV): utilization and coverage 2009–2013, Alberta, Canada," *BMC Public Health*, vol. 14, no. 1, p. 1098, 2014.

[8] Government of Ontario, "Ontario's routine immunization schedule Ontario 2017," September 2017, http://www.health. gov.on.ca/en/public/programs/immunization/static/immunization_tool.html-adult.

[9] GlaxoSmithKline Inc., "SHINGRIX approved in Canada as the first non-live adjuvanted vaccine to help protect against shingles," October 2017, http://ca.gsk.com/en-ca/media/press-releases/2017/shingrix-approved-in-canada-as-the-first-non-live-adjuvanted-vaccine-to-help-protect-against-shingles.

[10] F. Marra, M. Chong, and M. Najafzadeh, "Increasing incidence associated with herpes zoster infection in British Columbia, Canada," *BMC Infectious Diseases*, vol. 16, no. 1, p. 589, 2016.

[11] M. Brisson, W. J. Edmunds, B. Law et al., "Epidemiology of varicella zoster virus infection in Canada and the United Kingdom," *Epidemiology and Infection*, vol. 127, no. 2, pp. 305–314, 2001.

[12] M. Brisson, J. M. Pellissier, S. Camden, C. Quach, and P. De Wals, "The potential cost-effectiveness of vaccination against herpes zoster and post-herpetic neuralgia," *Human Vaccines*, vol. 4, no. 3, pp. 238–245, 2008.

[13] K. J. Friesen, S. Alessi-Severini, D. Chateau, J. Falk, and S. Bugden, "The changing landscape of antiviral treatment of herpes zoster: a 17-year population-based cohort study," *ClinicoEconomics and Outcomes Research*, vol. 8, pp. 207–214, 2016.

[14] M. L. Russell, D. C. Dover, K. A. Simmonds, and L. W. Svenson, "Shingles in Alberta: before and after publicly funded varicella vaccination," *Vaccine*, vol. 32, no. 47, pp. 6319–6324, 2013.

[15] M. L. Russell, D. P. Schopflocher, L. Svenson, and S. N. Virani, "Secular trends in the epidemiology of shingles in Alberta," *Epidemiology and Infection*, vol. 135, no. 6, pp. 908–913, 2007.

[16] B. M. McDonald, D. C. Dover, K. A. Simmonds, C. A. Bell, L. W. Svenson, and M. L. Russell, "The effectiveness of shingles vaccine among Albertans aged 50 years or older: a retrospective cohort study," *Vaccine*, vol. 35, no. 50, pp. 6984–6989, 2017.

[17] P. Tanuseputro, B. Zagorski, K. J. Chan, and J. C. Kwong, "Population-based incidence of herpes zoster after introduction of a publicly funded varicella vaccination program," *Vaccine*, vol. 29, no. 47, pp. 8580–8584, 2011.

[18] T. Antoniou, H. Zheng, S. Singh, D. N. Juurlink, M. M. Mamdani, and T. Gomes, "Statins and the risk of herpes zoster: a population-based cohort study," *Clinical Infectious Diseases*, vol. 58, no. 3, pp. 350–356, 2014.

[19] J. A. Queenan, P. Farahani, B. Ehsani-Moghadam, and R. V. Birtwhistle, "The prevalence and risk for herpes zoster infection in adult patients with diabetes mellitus in the Canadian primary care Sentinel surveillance Network," *Canadian Journal of Diabetes*, vol. 42, no. 5, pp. 465–469, 2017.

[20] K. Kawai, B. G. Gebremeskel, and C. J. Acosta, "Systematic review of incidence and complications of herpes zoster: towards a global perspective," *BMJ Open*, vol. 4, no. 6, article e004833, 2014.

[21] S. Pinchinat, A. M. Cebrián-Cuenca, H. Bricout, and R. W. Johnson, "Similar herpes zoster incidence across Europe: results from a systematic literature review," *BMC Infectious Diseases*, vol. 13, no. 1, p. 170, 2013.

[22] J. Leung, R. Harpaz, N.-A. Molinari, A. Jumaan, and F. Zhou, "Herpes zoster incidence among insured persons in the United States, 1993-2006: evaluation of impact of varicella vaccination," *Clinical Infectious Diseases*, vol. 52, no. 3, pp. 332–340, 2011.

[23] M. Papagianni, S. Metallidis, and K. Tziomalos, "Herpes zoster and diabetes mellitus: a review," *Diabetes Therapy*, vol. 9, no. 2, pp. 545–550, 2018.

[24] M. J. Levin, E. Bresnitz, Z. Popmihajlov et al., "Studies with herpes zoster vaccines in immune compromised patients," *Expert Review of Vaccines*, vol. 16, no. 12, pp. 1217–1230, 2017.

[25] B. P. Yawn, P. Saddier, P. C. Wollan, J. L. St Sauver, M. J. Kurland, and L. S. Sy, "A population-based study of the incidence and complication rates of herpes zoster before zoster vaccine introduction," *Mayo Clinic Proceedings*, vol. 82, no. 11, pp. 1341–1349, 2007.

[26] J. P. Mullooly, K. Riedlinger, C. Chun, S. Weinmann, and H. Houston, "Incidence of herpes zoster, 1997–2002," *Epidemiology and Infection*, vol. 133, no. 2, pp. 245–253, 2005.

[27] M. Klompas, M. Kulldorff, Y. Vilk, S. R. Bialek, and R. Harpaz, "Herpes zoster and postherpetic neuralgia surveillance using structured electronic data," *Mayo Clinic Proceedings*, vol. 86, no. 12, pp. 1146–1153, 2011.

[28] K. Shiraki, N. Toyama, T. Daikoku, and M. Yajima, "Herpes zoster and recurrent herpes zoster," *Open Forum Infectious Diseases*, vol. 4, no. 1, article ofx007, 2017.

20

Evaluating the Contribution of *Nocardia* spp. and *Mycobacterium tuberculosis* to Pulmonary Infections among HIV and Non-HIV Patients at the Komfo Anokye Teaching Hospital, Ghana

Samuel Asamoah Sakyi (iD),[1] Kwabena Owusu Danquah,[2] Richard Dadzie Ephraim (iD),[3] Anthony Enimil,[4] Venus Frimpong,[2] Linda Ahenkorah Fondjo (iD),[1] and Esther Love Darkoh (iD)[5]

[1]*Department of Molecular Medicine, School of Medical Sciences,*
Kwame Nkrumah University of Science and Technology (KNUST), Kumasi, Ghana
[2]*Department of Medical Laboratory Technology, Faculty of Allied Health Sciences,*
Kwame Nkrumah University of Science and Technology (KNUST), Kumasi, Ghana
[3]*Department of Medical Laboratory Technology, School of Allied Health Sciences, University of Cape Coast (UCC),*
Cape Coast, Ghana
[4]*Department of Child Health, School of Medical Sciences, Kwame Nkrumah University of Science and Technology (KNUST),*
Kumasi, Ghana
[5]*Department of Theoretical and Applied Biology, College of Science,*
Kwame Nkrumah University of Science and Technology (KNUST), Kumasi, Ghana

Correspondence should be addressed to Samuel Asamoah Sakyi; samasamoahsakyi@yahoo.co.uk

Academic Editor: Jorge Garbino

Tuberculosis (TB) is a major cause of human mortality particularly in association with the human immunodeficiency virus (HIV). *Nocardia* spp. has emerged as an opportunistic infection especially in HIV patients. The high prevalence of TB and HIV coupled with the lack of a definitive laboratory diagnosis for *Nocardia* spp. could lead to misdiagnosed pulmonary TB. This study determined the prevalence of pulmonary infections due to *Nocardia* spp. and *Mycobacterium tuberculosis* in sputum of HIV and non-HIV patients with suspected pulmonary tuberculosis at KATH. A total of sixty sputum samples were obtained from HIV and non-HIV patients with suspected pulmonary tuberculosis. Samples were examined by fluorescence based Ziehl–Neelsen staining, culture, and PCR methods. The prevalence of *Nocardia* spp. and *Mycobacterium tuberculosis* was 18.3% and 20%, respectively, with the latter having the highest rate among patients aged 21–40 years ($P = 0.075$). The prevalence of *Nocardia* spp. among HIV patients was 90.9% whilst 16.7% of the patients had HIV/*Nocardia* spp. coinfection. Detection of *Mycobacterium tuberculosis* by fluorescence-based Ziehl–Neelsen staining, culture, and PCR yielded 9 (15%), 11 (18.3%), and 12 (20%), respectively. There is a high prevalence of nocardiosis especially in HIV patients. PCR is a better diagnostic method that detects both *Nocardia* spp. and *Mycobacterium tuberculosis* and should be incorporated into routine diagnosis for pulmonary infections.

1. Introduction

Tuberculosis remains a major cause of human mortality and morbidity, threatening the lives of one-third of the world's popu [1]. It is caused by *Mycobacterium tuberculosis* complex such as *Mycobacterium bovis, M. africanum, M. bovis bacillus* Calmette–Guerin, *and M. tuberculosis* [2, 3]. The latter, however, is responsible for most tuberculosis (TB) infections in humans [4]. An estimated 7–9 million cases of TB are reported annually resulting in 1.5–2 million deaths worldwide [5]. According to the WHO [6], TB is endemic in sub-Saharan Africa with about 1.5 million cases reported annually. This high prevalence of TB in developing countries is due to poverty, overcrowding, and HIV infection.

In Ghana, the disease plaques all segments of the society and over 46,000 new cases of TB are reported annually [6]. A study conducted in Ghana on the burden of HIV on TB patients showed that 1633 (92.2%) tested positive to HIV from 1772 TB patients [7].

Nocardia asteroides is the most common causative agent of pulmonary nocardiosis, accounting for 85% of all cases [8]. It is contracted through inhalation into the respiratory tract. The pulmonary event in humans may either be self-limiting, transient, or subclinical, or it may progress to an acute, subacute, or chronic process mimicking tuberculous (TB) or mycotic infection or a malignancy. The infection is more common in immunocompromised hosts [9–11] especially those with impaired cell-mediated immunity such as patients with HIV infection, those on long-term corticosteroid exposure, malignancy, chronic alcoholism, and diabetes mellitus, and patients with a history of solid organ transplantation [8, 12–17].

The laboratory diagnosis and clinical manifestation of TB and nocardiosis are similar and requires accurate laboratory test in order to distinguish one from the other. The lack of a definitive laboratory diagnosis of nocardiosis has often led to misdiagnosis and hence mistreatment [18]. Additionally, cases of pulmonary nocardiosis in HIV-infected persons have also been diagnosed as pulmonary TB [19]. Moreover, little is known about the coinfection of pulmonary nocardiosis and tuberculosis in HIV and non-HIV patients in Ghana. Accurate identification of *Nocardia* species is burdened by its characteristic branching on Gram staining, which makes it seem acid fast and mimics *Mycobacterium tuberculosis*. Besides, conventional methods involve long-term culture, the identification of growth characteristics of colonies, assessment of microscopic morphology of colonies, and biochemical and susceptibility testing. This method therefore carries a high risk of contamination from other bacteria and fungi from the environment.

In as much as nocardiosis resembling tuberculosis, first-line antituberculous drugs are not efficient for its treatment. Moreover, optimal therapeutic strategies depend on rapid and accurate identification of *Nocardia* spp. As such, the use of molecular methods for identification, such as PCR with high sensitivity and specificity, is necessary to improve the accuracy of diagnosis of nocardiosis. Therefore, the suggested approach to overcome this problem is molecular techniques, since they are more specific, sensitive, and rapid as compared to conventional diagnostic methods. Consequently, unraveling the prevalence of pulmonary infections due to *Nocardia* species and *Mycobacterium tuberculosis* is important in mitigating misdiagnosis of pulmonary infections especially among HIV/AIDS patients and ultimately ensure accurate diagnosis and treatment.

2. Materials and Methods

2.1. Study Design. This hospital-based cross-sectional study was conducted at the Komfo Anokye Teaching Hospital (KATH) in Kumasi from March to July, 2017.

2.2. Study Area. The study was conducted at KATH which is located in the Kumasi metropolis. The metropolis is one of the 27 districts in Ashanti region, with a population of about 1,730,249. The hospital is one of the largest health facilities serving both as the first consultation point and as a referral centre for the Northern and middle belt of Ghana.

2.3. Ethical Considerations. Ethical approval was sought from the Committee on Human Research, Publication and Ethics (CHRPE) of the School of Medical Sciences, Kwame Nkrumah University of Science and Technology (CHRPE/AP/564/17). All participants gave their written informed consent after the aim and objectives of the study had been explained to them.

2.4. Inclusion and Exclusion Criteria. HIV and non-HIV patients suspected with pulmonary tuberculosis with laboratory request by clinicians to undergo pulmonary tuberculosis investigations were recruited as subjects. However, HIV and non-HIV patients without any clinical suspicion of pulmonary infection were excluded. A total of 60 patients aged between 4 and 80 years were recruited into the study.

2.5. Sputum Collection and Questionnaire Administration. Structured questionnaires were administered to all study participants to collect demographic information and medical history and HIV infection status as well as information on the use of steroids and previous transplantation history. Two milliliter of early morning and on-spot sputum specimens were collected from each participant with suspected pulmonary tuberculosis. The participant was requested to cough so that expectoration comes from as deep down the chest as possible and spat into a sterile, wide mouth, and leak-proof specimen containers.

2.6. Sputum Decontamination and Processing. The obtained sixty sputum samples were decontaminated immediately according to standardized routine diagnosis procedures by the NaOH/N-acetyl-L-cysteine (NALC) method. The concentrated specimen was then used for culture, smear preparation, and PCR assays for *Mycobacterium tuberculosis* and *Norcadia* spp. [20]. For the culture, 250 μl of each of the concentrated sputum was inoculated onto Löwenstein–Jensen media and incubated at 37°C. *Nocardia* spp. are acid fast, can withstand the decontamination with NaOH as well as NALC method, and thereby can grow on Löwenstein–Jensen media. Colonies that were suspicious were examined using acid-fast and Gram-staining method while cultures that did not show any growth after some weeks were reported as negative.

Prior to microscopic examination, a drop of the sediment of the sputum sample was spread on each clean microscopic slide using a Pasteur pipette. Slides were allowed to dry, fixed by heat, and stained using Ziehl–Neelsen acid-fast staining.

2.7. DNA Extraction and PCR Assay. After decontamination, the genomic DNA was extracted using GenoLyse Kit (VER

1.0, Hain Lifesciences, Germany) following the manufacturer's instructions. Primers for *Norcadia asteroides* ATCC 19247 and *Mycobacterium tuberculosis* H37RV were synthesized and purchased from inqaba biotec, South Africa. The isolated DNA was amplified using specific pairs of primers IS1 (5′CTCGTCCAGCGCCGCTTCGG3′) and IS2 (5′CCTGCGAGCGTAGGCGGTGG3′) for *Mycobacterium tuberculosis* complex. The PCR protocols were optimized to 30 cycles consisting of 5 minutes at 96°C for initial heat activation, 1 minute at 95°C for denaturation, 1 minute at 65°C for annealing, and 1 minute at 72°C for extension, whereas the final extension was done for 1 minute at 72°C.

Primers NG1 (5′CTCGTCCAGCGCCGCTTCGG3′) and NG2 (5′CCTGCGAGCGTAGGCGGTGG3′) were used to amplify a *Nocardia* genus-specific 590 bp fragment of 16S rRNA. The PCR protocols were optimized to 30 cycles consisting of 10 minutes at 94°C for initial denaturation, 1 minute at 94°C for denaturation, 20 seconds at 55°C for annealing, and 1 minute at 72°C for extension. The final extension was done for 10 minutes at 72°C.

Amplification with these primers was observed by electrophoresis on 2% (w/v) agarose gel stained with ethidium bromide as shown in Figures 1 and 2. The *Nocardia asteroides* ATCC 19247 and *Mycobacterium tuberculosis* H37RV were used as positive reference strains. Two PCRs for each sample were performed in separate tubes with two pairs of primers. One set was dedicated to the *Mycobacterium tuberculosis* complex, whereas the other set was for *Nocardia* spp. For each round of PCR, ddH$_2$O was used as the negative template.

3. Analysis

Data analysis was carried out using the Statistical Package for the Social Sciences (SPSS, version 23). The chi-square test was used to determine the significance differences between variables, and the level of significance was set at $P < 0.05$.

4. Results

4.1. Demographic Characteristics/Prevalence of Pulmonary Infections. Of the 60 participants that were recruited into the study, 56.7% (34/60) were males whilst 43.3% (26/60) were females with ages ranging from 4–80 years, whereas the mean age of the study population was 43.9 ± 19.0 years. Additionally, 25% were HIV positive whereas 75% of the participants were HIV negative (Table 1).

Prevalence of *Nocardia* spp. and *Mycobacterium tuberculosis* was 18.3% and 20%, respectively. Though males had higher number of infections caused by *Mycobacterium tuberculosis* than females, this difference was not statistically significant ($P = 0.896$). Moreover, pulmonary infection caused by *Nocardia* spp. ($P = 0.087$) and *Mycobacterium tuberculosis* ($P = 0.075$) between ages showed no significant difference as presented in Table 2.

It was also observed from the study that the prevalence of *Nocardia* spp. was higher in the HIV patients (90.9%) as compared to the HIV-negative group (12.2%), and the

difference was statistically significant ($\chi^2 = 26.181$; $P = 0.000$) as shown in Figure 3.

With regards to coinfection, study participants harbored two or more diseases, and of the total study sample size (60), coinfection of HIV and *Nocardia* spp. was observed in 10 (16.7%) participants while 5 (8.3%) had both HIV and tuberculosis (Figure 4).

Findings from fluorescence-based Ziehl–Neelsen examination indicated that *Mycobacterium tuberculosis* was found in 9 (15%) samples, and culture identified 11 (18.3%) positives whereas PCR analysis identified 12 (20%) positives for *Mycobacterium tuberculosis*. Moreover, based on the area under the receiver operating characteristic (ROC) curve, the use of microscopy in diagnosing TB was 71.9% (Figure 5).

5. Discussion

This study determined the prevalence of *Nocardia* spp. and *Mycobacterium tuberculosis* in sputum samples of patients with suspected pulmonary infections. Gender is an important factor for determining pulmonary infection according to Gupta et al. [21] and Gajbhare et al. [22]. The current study revealed that pulmonary infections were higher in males than females and were common in the age group of 21–40 years (10.6%). This affirms the findings of Codlin et al. [23] who reported higher prevalence of tuberculosis in males than in females. A related study conducted by Muniyandi et al. [24] on socioeconomic dimensions of tuberculosis control showed that 73% of the study population were males. This could be due to the fact that more males are likely to involve in activities that will predispose them to reduced immunity. Moreover, socioeconomic reasons may further subject them to poor diet and overall poor health conditions. In the developing countries, men are seen as the head of the family, and they tend to engage in various job-related activities with its associated hazards, which expose them to pulmonary infections. This study further observed that majority of the study participants that had pulmonary infections were HIV positive. This corroborates the studies by Kherad et al. [25] and Luetkemeyer [26] who also reported high coinfection in tuberculosis and HIV patients. This is due to the fact that individuals with HIV infection are immunocompromised and that predisposes them to TB infection. Contrary to the high prevalence of TB infection among HIV patients in our study, Sharma et al. [27] reported low tuberculosis infection in India. The low TB observed in this study could be due to overall low prevalence of TB in the study area.

Opportunistic microorganisms like *Nocardia* spp. can mimic pulmonary tuberculosis in HIV/AIDS and non-HIV patients and can be fatal if untreated [28]. Some investigators have previously reported incidence of pulmonary nocardiosis and tuberculosis in HIV-infected patients [16, 29]. Ekrami et al. [28] reported concomitant pulmonary nocardiosis and tuberculosis in HIV patients. It was found in their study that the coincidence of pulmonary tuberculosis and nocardiosis was 1% for their entire study population and 6.25% among HIV-infected patients. In another study, pulmonary nocardiosis in HIV-infected patients with suspected pulmonary

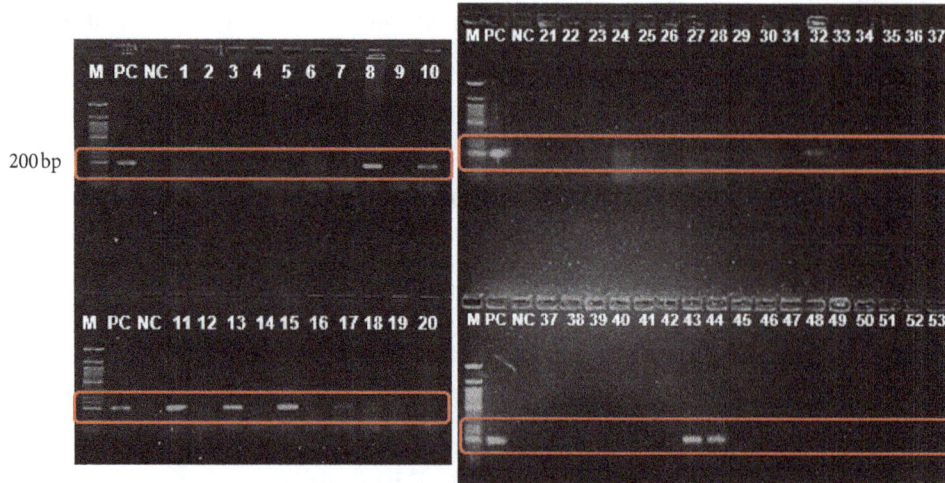

FIGURE 1: Amplification of TB with IS6110 primers. M: molecular weight marker, PC: positive control, NC: negative control, bp: base pairs (expected base pairs of *Mycobacterium tuberculosis*, 200 bp).

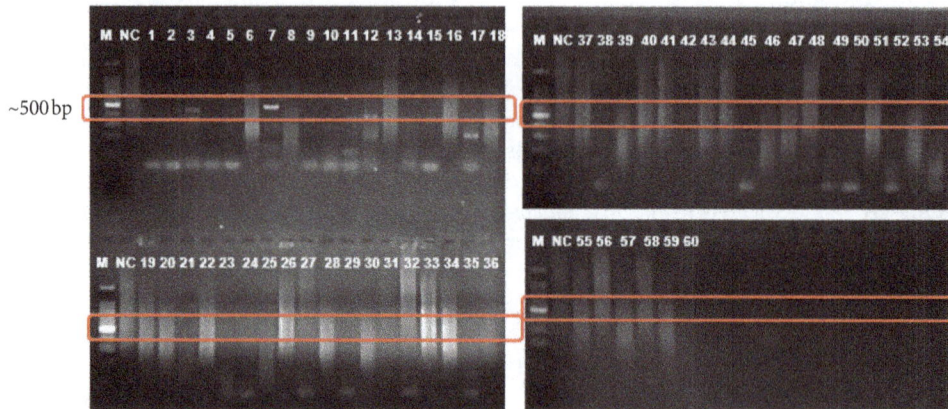

FIGURE 2: Amplification of *Nocardia* with IS1&2 primers: M: molecular weight marker, PC: positive control, NC: negative control, bp: base pairs (expected base pairs of *Nocardia asteroides*, 500 bp).

TABLE 1: Sociodemographic characteristics of study participants.

Variables	Frequency	Percentage (%)
Ages		
<20	7	11.7
21–40	18	30.0
41–60	25	41.7
≥61	10	16.7
Gender		
Male	34	56.7
Female	26	43.3
HIV status		
Positive	15	25.0
Negative	45	75.0

TABLE 2: Prevalence of *Nocardia* spp. and *Mycobacterium tuberculosis*.

Variable	Number infected	Prevalence (%)	Chi-square value (χ^2)	P value
Infections due to *Mycobacterium tuberculosis*				
Gender				
Male	7	11.7	0.016	0.896
Female	5	8.3		
Ages				
≤20	1	8.3		
21–40	7	58.3	6.907	0.075
41–60	4	41.7		
≥61	—	—		
Nocardia spp.				
Gender				
Male	9	81.8	3.470	0.062
Female	2	18.2		
Ages				
≤20	—	—		
21–40	6	54.5	6.568	0.087
41–60	5	45.5		
≥61	—	—		

tuberculosis was reported to be 3% by Alnaum et al. [30]. In our study, however, 90.9% of *Nocardia* spp. was from HIV patients whereas 6.7% had tuberculosis, HIV, and nocardiosis coinfection and may be attributed to suppression of cell-mediated immunity [31]. In addition, epidemiological data on the prevalence of AIDS-associated nocardiosis are scarce; nevertheless, based on initial studies from other parts of the

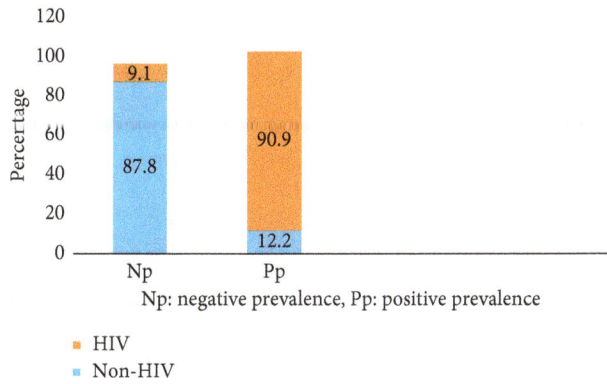

Figure 3: Prevalence of *Nocardia* spp. in HIV and non-HIV patients.

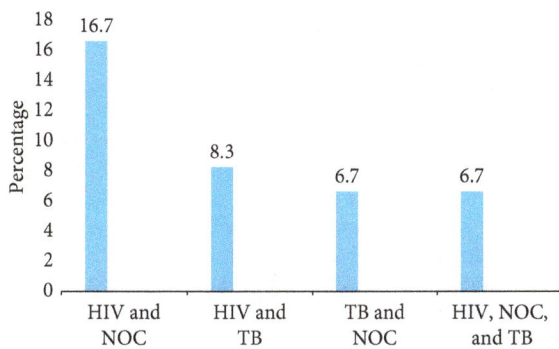

Figure 4: HIV, TB, and *Nocardia* spp. coinfection among study participants. NOC, *Nocardia*.

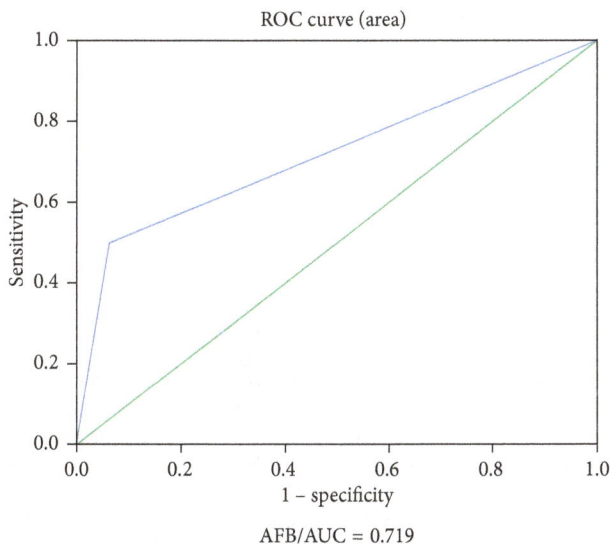

Figure 5: ROC of AFB in diagnosing TB.

world, nocardiosis has been regarded as an unusual complication of HIV infection. The reason for this apparently high prevalence of HIV-associated nocardiosis is unclear and probably multifactorial. Though previous studies have reported that between 57% and 68% of patients have AIDS-defining criteria at the time of diagnosis of *Nocardia* infection [12, 18]. The disease may still be underreported [32].

Diagnosis of tuberculosis using molecular techniques like the PCR has been more efficient than the conventional methods [33, 34]. In the current study, we detected 20.0% and 15% of *Mycobacterium tuberculosis* in participants with the use of polymerase chain reaction (PCR) and acid-fast bacilli (AFB) correspondingly. Nonetheless, *Nocardia* was not distinguished in sputum specimens using conventional methods in this study, but positive samples that yielded a result of 18.3% were determined using the PCR assay. The prevalence of *Nocardia* in this study was significantly lower than a prevalence of 37.5% from Dawar et al. [35] on epidemiology of nocardiosis—a six-year study from Northern India. The difference in prevalence may be due to differences in methodology, as most of the other studies used microscopy, whilst this study used polymerase chain reaction. Another reason could be due to sampling technique as this current study concentrated on patients with suspected TB whilst the other studies ranged from immunocompromised patients to patients from the general population.

This result is very significant because previous laboratory-based data had not isolated any *Nocardia* in the chest clinic of the Komfo Anokye Teaching Hospital. *Nocardia* spp. is one of the opportunistic infections in the HIV/AIDS patients just as tuberculosis is and can be fatal if untreated. Untreated pulmonary nocardiosis is very similar to tuberculosis particularly in immunocompromised patients and could be mistaken for other bacterial infections and underestimated. Also, as much as nocardiosis resembles tuberculosis, first-line antituberculous drugs are not efficient for its treatment. Moreover, optimal therapeutic strategies depend on rapid and accurate identification of *Nocardia* spp. This means that the chest clinic at the Komfo Anokye Teaching Hospital must put in measures to diagnose *Nocardia*, since it is likely that a lot more patients are being missed and runs a risk of complications due to the nontreatment.

6. Conclusions

The prevalence of *Mycobacterium tuberculosis* in the study population was 20% whilst *Nocardia* spp. was 18.3%. The most prevalent coinfection observed was HIV and *Nocardia* spp. with an occurrence of 16.7%. Hence, in Ghana, a better diagnostic method with high sensitivity and specificity should be employed to improve the accuracy of diagnosis of nocardiosis. Moreover, *Nocardia* diagnosis should be incorporated into routine diagnosis for pulmonary infections in patients and especially those who fail to respond to anti-TB treatment in Ghana.

Acknowledgments

We are grateful to Mr. Ishmael Kwabena Tetteh and Mr. Festus Adongo at the Microbiology and Tuberculosis laboratory of the Komfo Anokye Teaching Hospital for their immense support during the data acquisition. Funding for this project was sought from the KNUST research fund (kref-0-2016).

References

[1] D. Schlossberg, *Tuberculosis and Non-Tuberculosis Mycobacterial Infections*, McGraw-ill Professional, New York City, NY, USA, 5th edition, 2006, https://www.scribd.com/document/245948024/Tuberculosis-and-Nontuberculosis-Mycobacterial-Infections-5th-Edition-McGraw-Hill-Professional-2005.

[2] D. van – Soolingen, T. Hoogenboezem, P. E. De Haas et al., "Novel pathogenic taxon of *Mycobacterium tuberculosis* complex, Canetti: characterization of an exceptional isolate from Africa," *International Journal of Systematic Bacteriology*, vol. 47, pp. 1236–1245, 1997.

[3] D. Cousins, R. Bastida, A. Cataldi, V. Quse, S. Redrobe, and S. Dow, "Tuberculosis in seals caused by a novel member of the *Mycobacterium tuberculosis* complex: *Mycobacterium pinnipedii* sp," *International Journal of Systematic and Evolutionary Microbiology*, vol. 53, no. 5, pp. 1305–1314, 2003.

[4] R. Skolnik, *Global Health 101*, Jones & Bartlett Publishers, Burlington, MA, USA, 2011, ISBN: 1449675530, 9781449675530.

[5] S. D. Lawn and A. I. Zumla, "Tuberculosis," *The Lancet*, vol. 378, no. 9785, pp. 57–72, 2011.

[6] World Health Organization, *Global Tuberculosis Control Report*, World Health Organization, Geneva, Switzerland, 2005, http://library.cphs.chula.ac.th/Ebooks/AnnualReport/TB/TB2005.pdf.

[7] E. Osei, J. Der, R. Owusu, P. Kofie, and W. K. Axame, "The burden of HIV on Tuberculosis patients in the volta region of Ghana from 2012 to 2015: implication for tuberculosis control," *BMC Infectious Diseases*, vol. 17, no. 1, p. 504, 2017.

[8] R. Martinez, S. Reyes, and R. Menéndez, "Pulmonary nocardiosis: risk factors, clinical features, diagnosis and prognosis," *Current Opinion in Pulmonary Medicine*, vol. 14, no. 3, pp. 219–227, 2008.

[9] M. Neibecker, C. Schwarze-Zander, J. K. Rockstroh, U. Spengler, and J. T. Blackard, "Evidence for extensive genotypic diversity and recombination of GB virus C (GBV-C) in Germany," *Journal of Medical Virology*, vol. 83, no. 4, pp. 685–694, 2011.

[10] D. Gupta and G. Dutta, "Pulmonary nocardiosis mimicking tuberculosis- a case report," *International Journal of Contemporary Medicine*, vol. 1, no. 1, pp. 24–28, 2013.

[11] World Health Organization, *Global Tuberculosis Report*, World Health Organization, Geneva, Switzerland, 2014, http://www.who.int/tb/publications/global_report/en/pdf.

[12] R. B. Uttamchandani, G. L. Daikos, R. R. Reyes et al., "Nocardiosis in 30 patients with advanced human immunodeficiency virus infection: clinical features and outcome," *Clinical Infectious Diseases*, vol. 18, no. 3, pp. 348–353, 1994.

[13] S. Husain, K. McCurry, J. Dauber, N. Singh, and S. Kusne, "Nocardia infection in lung transplant recipients," *Journal of Heart and Lung Transplantation*, vol. 21, no. 3, pp. 354–359, 2002.

[14] M. Narushima, H. Suzuki, T. Kasai et al., "Pulmonary nocardiosis in a patient treated with corticosteroid therapy," *Respirology*, vol. 7, no. 1, pp. 87–89, 2002.

[15] A. S. Daly, A. McGeer, and J. H. Lipton, "Systemic nocardiosis following allogeneic bone marrow transplantation," *Transplant Infectious Disease*, vol. 5, no. 1, pp. 16–20, 2003.

[16] V. Pintado, E. Gómez-Mampaso, J. Cobo et al., "Nocardial infection in patients infected with the human immunodeficiency virus," *Clinical Microbiology and Infection*, vol. 9, no. 7, pp. 716–720, 2003.

[17] M. A. Saubolle and D. Sussland, "Nocardiosis: review of clinical and laboratory experience," *Journal of Clinical Microbiology*, vol. 41, no. 10, pp. 4497–4501, 2003.

[18] S. B. Lucas, A. Hounnou, C. Peacock, A. Beaumel, A. Kadio, and K. M. De Cock, "Nocardiosis in HIV- positive patients: an autopsy study in West Africa," *Tuberculosis and Lung Disease*, vol. 75, no. 4, pp. 301–307, 1994.

[19] V. Kandi, "Human nocardia infections: a review of pulmonary nocardiosis," *Cureus*, vol. 7, no. 8, p. e304, 2015.

[20] R. C. Read, "Nocardiosis and actinomycosis," *Medicine*, vol. 37, no. 12, pp. 657–659, 2009.

[21] D. Gupta, K. Das, T. Balamughesh, A. N. Aggarwal, and S. K. Jindal, "Role of socio- economic factors in tuberculosis prevalence," *Indian Journal of Tuberculosis*, vol. 51, no. 1, pp. 27–32, 2004.

[22] D. M. Gajbhare, R. C. Bedre, and H. M. Solanki, "A study of socio-demographic profile and treatment outcome of tuberculosis patients in an urban slum of Mumbai, Maharashtra," *Indian Journal of Basic and Applied Medical Research*, vol. 4, no. 1, pp. 50–57, 2014.

[23] A. J. Codlin, S. Khowaja, Z. Chen et al., "Gender differences in tuberculosis notification in Pakistan," *American Journal of Tropical Medicine and Hygiene*, vol. 85, no. 3, pp. 514–517, 2011.

[24] M. Muniyandi, R. Ramachandran, R. Balasubramanian, and P. R. Narayanan, "Socio-economic dimensions of tuberculosis control: review of studies over two decades from Tuberculosis Research Center," *Journal of Communicable Diseases*, vol. 38, no. 3, pp. 204–215, 2006.

[25] O. Kherad, F. R. Herrmann, J.-P. Zellweger, T. Rochat, and J.-P. Janssens, "Clinical presentation, demographics and outcome of tuberculosis (TB) in a low incidence area: a 4- year study in Geneva, Switzerland," *BMC Infectious Diseases*, vol. 9, no. 1, p. 217, 2009.

[26] A. Luetkemeyer, *Tuberculosis and HIV*, University of California, San Francisco, CA, USA, 2013, http://hivinsite.ucsf.edu/InSite?page=kb-05-01- 06#S1X.

[27] S. K. Sharma, P. K. Saha, Y. Dixit, N. H. Siddarmaiah, P. Seth, and J. N. Pande, "HIV seropositivity among adult tuberculosis patients in Delhi," *Indian Journal of Chest Diseases and Allied Sciences*, vol. 42, no. 3, pp. 157–160, 2000.

[28] A. Ekrami, A. D. Khosravi, A. R. Samarbaf Zadeh, and M. Hashemzadeh, "Nocardia co- infection in patients with pulmonary tuberculosis," *Jundishapur Journal of Microbiology*, vol. 7, no. 9, 2014.

[29] M. Singh, R. S. Sandhu, H. S. Randhawa, and B. M. Kallan, "Prevalence of pulmonary nocardiosis in a tuberculosis

hospital in Amritsar, Punjab," *Indian Journal of Chest Diseases and Allied Sciences*, vol. 42, no. 4, pp. 325–340, 2000.

[30] H. M. Alnaum, M. M. Elhassan, F. Y. Mustafa, and M. E. Hamid, "Prevalence of nocardia species among HIV-positive patients with suspected tuberculosis," *Tropical Doctor*, vol. 41, no. 4, pp. 224–226, 2011.

[31] G. A. Filice, "Nocardiosis in persons with human immunodeficiency virus infection, transplant recipients, and large, geographically defined populations," *Journal of Laboratory and Clinical Medicine*, vol. 145, no. 3, pp. 156–162, 2005.

[32] K. Javaly, H. W. Horowitz, and G. P. Wormser, "Nocardiosis in patients with human immunodeficiency virus infection report of 2 cases and review of the literature," *Medicine*, vol. 71, no. 3, pp. 128–138, 1992.

[33] A. Mohan, S. K. Sharma, V. K. Arora, S. Sharma, and J. Prakash, "Concurrent pulmonary Aspergillosis and Nocardiosis in an old tubercular cavity masquerading as malignancy in an immunocompetent individual," *Respiratory Medicine CME*, vol. 1, no. 3, pp. 231–234, 2008.

[34] J. Ambrosioni, D. Lew, and J. Garbino, "Nocardiosis: updated clinical review and experience at a tertiary center," *Infection*, vol. 38, no. 2, pp. 89–97, 2010.

[35] R. Dawar, R. Girotra, S. Quadri et al., "Epidemiology of nocardiosis-a six years study from Northern India," *Journal of Microbiology & Infectious Diseases*, vol. 6, no. 2, 2016.

21

The Role of Adjunctive Therapies in Septic Shock by Gram Negative MDR/XDR Infections

Stefano Busani, Erika Roat, Giulia Serafini, Elena Mantovani, Emanuela Biagioni, and Massimo Girardis

Intensive Care Unit, Modena University Hospital, L.go del Pozzo 71, 41100 Modena, Italy

Correspondence should be addressed to Massimo Girardis; girardis.massimo@unimo.it

Academic Editor: Alessandra Oliva

Patients with septic shock by multidrug resistant microorganisms (MDR) are a specific sepsis population with a high mortality risk. The exposure to an initial inappropriate empiric antibiotic therapy has been considered responsible for the increased mortality, although other factors such as immune-paralysis seem to play a pivotal role. Therefore, beyond conventional early antibiotic therapy and fluid resuscitation, this population may benefit from the use of alternative strategies aimed at supporting the immune system. In this review we present an overview of the relationship between MDR infections and immune response and focus on the rationale and the clinical data available on the possible adjunctive immunotherapies, including blood purification techniques and different pharmacological approaches.

1. Introduction

Since early 90s, the American College of Chest Physicians and Society of Critical Care Medicine Consensus Conference has placed great emphasis to sepsis and its definition [1]. The Third International Consensus Definitions for Sepsis and Septic Shock (Sepsis-3) revised the definitions emphasizing the role of the host response and the related pathophysiological mechanisms inducing organ dysfunction [2]. The change of perspective from invading pathogens to the host response has radically transformed the vision of sepsis pathobiology in the last decades. The current concepts indicate that sepsis progress on a double track sustained by products of infecting microorganisms and by endogenous mediators derived from complement activation and by specific cell-surface receptors expressed on immune, epithelial, and endothelial cells. A complex system of intracellular signals is created by the binding of pathogen-associated molecular patterns (PAMPs) and damage-associated molecular patterns (DAMPs) that lead to the expression of several common gene classes involved in inflammation, adaptive immunity, and cellular metabolism [3]. Specifically, the recognition of PAMPs and DAMPs produces the recruitment of proinflammatory intermediates that initiate the expression of early activation genes [4].

2. Sepsis Related Immune-Paralysis

Recent data on septic patients clarified that host response may be hyper- or hyporeactive with an overwhelming inflammation associated with a boost of proinflammatory cytokines in the former and an immune-paralysis with the prevalence of anti-inflammatory cytokines and cellular apoptosis in the latter. Although proinflammatory and anti-inflammatory responses occur simultaneously, early phases of sepsis are usually characterized by hyperinflammatory processes associated with classical clinical signs ranging from slight to severe impairment of organ function, including shock appearance [5]. On the other hand, immune-suppressive state becomes predominant in later stages of sepsis producing the so-called persistent inflammation/immunosuppression and catabolism syndrome (PICS) [6]. The hypothesis for explaining PICS developing are mainly two: (i) a persistent and dysregulated activity of PAMPs, DAMPs, inflammasomes, and tissue "alarmins" and (ii) the role of opportunistic infections (e.g., viral reactivation, infection *Acinetobacter* spp), changes in the host microbiota, and invasive procedures performed in critically ill patients [4]. Sepsis related immunosuppression causes profound changes in both the innate and adaptive immunity [7, 8] with persistent lymphopenia and high level of immature forms of myeloid cells. The sepsis induced immune dysfunction makes critically ill patient highly susceptible to colonization and secondary infections, including break-through infections, by opportunistic nosocomial multidrug resistant (MDR) bacteria. Therefore, patients carrying MDR bacteria might be considered a special population requiring specific strategies directed to supported immune system beyond the appropriate antibiotic therapy and standard supportive treatments.

3. Patients with MDR Bacteria: Why Are They a Special Population?

Sepsis and septic shock related to MDR bacteria are progressively increasing in the last decades with gram negative pathogens responsible for the majority of cases [9]. International guidelines define MDR bacteria as microorganisms nonsusceptible in vitro to at least three different antimicrobial categories (previously excluding intrinsic resistance), XDR as nonsusceptible to at least one agent in all but two or fewer antimicrobial categories, and PDR as resistant to any agents in all antimicrobial classes tested [10]. The burden of infections sustained by MDR bacteria is variable in different areas: world data show a lower incidence in northwest of Europe, USA, and Canada and a higher incidence in southeast of Europe, Latin America, and Asia Pacific [11]. According to recent studies, around one-third of the intensive care unit (ICU) acquired infections are sustained by MDR bacteria most of whom are *Acinetobacter* spp., *Klebsiella pneumoniae*, and *Pseudomonas* spp. isolates [12]. The capability of these bacteria to survive for prolonged time in the hospital environment, the high risk of transfer among patients and healthcare staff, and the antibiotic resistance are responsible for their increasing widespread. Note that MDR strains are progressively increasing also in community acquired infections and the acquisition of these pathogens through travels in different world regions is becoming frequent.

MDR infections influences patients' outcome with higher mortality rates in metallo-β-lactamases *Enterobacteriaceae* and *Pseudomonas aeruginosa* and in carbapenem-resistant *Klebsiella pneumoniae*, likely due to the delay in the appropriate antimicrobial therapy [13]. The Centre for control of Diseases calculates that gram negative MDR infections are responsible for approximately 40,000 cases and more than 2,800 deaths in the United States (CDC 2013 Threat report). It is well known that the administration of an appropriate antimicrobial therapy within the first hour of diagnosis is strongly recommended in the management of patients septic shock and that an initial noneffective therapy is related to increased mortality [14]. In MDR infections the choice of an appropriate antimicrobial treatment is more complicated. In patients with bloodstream infections sustained by ESBL producing microorganisms, an appropriate antibiotic therapy reduced the 3-week mortality by 40% compared to a nonappropriate one [15].

The risk factors for acquisition of MDR infections are well known and related to both specific characteristics of patients and local epidemiology. The former includes specific conditions such as advanced age, diabetes, end-stage liver disease, immunosuppressive therapy, use of corticosteroids, malignancy, organ transplantation, recent surgery, recent exposure (<3 months) to antibiotic therapy, prior hospital admission, and MDR colonization [16]. It is noteworthy that the majority of these factors are related to a possible dysfunction of the immune response. In fact, advanced age is associated with a progressive dysfunction of immune system, both cell-mediated and humoral, defined as immunosenescence [17–19]. Similarly, in patients with malignancies, the growth of tumors takes place developing a condition of immunotolerance which allows cancer cells to escape from elimination [20, 21]. Tumors create an immunosuppressive microenvironment by producing mediators (IL-10, TGF-β, and VEGF) responsible for maturation and expansion of suppressive immune cells such as regulatory T cells, immature dendritic cells, and tumor associated macrophages [22]. Due to their immunocompromised condition, also cirrhotic patients have a high risk of developing infections. In these patients the magnitude of cellular immune depression is comparable to patients with severe sepsis with defects in innate immunity caused by a persistent activation of compensatory anti-inflammatory mechanisms to counteract the high burden of proinflammatory mediators occurring in end-stage liver disease [23, 24].

The relationship between MDR infections and the host immune response is so far unclear. A recent study described the interactions between different clones and resistance phenotypes of *Klebsiella pneumoniae* and innate immune response. In vitro stimulation of human peripheral blood mononuclear cells (PBMCs) with different heat-killed isolates of *K. pneumoniae* led to different patterns of TNF-α production. In particular, the highly virulent KPC-producing isolates of the ST17 clones are associated with low release of both TNF-α and IL-17 mediated by toll like receptor 9 that may contribute to a state of immunosuppression [25]. A similar work on *P. aeruginosa* showed that antibiotic susceptible isolates induce a significantly higher production of IL-1β and IL-6 and by human monocytes compared to MDR ones [26]. These results suggest that multidrug resistance could play a role in the modulation of host both innate and adaptive immune response. However, further studies are needed to better understand these complex relationships and the potential relevance of a specific immunomodulatory therapy in these infections.

4. The Role of Immune Adjuvant Therapies in MDR Infections

As described above, immune-paralysis is a hallmark of patients colonized or infected by MDR bacteria and, therefore, the development of treatments directed to restore the function of immune response may be useful to support

TABLE 1: The rationale and the possible adverse reactions of adjunctive immune-modulatory therapies in patients with sepsis.

	Potential advantages	Potential adverse effects
Extracorporeal blood purification techniques	(i) Removal of endotoxin (ii) Removal of middle molecular weight molecules (e.g., cytokines) (iii) Increase in HLA-DR expression on monocytes (iv) Restoration of TNF-α production	(i) Decrease of blood pressure (ii) Bleeding due to anticoagulant use (iii) Removal of drugs (e.g., amines, antibiotics) (iv) Possible removal of useful molecules (e.g., immune mediators)
Granulocytes-macrophage colony stimulating factor Interferon-γ	(i) Proliferation and maturation of granulocyte and monocyte precursor cells (ii) Stimulation of antigen presenting cells (iii) Increase in mHLA-DR expression (iv) Production of proinflammatory cytokines	(i) Fever (ii) Headache (iii) Edema (iv) Bone pain (v) Shortness of breath
PD-1/PD-L pathway	(i) Antiapoptotic effect (ii) Blockade of negative regulatory molecules	(i) Rare autoimmune reactions for long-term administration
Interleukin-7	(i) Stimulation of proliferation, maturation, and survival of T cells (ii) Increase of TCR repertoire diversity (iii) Production of proinflammatory cytokines	(i) Rare induction of fever and capillary leak syndrome
Interleukin-15	(i) Antiapoptotic effect on T cells and NK cells (ii) Expansion and activation of NK cells and CD8 memory T cells (iii) Stimulation of NK cells-dendritic cells crosstalk (iv) Antiapoptotic effect on dendritic cells (v) Production of proinflammatory cytokines	(i) Fever (ii) Rigor (iii) Hypotension (iv) Capillary leak syndrome (v) Nausea
Intravenous immunoglobulins	(i) Pathogen and apoptotic cells clearance (ii) Scavenging of toxins and mediators (iii) Anti-inflammatory effects (iv) Antiapoptotic effects on immune cells	(i) Rare allergic reactions

antibiotic therapy in this specific population. Although many immune therapies have been investigated on animal models of sepsis, only few of them have been properly evaluated in patients (Table 1).

4.1. Extracorporeal Blood Purification Techniques. Different extracorporeal blood purification techniques have been recently developed and used during sepsis to remove endotoxins and proinflammatory mediators that play a substantial role in the inflammatory response of the host. Unfortunately, the effects of these treatments on the patient's immune response are unknown, particularly the long-term effects on the mechanisms leading to immune-paralysis. As regards impact on clinical outcome, two meta-analyses showed no benefits by the use of high volume hemofiltration [27, 28] as well as of cascade hemofiltration, despite promising results in an animal model [29, 30]. The use of hemoperfusion with polymyxin-B (PMX-B) for endotoxin blood removal showed contrasting results but a potential benefit in patients after emergency abdominal surgery seems to be plausible [31–33]. The just completed EUPHRATES trial will clarify better the role of this technique in septic patients with

endotoxemia [34]. Interestingly, beyond endotoxin removal, immune-modulatory effects of PMX-B hemoperfusion has been also postulated with possible positive effects on the prevention of immune-paralysis [35]. Similarly, the association between plasma filtration and adsorption (CPFA) seems to have positive effects on the immune response with an increase in HLA-DR expression on monocytes and a restored lipopolysaccharide induced TNF-α production [36]. Unfortunately, a recent randomized control trial in patients with septic shock did not show significant benefits by the use of CPFA [37]. Highly adsorptive membranes and high cut-off membranes can also be used to obtain a blood purification and the progressive optimization of these techniques will lead to preservation of useful molecules and a more selective removal of inflammatory mediators [38]. However, so far evidences are only anecdotal and they should be used only for research purposes or compassionate use.

4.2. Pharmacological Approaches. The use of different molecules able to modulate the immune system has been also proposed in septic patients. Granulocytes-macrophage colony stimulating factor (GM-CSF) and interferon-γ

(INF-γ) have been tested because of their effects on antigen presenting cells whose function in septic shock is deeply impaired. A meta-analysis of randomized trials in septic shock patients showed a better infection clearance in treated patients but no improvement in 28-day mortality [39]. It is notable that when GM-CSF was administered in patients with immune dysfunction (i.e., low mHLA-DR expression), its use was associated with prompt restoring of immune functioning and to reduced mechanical ventilation time and hospital length of stay [40]. INF-γ has been also administrated in subjects with trauma and burns with contradictory results. Again, it is to underline that, in burn patients with significant reduction of HLA-DR expression on monocytes, its use concomitant to GM-CSF was able to increase HLA-DR and to restore TNF-α secretion in ex vivo stimulated PBMCs [41].

Another potential target is the PD-1/PD-L pathway. Septic patients show an increased expression of PD-1 on T cells which leads to inhibition of cell proliferation, induction of IL-10 secretion, apoptosis, and anergy. Different studies have observed that block of this axis is able to improve survival in murine models of sepsis. In human antibodies anti-PD-1 and anti PD-L have been tested only to treat different types of cancer inducing a restoration of T cell activity [42]. In septic shock the PD-1 expression on T cells and/or PD-L expression on antigen presenting cells could be used as biomarkers of T cell exhaustion to drive anti-PD-1 and anti PD-L antibody administration. Other inhibitory receptors on T cell surface, such as TIM-3, LAG-3, CTLA-4, and BTLA, could be used for the same purpose in sepsis and septic shock but clinical trials are still lacking [43].

The use of recombinant interleukins in order to improve lymphocytes survival and function has been only experimented in HIV and cancer patients, but the potential benefits of these pleiotropic molecules have been demonstrated in animal models of septic shock. IL-7 has an antiapoptotic effect on T cell and is a crucial factor for lymphocyte production, maturation, and proliferation [44]. In different murine models of sepsis, the use of IL-7 is able to restore depleted T cells in lymphoid organs and induce T cell proliferation and INF-γ secretion leading to a significant improvement in survival [45]. IL-15 appears also as an interesting option because it promotes survival of dendritic cells and contributes to natural killer-dendritic cell interactions combined with antiapoptotic and function-enhancing properties on lymphocytes [46].

Compared to the above therapies, more data exists on the effects of intravenous immunoglobulins (IVIG) administration. Two preparations obtained from plasma of healthy donors are available: polyclonal standard IgG and IgM-enriched preparation. Both preparations are able to determine pathogen clearance but the higher killing on gram negative bacteria is obtained with IgM preparation because of specific proprieties of IgM fraction in neutralization and clearance of toxins [47, 48]. Beyond pathogen and toxin clearance, the pleiotropic effects on the immune response of endogenous immunoglobulins combined to the reduction of circulating IgG and IgM in nonsurvivors make the use of IVIG in patients with sepsis attractive [49, 50]. A recent meta-analysis of 18 trials in septic patients reveals a reduction in mortality using IVIG compared to control arm, in particular by using IgM-enriched formulation [49]. However, the heterogeneity in terms of type of preparation, dosage, and duration hinders the significance of the positive results observed. Unfortunately, in IVIG studies, neither patient's Ig plasma concentration nor other immunological markers have been ever used to identify patient at risk for immune failure. The use of specific biomarkers to identify patient who could benefit from immune therapy appears to be fundamental. In this light, the measurement of immunoglobulin plasma levels and their kinetic may be considered an appropriate guide to decide the use and to titrate the dose of IVIG [51].

5. Conclusions

The management of septic shock in patients suffering from infection caused by MDR/XDR bacteria is a true challenge. Taking into account the fact that multiresistant microorganisms are spreading worldwide, the probability to face such a patient is no longer an extraordinary event. The application of the Surviving Sepsis Campaign guidelines [52] and timely administration of antibiotics are often ineffective in these patients due to their frailty and poor immunological status [41]. Therefore, the use of adjunctive therapies for restoring immune function seems to be very promising but, unfortunately, sound evidences are not yet available. Waiting for the results of the ongoing trials, we believe that in patients with sepsis by MDR/XDR infections the capability of immune response should be carefully monitored by appropriate biomarkers.

References

[1] R. C. Bone, W. J. Sibbald, and C. L. Sprung, "The ACCP-SCCM consensus conference on sepsis and organ failure," *Chest*, vol. 101, no. 6, pp. 1481–1483, 1992.

[2] C. W. Seymour, V. X. Liu, and T. J. Iwashyna, "The third international consensus definitions for sepsis and septic shock (Sepsis-3)," *The Journal of the American Medical Association*, vol. 315, no. 8, pp. 762–774, 2016.

[3] D. Tang, R. Kang, C. B. Coyne, H. J. Zeh, and M. T. Lotze, "PAMPs and DAMPs: signal 0s that spur autophagy and immunity," *Immunological Reviews*, vol. 249, no. 1, pp. 158–175, 2012.

[4] R. S. Hotchkiss, L. L. Moldawer, S. M. Opal, K. Reinhart, I. R. Turnbull, and J. Vincent, "Sepsis and septic shock," *Nature Reviews Disease Primers*, vol. 2, p. 16045, 2016.

[5] R. S. Hotchkiss, G. Monneret, and D. Payen, "Sepsis-induced immunosuppression: from cellular dysfunctions to immunotherapy," *Nature Reviews Immunology*, vol. 13, no. 12, pp. 862–874, 2013.

[6] J. C. Mira, L. F. Gentile, B. J. Mathias et al., "Sepsis pathophysiology, chronic critical illness, and persistent inflammation-immunosuppression and catabolism syndrome," *Critical Care Medicine*, vol. 45, no. 2, pp. 253–262, 2016.

[7] A. Drewry, N. Samra, L. Skrupky, B. Fuller, S. Compton, and R. Hotchkiss, "Persistent lymphopenia after diagnosis of sepsis predicts mortality," *Shock*, vol. 42, no. 5, pp. 383–391, 2014.

[8] M. J. Delano, P. O. Scumpia, J. S. Weinstein et al., "MyD88-dependent expansion of an immature GR-1 +CD11b+ population induces T cell suppression and Th2 polarization in sepsis," *Journal of Experimental Medicine*, vol. 204, no. 6, pp. 1463–1474, 2007.

[9] G. Cornaglia, H. Giamarellou, and G. M. Rossolini, "Metallo-β-lactamases: a last frontier for β-lactams?" *The Lancet Infectious Diseases*, vol. 11, no. 5, pp. 381–393, 2011.

[10] A.-P. Magiorakos, A. Srinivasan, R. B. Carey et al., "Multidrug-resistant, extensively drug-resistant and pandrug-resistant bacteria: an international expert proposal for interim standard definitions for acquired resistance," *Clinical Microbiology and Infection*, vol. 18, no. 3, pp. 268–281, 2012.

[11] R. N. Jones, "Resistance patterns among nosocomial pathogens: trends over the past few years," *Chest*, vol. 119, no. 2, pp. 397S–404S, 2001.

[12] A. Tabah, D. Koulenti, K. Laupland et al., "Characteristics and determinants of outcome of hospital-acquired bloodstream infections in intensive care units: the EUROBACT international cohort study," *Intensive Care Medicine*, vol. 38, no. 12, pp. 1930–1945, 2012.

[13] N. Gupta, B. M. Limbago, J. B. Patel, and A. J. Kallen, "Carbapenem-resistant enterobacteriaceae: epidemiology and prevention," *Clinical Infectious Diseases*, vol. 53, no. 1, pp. 60–67, 2011.

[14] R. Ferrer, A. Artigas, D. Suarez et al., "Effectiveness of treatments for severe sepsis: a prospective, multicenter, observational study," *American Journal of Respiratory and Critical Care Medicine*, vol. 180, no. 9, pp. 861–866, 2009.

[15] M. Tumbarello, M. Sanguinetti, E. Montuori et al., "Predictors of mortality in patients with bloodstream infections caused by extended-spectrum-beta-lactamase-producing Enterobacteriaceae: importance of inadequate initial antimicrobial treatment," *Antimicrob Agents Chemother*, vol. 51, pp. 1987–1994, 2007.

[16] M. Bassetti, A. Carnelutti, and M. Peghin, "Patient specific risk stratification for antimicrobial resistance and possible treatment strategies in gram-negative bacterial infections," *Expert Review of Anti-infective Therapy*, vol. 15, no. 1, pp. 55–65, 2016.

[17] D. Weiskopf, B. Weinberger, and B. Grubeck-Loebenstein, "The aging of the immune system," *Transplant International*, vol. 22, no. 11, pp. 1041–1050, 2009.

[18] J. Chen, "Senescence and functional failure in hematopoietic stem cells," *Experimental Hematology*, vol. 32, no. 11, pp. 1025–1032, 2004.

[19] L. Ginaldi, M. De Martinis, A. D'Ostilio, L. Marini, M. F. Loreto, and D. Quaglino, "The immune system in the elderly: III. Innate immunity," *Immunologic Research*, vol. 20, no. 2, pp. 117–126, 1999.

[20] R. Nurieva, J. Wang, and A. Sahoo, "T-cell tolerance in cancer," *Immunotherapy*, vol. 5, no. 5, pp. 513–531, 2013.

[21] F. M. Marincola, E. M. Jaffee, D. J. Hicklin, and S. Ferrone, "Escape of human solid tumors from T-cell recognition: molecular mechanisms and functional significance," *Advances in Immunology*, vol. 74, pp. 181–273, 1999.

[22] D. Gabrilovich, "Mechanisms and functional significance of tumour-induced dendritic-cell defects," *Nature Reviews Immunology*, vol. 4, no. 12, pp. 941–952, 2004.

[23] H. E. Wasmuth, D. Kunz, E. Yagmur et al., "Patients with acute on chronic liver failure display 'sepsis-like' immune paralysis," *Journal of Hepatology*, vol. 42, no. 2, pp. 195–201, 2005.

[24] C. G. Antoniades, P. A. Berry, J. A. Wendon, and D. Vergani, "The importance of immune dysfunction in determining outcome in acute liver failure," *Journal of Hepatology*, vol. 49, no. 5, pp. 845–861, 2008.

[25] I.-M. Pantelidou, I. Galani, M. Georgitsi, G. L. Daikos, and E. J. Giamarellos-Bourboulis, "Interactions of klebsiella pneumoniae with the innate immune system vary in relation to clone and resistance phenotype," *Antimicrobial Agents and Chemotherapy*, vol. 59, no. 11, pp. 7036–7043, 2015.

[26] E. J. Giamarellos-Bourboulis, D. Plachouras, A. Tzivra et al., "Stimulation of innate immunity by susceptible and multidrug-resistant Pseudomonas aeruginosa: An in vitro and in vivo study," *Clinical and Experimental Immunology*, vol. 135, no. 2, pp. 240–246, 2004.

[27] E. Clark, A. O. Molnar, O. Joannes-Boyau, P. M. Honoré, L. Sikora, and S. M. Bagshaw, "High-volume hemofiltration for septic acute kidney injury: a systematic review and meta-analysis," *Critical Care*, vol. 18, no. 1, p. R7, 2014.

[28] E. M. J. Borthwick, C. J. Hill, K. S. Rabindranath, A. P. Maxwell, D. F. McAuley, and B. Blackwood, "High-volume haemofiltration for sepsis," *Cochrane Database of Systematic Reviews*, vol. 2013, no. 1, Article ID CD008075, 2013.

[29] T. Rimmele, D. Hayi-Slayman, M. Page, H. Rada, M. Monchi, and B. Allaouchiche, "Cascade hemofiltration: principle, first experimental data," *Annales Francaises D'Anesthesie Et De Reanimation*, vol. 28, no. 3, pp. 249–252, 2009.

[30] J.-P. Quenot, C. Binquet, C. Vinsonneau et al., "Very high volume hemofiltration with the Cascade system in septic shock patients," *Intensive Care Medicine*, vol. 41, no. 12, pp. 2111–2120, 2015.

[31] F. Zhou, Z. Peng, R. Murugan, and J. A. Kellum, "Blood purification and mortality in sepsis: a meta-analysis of randomized trials," *Critical Care Medicine*, vol. 41, no. 9, pp. 2209–2220, 2013.

[32] D. M. Payen, J. Guilhot, Y. Launey et al., "Early use of polymyxin B hemoperfusion in patients with septic shock due to peritonitis: a multicenter randomized control trial," *Intensive Care Medicine*, vol. 41, no. 6, pp. 975–984, 2015.

[33] D. N. Cruz, M. Antonelli, R. Fumagalli et al., "Early use of polymyxin B hemoperfusion in abdominal septic shock: the EUPHAS randomized controlled trial," *the Journal of the American Medical Association*, vol. 301, no. 23, pp. 2445–2452, 2009.

[34] D. J. Klein, D. Foster, C. A. Schorr, K. Kazempour, P. M. Walker, and R. P. Dellinger, "The EUPHRATES trial (evaluating the use of polymyxin B hemoperfusion in a randomized controlled trial of adults treated for endotoxemia and septic shock): study protocol for a randomized controlled trial," *Trials*, vol. 15, no. 1, article 218, 2014.

[35] E. Esteban, R. Ferrer, L. Alsina, and A. Artigas, "Immunomodulation in sepsis: the role of endotoxin removal by polymyxin B-immobilized cartridge," *Mediators of Inflammation*, vol. 2013, Article ID 507539, 12 pages, 2013.

[36] H. Mao, S. Yu, X. Yu et al., "Effect of coupled plasma filtration adsorption on endothelial cell function in patients with multiple organ dysfunction syndrome," *The International Journal of Artificial Organs*, vol. 32, no. 1, pp. 31–38, 2009.

[37] S. Livigni, G. Bertolini, C. Rossi et al., "Efficacy of coupled plasma filtration adsorption (CPFA) in patients with septic shock: a multicenter randomised controlled clinical trial," *BMJ Open*, vol. 4, no. 1, Article ID e003536, 2014.

[38] M. Haase, R. Bellomo, I. Baldwin et al., "Hemodialysis membrane with a high-molecular-weight cutoff and cytokine levels in sepsis complicated by acute renal failure: a phase 1 randomized trial," *American Journal of Kidney Diseases*, vol. 50, no. 2, pp. 296–304, 2007.

[39] L. Bo, F. Wang, J. Zhu, J. Li, and X. Deng, "Granulocyte-colony stimulating factor (G-CSF) and granulocyte-macrophage colony stimulating factor (GM-CSF) for sepsis: a meta-analysis," *Critical Care*, vol. 15, no. 1, article R58, 2011.

[40] C. Meisel, J. C. Schefold, R. Pschowski et al., "Granulocyte-macrophage colony-stimulating factor to reverse sepsis-associated immunosuppression: a double-blind, randomized, placebo-controlled multicenter trial," *American Journal of Respiratory and Critical Care Medicine*, vol. 180, no. 7, pp. 640–648, 2009.

[41] W. Döcke, F. Randow, U. Syrbe et al., "Monocyte deactivation in septic patients: restoration by IFN-γ treatment," *Nature Medicine*, vol. 3, no. 6, pp. 678–681, 1997.

[42] S. L. Topalian, F. S. Hodi, J. R. Brahmer et al., "Safety, activity, and immune correlates of anti-PD-1 antibody in cancer," *The New England Journal of Medicine*, vol. 366, no. 26, pp. 2443–2454, 2012.

[43] S. Sierro, P. Romero, and D. E. Speiser, "The CD4-like molecule LAG-3, biology and therapeutic applications," *Expert Opinion on Therapeutic Targets*, vol. 15, no. 1, pp. 91–101, 2011.

[44] A. Ma, R. Koka, and P. Burkett, "Diverse functions of IL-2, IL-15, and IL-7 in lymphoid homeostasis," *Annual Review of Immunology*, vol. 24, pp. 657–679, 2006.

[45] K. R. Kasten, P. S. Prakash, J. Unsinger et al., "Interleukin-7 (IL-7) treatment accelerates neutrophil recruitment through γδ T-cell IL-17 production in a murine model of sepsis," *Infection and Immunity*, vol. 78, no. 11, pp. 4714–4722, 2010.

[46] T. Hiromatsu, T. Yajima, T. Matsuguchi et al., "Overexpression of interleukin-15 protects against Escherichia coli-induced shock accompanied by inhibition of tumor necrosis factor-α-induced apoptosis," *Journal of Infectious Diseases*, vol. 187, no. 9, pp. 1442–1451, 2003.

[47] F. S. Rossmann, A. Kropec, D. Laverde, F. R. Saaverda, D. Wobser, and J. Huebner, "In vitro and in vivo activity of hyperimmune globulin preparations against multiresistant nosocomial pathogens," *Infection*, vol. 43, no. 2, pp. 169–175, 2015.

[48] M. Trautmann, T. K. Held, M. Susa et al., "Bacterial lipopolysaccharide (LPS)-specific antibodies in commercial human immunoglobulin preparations: Superior antibody content of an IgM- enriched product," *Clinical and Experimental Immunology*, vol. 111, no. 1, pp. 81–90, 1998.

[49] S. Busani, E. Damiani, I. Cavazzuti, A. Donati, and M. Girardis, "Intravenous immunoglobulin in septic shock: review of the mechanisms of action and meta-analysis of the clinical effectiveness," *Minerva Anestesiologica*, vol. 82, no. 5, pp. 559–572, 2016.

[50] J. F. Bermejo-Martín, A. Rodriguez-Fernandez, R. Herrán-Monge et al., "Immunoglobulins IgG1, IgM and IgA: A synergistic team influencing survival in sepsis," *Journal of Internal Medicine*, vol. 276, no. 4, pp. 404–412, 2014.

[51] S. Dietz, C. Lautenschläger, U. Müller-Werdan et al., "Serum IgG levels and mortality in patients with severe sepsis and septic shock: The SBITS data," *Medizinische Klinik Intensivmedizin und Notfallmedizin*, pp. 1–9, 2016.

[52] R. P. Dellinger, M. M. Levy, and A. Rhodes, "Surviving Sepsis Campaign: International Guidelines for Management of Sepsis and Septic Shock: 2016," *Intensive Care Medicine*, vol. 42, no. 1, pp. 580–637, 2017.

22

Inflammasomes in *Mycobacterium tuberculosis*-Driven Immunity

Sebastian Wawrocki and Magdalena Druszczynska

Division of Cell Immunology, Department of Immunology and Infectious Biology, Institute of Microbiology, Biotechnology and Immunology, Faculty of Biology and Environmental Protection, University of Lodz, Banacha 12/16, 90-237 Lodz, Poland

Correspondence should be addressed to Sebastian Wawrocki; sebastian.wawrocki@biol.uni.lodz.pl

Academic Editor: Maria L. Tornesello

The development of effective innate and subsequent adaptive host immune responses is highly dependent on the production of proinflammatory cytokines that increase the activity of immune cells. The key role in this process is played by inflammasomes, multimeric protein complexes serving as a platform for caspase-1, an enzyme responsible for proteolytic cleavage of IL-1β and IL-18 precursors. Inflammasome activation, which triggers the multifaceted activity of these two proinflammatory cytokines, is a prerequisite for developing an efficient inflammatory response against pathogenic *Mycobacterium tuberculosis* (*M.tb*). This review focuses on the role of NLRP3 and AIM2 inflammasomes in *M.tb*-driven immunity.

1. Introduction

Mycobacterium tuberculosis (*M.tb*), the causative agent of tuberculosis (TB), is a facultative intracellular bacterium that can survive and replicate within host macrophages [1, 2]. By avoiding critical components of macrophage-killing repertoire such as phagosome-lysosome fusion, phagosome acidification, activity of lysosomal enzymes or reactive oxygen, and nitrogen intermediates, *M.tb* evades killing and eradication [3]. In addition to phagocytic activity and ability to present antigens to T-cells, macrophages are key cells that regulate the antimycobacterial immune response via secreted cytokines. The functional capacity of macrophages in fighting infection depends on the degree of their activation. Inactive macrophages have limited ability to inhibit the growth of ingested mycobacteria, thereby serving as a safe life niche. After activation by interferon-gamma (IFN-γ) that is secreted by T-cells, macrophages acquire enhanced bactericidal strength enabling them to kill mycobacteria growing intracellularly [4]. The IFN-γ-driven antimicrobial properties of phagocytes are augmented by IL-18 and IL-1β, two proinflammatory cytokines processed by caspase-1 that are recruited to the inflammasomes, multiprotein platforms composed inter alia of intracellular sensors for pathogen- or host-derived molecules. IL-18, belonging to the IL-1 family, is produced by a wide range of immune and nonimmune cells [5–7]. The IL-18 precursor (pro-IL-18) is converted by caspase-1 into an active molecule, which forms a signaling complex with IL-18R [8, 9]. The receptor is composed of two chains: alpha (IL-18Ra) and beta (IL-18Rb). IL-18Rb is a signal transduction chain, essential for the formation of a high affinity complex and cell activation. The primary role of IL-18 is to induce IFN-γ production in cooperation with IL-12 or IL-15, although immunological effects exerted by IL-18 are dependent on the cytokine microenvironment. IL-18 is able to polarize T lymphocyte response towards Th1, induce T-cell proliferation, activate NK cells, enhance CD8(+) T cytolytic activity, and augment, apart from IFN-γ, the production of varied cytokines including tumor necrosis factor-α (TNF-α), interleukin- (IL-) 4, IL-5, IL-13, IL-17, and granulocyte-macrophage colony stimulating factor (GM-CSF) [8, 10, 11]. Thus, the multifaceted activity of IL-18 seems to play a prominent role in host defense against both extracellular and intracellular pathogens, including *M.tb*. However, an excessive IL-18 response might contribute to the induction of pathomechanisms leading to the damage of cells and tissues [12, 13]. Therefore, the proinflammatory activity of IL-18 is balanced by a constitutively secreted IL-18 binding protein (IL-18BP), whose binding to IL-18 decreases the production of IFN-γ and other cytokines, thereby reducing the risk of immunopathology [14]. The other inflammasome-dependent cytokine, IL-1β, which is mainly produced by monocytes and macrophages, plays an important role in inflammation and host immune response by affecting the function of various cells, either alone or in combination with other cytokines [15–17]. The activity of IL-1β is tightly regulated at the levels of its transcription and release. The production of IL-1β is regulated by several proteins including pyrin, PI-9 (the caspase-1 inhibitor proteinase inhibitor 9), and some CARD-containing proteins, which interfere with the recruitment of caspase-1 or directly neutralize its activity [18]. The effects of IL-1β are exerted via binding specific cell surface receptors—IL-1RI and IL-1RII [19]. As in the mature IL-18 form, active IL-1β is created after the proteolytic cleavage of its precursor by inflammasome-dependent caspase-1. Mature IL-1β plays important homeostatic functions in organisms and is implicated in the initiation of antimicrobial immunity via the induction of TNF-α and IL-6 release and polarization of Th17 response, which improve protective mucosal host defense by the secretion of IL-17 and IL-22 [20, 21]. The proinflammatory role of IL-1β in the resistance against *M.tb* has been confirmed by the observation that IL-1β or IL-1R knockout mice were found to be more susceptible to TB showing high mortality and increased bacterial burden in the lungs [22]. Additionally, double-deficient IL-1α/β mice had significantly larger granulomas, and their alveolar macrophages produced less nitric oxide than the cells from wild-type animals [23].

2. Inflammasomes—Mediators of Inflammation

Inflammation is an evolutionarily conserved protective response to noxious stimuli mounted by the innate immune system of the host. Immune deficiencies leading to insufficient development of inflammation processes may result in severe and recurrent infections, although overly intense activation of the inflammation cascade may be a cause of chronic systemic inflammatory disorders [24, 25]. The development of innate immunity starts from the recognition of conservative antigenic structures called DAMPs (danger-associated molecular patterns) and PAMPs (pathogen-associated molecular patterns) by pattern recognition receptors (PRRs) presented on the surface of first-line defense immune cells—macrophages and neutrophils. Activation of these receptors triggers a cascade of signals that results in the induction of multiple proinflammatory cytokines. The final step of the activation is the production of oxygen and nitrogen radicals, essential elements of the intracellular killing system. The secretion of these radicals is under strict control of a variety of monocyte/macrophage-derived cytokines such as IL-1β and IL-18. The key role in this process is played by structures called inflammasomes, multimeric protein complexes that control many aspects of innate and adaptive immunity. Through their cooperation with PRRs, inflammasomes activate host defense pathways resulting in clearance of various viral and bacterial infections, including those caused by mycobacteria. They function as an activating scaffold for inflammatory caspases that play an essential role in the maturation and secretion of proinflammatory cytokines as well as in pyroptosis, an inflammatory death of infected cells [26, 27]. Caspases are produced as inactive proenzymes that dimerize and undergo cleavage to form active molecules. Assembly into dimers, facilitated by various adaptor proteins binding to specific regions of their precursor forms—procaspases, is achieved through inflammasome formation [28]. Activated inflammatory caspases, typically caspase-1, lead to the generation of active IL-1β, IL-18, and IL-33 from their proprotein precursors. The mature cytokines are engaged in the recruitment of immune cells to the sites of infection and enhancement of the host's defensive responses against invading pathogens [26].

The inflammasomes are activated by multiple recognition receptors, which determine their structure and function. The canonical inflammasome sensors are nucleotide-binding domain–like (NLR) proteins and absent in melanoma 2–like (ALR) proteins and PYRIN. All of them have the ability to assemble inflammasomes and activate the inflammatory caspase-1.

The NLR family contains the NLRPs (or NALPs) and the IPAF (ICE-protease-activating factor) subfamilies [29, 30]. Each NLR molecule (NLRP1, NLRP3, NLRP6, NLRP7, NLRP12, or NAIP/NLRC4) recognizes specific ligands that activate the assembly of the inflammasome. NLR proteins consist of the conserved nucleotide-binding and oligomerization domain (NACHT or NOD), an N-terminal caspase recruitment domain (CARD) or pyrin domain (PYD) or baculovirus inhibitor repeat- (BIR-) like domain, and C-terminal leucine rich repeats (LRRs) [26, 31–35]. LRRs are responsible for the recognition of PAMPs, while the NACHT domain activates proinflammatory cytokine pathways via ATP-dependent oligomerization [26, 29]. The NLRP1 inflammasome has a CARD that activates caspase-1 [36, 37], and therefore the recruitment of ASC is not required to interact directly with procaspase-1. However, it has been shown that the participation of ASC in the process enhanced the activation of the enzyme. In contrast, NLRP3 contains no typical CARD domain that contributes to the activation of caspase-1 through the interaction of the PYD domain of NLRP3 with ASC [25]. Compared with NLRP1 and NLRP3, the IPAF protein does not contain a PYD but instead has a CARD that interacts directly with procaspase-1 without the need for ASC [38].

The members of the ALR group (known as the PYHIN family) are characterized by the presence of the pyrin domain (PYD) and one or two hematopoietic IFN-inducible nuclear antigens with 200 amino acid repeat (HIN-200) domains [26]. The PYD recruits proteins for the formation of inflammasomes, while the HIN domain recognizes and binds to DNA that can be found in the cytosol [26]. The best-known ALRs, absent in melanoma 2 (AIM2) and IFN-γ inducible protein 16 (IFI16), function as intracellular immune sensors that detect microbial DNA. The PYHIN proteins differ in their localization in the cell compartments; AIM2 can be found in the cytosol, whereas IFI16 is usually localized in the nucleus [39].

PYRIN, another canonical inflammasome-activating protein, is composed of an N-terminal PYD followed by two central B-box zinc finger and coiled-coil domains and in humans, a C-terminal B30.2/rfp/SPRY domain [40]. PYRIN associates through a PYD-PYD interaction with ASC protein, leading to its oligomerization that results in caspase-1 activation and interleukin-1β processing [40]. The activation of the PYRIN inflammasome is induced by the inactivation of RhoA GTPase by bacterial toxins [26, 41]. The process of activation has been detected in both mice and humans, suggesting that the B30.2/rfp/SPRY domain is not necessary for its initiation.

3. Inflammasomes in *Mycobacterium tuberculosis* Infection

The inflammasomes have been found to play important roles in host immunity against mycobacteria since it has been found that mice deficient in IL-18, IL-1β, or IL-1 receptor type I (IL-1R1) are more susceptible to *M.tb* infection [42–46]. Two inflammasomes, containing NLRP3 and AIM2 molecules as sensor proteins, were found to play a crucial role in *M.tb*-induced immunity (Figure 1) [20, 47, 48].

The NLRP3-containing inflammasome can be activated by a wide group of stimuli including whole mycobacterial cells, as well as viruses, fungi, environmental chemical irritants, and host-derived molecules such as extracellular ATP, fibrillar amyloid-β peptide, and hyaluronan [22, 49–53]. The NLRP3 inflammasome-activated responses result in the release of significant amounts of caspase-1, which leads to maturation and secretion of IL-1β and IL-18 and activation of pyroptosis [26]. The process of NLRP3 activation is triggered by at least two signals: (1) a priming signal eliciting the expression of NLRP3, pro-IL-1β, and pro-IL-18 genes after TLR stimulation and (2) an activation signal leading to the autocatalytic activation of procaspase-1 and proteolytic cleavage of pro-IL-1β and pro-IL-18. In most cell types, NLRP3 priming is a prerequisite for deubiquitination and assembly of the NLRP3 inflammasome. Relocalization of NLRP3 to the mitochondria is followed by the secretion of mitochondrial factors into the cytosol, potassium efflux through membrane ion channels, and release of cathepsin resulting in destabilization of lysosomal membranes. Apoptosis-associated speck-like protein (ASC) plays an important role in the formation of an effective inflammasome. ASC recruits procaspase-1 through its C-terminal caspase recruitment domain (CARD) and interacts with NLRP3 via its pyrin domain (PYD), serving as a bridge between these two molecules. The autocatalysis of procaspase-1 results in its cleavage and transformation into active caspase-1, which in turn cleaves the precursors of two proinflammatory cytokines, IL-1β and IL-18, leading to their secretion into the cytoplasm or induction [24, 25, 48, 54, 55]. However, the mechanism of triggering the NLRP3 inflammasome

complex activation cascade is still a subject of debate, and at least three models for the process have been proposed. The first suggestion is that the activation mechanism is associated with an efflux of potassium ions out of the cell and a reduction in their intracellular concentration. Such a model of activation occurs in monocytes/macrophages after stimulation with numerous stimuli including ATP, nigericin, bacterial cells, or their components [56, 57]. Recently, NEK7 protein, a member of the family of NIMA-related kinases (NEK proteins), has been identified as an NLRP3-binding protein that acts downstream of potassium efflux to regulate NLRP3 assembly and activation [58]. He et al. demonstrated that in the absence of NEK7, caspase-1 activation and IL-1β release were abrogated in response to signals that activate NLRP3 [58]. According to the second suggested mechanism, inflammasome activation is a result of lysosomal membrane damage and release of the phagosome content into cytosol [22, 59]. The third and most accepted model assumes that the induction of the NLRP3 inflammasome complex is caused by mitochondrial reactive oxygen species (ROS) [60–63]. The common final step in all of these models is the release of cathepsins into the cytosol leading to the lysosomal destabilization and conversion of procaspase-1 into a biologically active caspase-1 form. It should also be mentioned that formation of the NLRP3 inflammasome and cytokine release occur independently of transcriptional upregulation [64]. Juliana et al. showed that TLR4 signaling through MyD88 nontranscriptionally primed the NLRP3 inflammasome by its deubiquitination. The mechanism was dependent on mitochondria-derived reactive oxygen species and was involved in the secretion of cytokines, such as IL-18, and other inflammatory mediators such as high-mobility group protein 1 (HMGB1) [64, 65].

The AIM2 (absent in melanoma 2) receptor, possessing a C-terminal HIN-200 domain and an N-terminal pyrin domain (PYD), triggers AIM2 inflammasome activation, inflammatory cell death (pyroptosis), and release of IL-1β and IL-18 in response to cytosolic double-stranded (ds) DNA [66, 67]. Studies of gene-targeted AIM2-deficient mice have shown that AIM2 inflammasomes play a role in host defense against viruses and intracellular bacterial pathogens such as listeriae and mycobacteria [68–70]. AIM2 inflammasomes can be activated by DNA sequences having at least 80 base pairs in length in a sequence-independent manner [71, 72]. The HIN-200 and PYD domains take part in forming a complex, which is maintained in an inactive state during homeostasis [71, 73]. Binding of dsDNA to HIN-200 facilitates oligomerization of AIM2, and the resulting conformational change exposes the N-terminal PYD to allow the recruitment of the adaptor protein ASC. The CARD of ASC binds the CARD of procaspase-1, that forms an active AIM2 platform. Upon autoactivation, caspase-1 directs maturation and secretion of proinflammatory cytokines [48, 55, 66, 68, 74].

The latest data suggest that NLRP3- or ASC-deficient animals are characterized by impaired inflammasome formation and increased susceptibility to TB [20, 54, 68, 75, 76]. However, NLRP3$^{-/-}$ and ASC$^{-/-}$ mice produced IL-18 and IL-1β levels comparable to those of wild-type mice, which

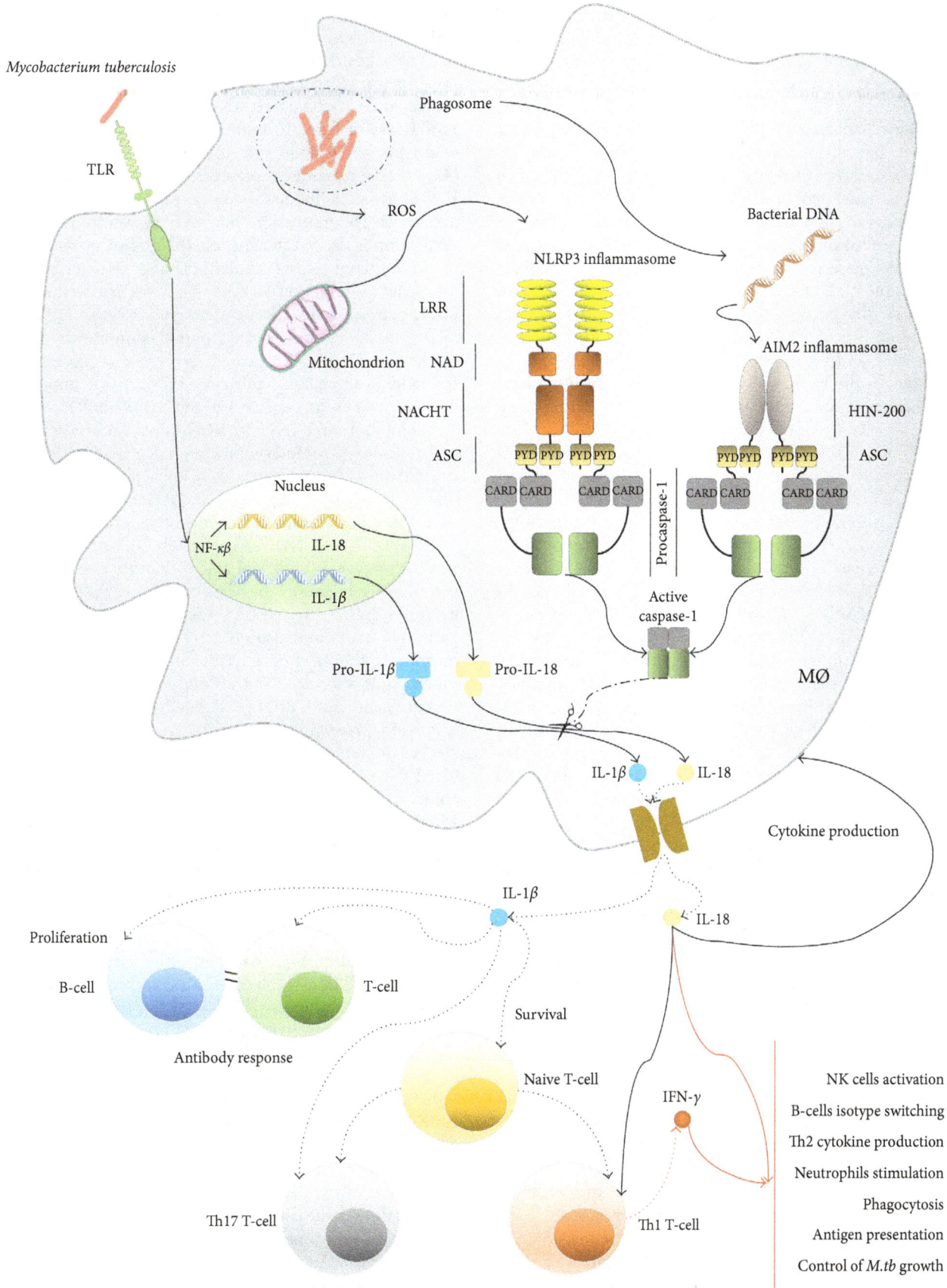

FIGURE 1: AIM2 and NLRP3 inflammasome activation pathways induced by *Mycobacterium tuberculosis*.

suggests the involvement of inflammasome-independent pathways in the secretion of these cytokines [21, 42, 47]. Many reports have demonstrated that a wide range of microorganisms are able to inhibit inflammasome activation and function. Viruses and many bacterial pathogens develop several mechanisms of repression of inflammasome folding; however, not all mechanisms are clearly understood. *Yersinia enterocolitica* produce YopE and YopT proteins that supress caspase-1 maturation, whereas YopK protein of *Y. pseudotuberculosis* binds to the type III secretion system, thereby preventing the recognition of the pathogen by host cell inflammasome. *Pseudomonas aeruginosa* mediates suppression of NLRC4-inflammasome by secreting ExoU and ExoS effectors, whose mechanism of action still needs elucidation. Virulent *M.tb* can inhibit the formation of AIM2 and NLRP3 inflammasomes both directly and indirectly, but the factors responsible for the inhibition have not been recognized thus far. One of the likely mechanisms is the activity of Zn-metalloprotease called ZMP1, which inhibits the activation of NLRP3 inflammasome and, as a consequence, leads to the reduction of caspase-1 activity [77–79]. Master et al. showed that infection of mice macrophages with zmp1-deleted *M.tb* induces activation of the inflammasome, resulting in enhanced maturation of phagosomes, increased IL-1β secretion, and better *M.tb* clearance in lungs [79]. It is probable that *M.tb* is able to restrain the activation of other inflammasome types, but evidence is needed to confirm this hypothesis. In addition to the induction of inflammasome activation via PRRs, *M.tb* antigens can modulate other innate immunity-associated functions. One recently identified protein, tyrosine phosphatase (Ptp) A, enters the nucleus of the host cells and regulates the transcription of many host genes involved in the mechanisms of innate immunity, cell proliferation, and migration [80]. The enzyme is also able to dephosphorylate certain host proteins (p-JNK, p-p38, and p-VPS33B), leading to inhibition of phagosome-lysosome fusion and blocking the acidification of phagosomes. Both activities are crucial for *M.tb* virulence in vivo through the promotion of *M.tb*'s intracellular survival in macrophages [80]. *M.tb* often escapes from the phagosome within a few days of the invasion of the host organism and creates difficulties in assessing the potential role of inflammasomes during the initial stages of mycobacterial infection. Moreover, the evaluation of IL-1β and IL-18 produced as a result of inflammasome activation is inadequate in revealing the significance of formed multiprotein platforms in the course of developing infection. The initiation of phagocytosis causes a decrease in the levels of potassium ions in macrophages, which have been found to be one of the crucial inflammasome activators during infections with *M.tb* and nontuberculous mycobacteria [81]. Other regulators such as thioredoxin-interacting proteins, activated by the increase in reactive oxygen species in cytosol, are thought to have minor effect on the formation of inflammasomes in *M.tb* infection [47]. The signaling cascade can also be activated by the mycobacterial type VII secretion system (ESX-1), which is responsible for translocation of extracellular DNA (eDNA) in cytosol and the production of IFN-β. Many studies have demonstrated that, at the molecular level, IFN-β regulates the AIM2 inflammasome activity [82, 83]. Some ESX-1-deficient *M. smegmatis* mutants have been shown to possess limited capacity for AIM2 inflammasome activation. However, in contrast to nontuberculous mycobacteria (NTM), *M.tb* mutants lacking ESX-1 system failed to inhibit AIM2 formation, while the wild-type strain inhibited the inflammasome activation [47, 84]. The suggested mechanism of inhibition involves the IFN-β-mediated induction of IL-10, which in turn suppresses IL-1β production [85, 86]. However, further investigation is needed to elucidate the molecular mechanism of *M.tb*-driven AIM2 inhibition and its consequences for bacterial virulence. *M. bovis* BCG vaccine strain, which does not possess the ESX-1 system, poorly activates multiple NLR and inflammasome complex components including caspase-1 [87]. The bacilli repress the expression of thioredoxin-interacting protein (TXNIP), an antioxidant inhibitor recruiting caspase-1 to the NLRP3 inflammasome. The inhibition of TXNIP by BCG limits NLRP3 activation and restrains pyroptosis following mycobacterial infection. Proinflammatory responses to BCG bacilli was found to be driven primarily through Toll-like receptors (TLRs), since BCG does not activate expression of genes downstream of TLR/MyD88- and NOD-2-driven NF-$\kappa\beta$ and AP-1 pathways. However, BCG is still able to induce moderate IL-1β secretion as measured by transcription of inflammasome network genes [87, 88]. Understanding BCG-induced pathways of inflammasome activation can be helpful in improving the existing vaccine or developing new antituberculous vaccines. The recombinant BCG ΔureC::hly vaccine candidate (VPM1002) has been shown to induce improved protection against TB over the parental BCG strain [4]. Saiga et al. demonstrated that VPM1002 activated the AIM2 inflammasome and caspase-1 through the ability of listeriolysin to perforate phagosome membranes, which is encoded by the *hly* gene integrated into BCG genome [4]. The perforation facilitates the release of mycobacterial DNA into the cytosol, in a way that is similar to the ESX-1 system of *M.tb*. Mice vaccinated with VPM1002 showed increased production of IL-1β and IL-18 as well as induction of the stimulator of IFN genes (STING)-dependent autophagy, which promotes delivery of BCG antigens to MHC molecules and improves their presentation to T-cells [4].

Apart from direct induction of proinflammatory cytokine secretion, the activated caspase-1 triggers the pyroptotic death of infected cells. The cytosolic protein Gasdermin D (GSDMS) is a key mediator of this process. The cleavage of GSDMD by activated caspase-1 results in the release of its N-terminal fragment (GSDMD-NT), which forms pores in the plasma membrane of the infected cell leading to the elimination of the pathogen [26, 89–91]. The pores disrupt cell membrane integrity allowing water influx, cell swelling, and osmotic lysis together with an efflux of small molecules, including proinflammatory cytokines. GSDMD-NT is able to kill both cell-free and intracellular microorganisms and can be thought as a new antibacterial agent. However, it is still not known whether GSDMD-NT is able to permeabilize the membrane of the phagosomes and kill the bacteria hidden within these organelles. So far, there is no evidence of such a function. It is probable that the inhibition of bacterial growth is mediated by other caspase components. Using single-cell analysis, Thurston et al. demonstrated that the replication of cytosolic *Salmonella typhimurium* was inhibited independently or prior to the onset of cell death, suggesting that caspase-1 and caspase-11 might have additional functions in the elimination of cytosolic bacteria [92].

4. Therapeutics Targeting Inflammasome Pathways

Biologic agents interfering with inflammasome activation may provide new means of therapeutical interventions for many diseases. These agents may target either upstream processes of inflammasome regulation or downstream IL-1 signaling [41]. Inappropriate activity of inflammasomes has been found to be involved in the pathogenesis of certain autoinflammatory skin disorders such as cryopyrin-associated periodic syndrome (CAPS) or familial Mediterranean fever (FMF) as well as a number of chronic inflammatory diseases such as multiple sclerosis, gouty arthritis (gout), atherosclerosis, type 2 diabetes, and obesity [29, 93, 94]. Moreover, mechanisms controlling the NLRP3 inflammasome arrangement have also been implicated in the development of lung, kidney, and liver diseases [95–97]. Colchicine, a drug used for treatment of gout, has been shown to inhibit macrophage NLRP3 inflammasome assembly and activation in vitro and in vivo [98]. Colchicine blocks monosodium urate crystal-induced NLRP3 inflammasome-driven caspase-1 activation and IL-1β processing and release, suppresses the expression of genes involved in cell regulation, and inhibits IL-1-induced L-selectin expression on neutrophils [99]. Other therapeutics that target inflammasome-driven end products include VX-765 (inhibitor of caspase-1 activation), Anakinra (recombinant form of IL-1 receptor antagonist), Canakinumab (monoclonal antibody against IL-1β), Rilonacept (IL-1 inhibitor), IL-18 binding protein, and anti-IL-18 receptors antibodies [8, 41, 100]. A number of new molecules have been identified as inhibitors of IL-1β processing (glyburide, parthenolide, CRID3, auranofin, isoliquiritigenin, β-hydroxybutyrate, and MCC950); however, confirming their clinical utility will require additional time and research [24].

5. Conclusion

Inflammasomes have been implicated as specialized signaling platforms critical for the regulation of both innate immunity and inflammation. *M.tb* has been shown to modulate the host innate immune response by delaying cell death systems of the host, thereby facilitating its own proliferation. Understanding the molecular mechanisms of inflammasome activation during intracellular pathogen infections such as with *M.tb*, and the evasive mechanisms employed by this evading pathogen, may lead to development of more potent therapies to combat the proliferation of *M.tb*.

Acknowledgments

This work was supported by the National Science Centre Grant nos. 2015/19/N/NZ6/01385 and 2016/21/B/NZ7/01771.

References

[1] A. Welin, D. Eklund, O. Stendahl, and M. Lerm, "Human macrophages infected with a high burden of ESAT-6-expressing *M. tuberculosis* undergo caspase-1- and cathepsin B-independent necrosis," *PLoS One*, vol. 6, no. 5, p. e20302, 2011.

[2] T. R. Lerner, S. Borel, and M. G. Gutierrez, "The innate immune response in human *tuberculosis*," *Cellular Microbiology*, vol. 17, no. 9, pp. 1277–1285, 2015.

[3] V. C. Korb, A. A. Chuturgoon, and D. Moodley, "*Mycobacterium tuberculosis*: manipulator of protective immunity," *International Journal of Molecular Sciences*, vol. 17, no. 3, p. 131, 2016.

[4] H. Saiga, N. Nieuwenhuizen, M. Gengenbacher et al., "The recombinant BCG ΔureC::hly vaccine targets the AIM2 inflammasome to induce autophagy and inflammation," *Journal of Infectious Diseases*, vol. 211, no. 11, pp. 1831–1841, 2015.

[5] H. E. Barksby, S. R. Lea, P. M. Preshaw, and J. J. Taylor, "The expanding family of interleukin-1 cytokines and their role in destructive inflammatory disorders," *Clinical & Experimental Immunology*, vol. 149, no. 2, pp. 217–225, 2007.

[6] D. Novick, S. Kim, G. Kaplanski, and C. A. Dinarello, "Interleukin-18, more than a Th1 cytokine," *Seminars in Immunology*, vol. 25, no. 6, pp. 439–448, 2013.

[7] C. A. Dinarello and F. Giamila, "Interleukin-18 and host defense against infection," *Journal of Infectious Diseases*, vol. 187, no. 2, pp. 370–384, 2003.

[8] C. A. Dinarello, D. Novick, S. Kim, and G. Kaplanski, "Interleukin-18 and IL-18 binding protein," *Frontiers in Immunology*, vol. 4, pp. 1–10, 2013.

[9] C. A. Dinarello, "Interleukin-1, interleukin-1 receptors and interleukin-1 receptor antagonist," *International Reviews of Immunology*, vol. 16, no. 5-6, pp. 457–499, 1998.

[10] R. Gutzmer, K. Langer, S. Mommert, M. Wittmann, A. Kapp, and T. Werfel, "Human dendritic cells express the IL-18R and are chemoattracted to IL-18," *Journal of Immunology*, vol. 171, no. 12, pp. 6363–6371, 2003.

[11] S. Gardella, C. Andrei, S. Costigliolo, A. Poggi, M. R. Zocchi, and A. Rubartelli, "Interleukin-18 synthesis and secretion by dendritic cells are modulated by interaction with antigen-specific T cells," *Journal of Leukocyte Biology*, vol. 66, no. 2, pp. 237–241, 1999.

[12] D. V. Pechkovsky, T. Goldmann, E. Vollmer, J. Müller-Quernheim, and G. Zissel, "Interleukin-18 expression by alveolar epithelial cells type II in tuberculosis and sarcoidosis," *FEMS Immunology & Medical Microbiology*, vol. 46, no. 1, pp. 30–38, 2006.

[13] S. El-Masry, M. Lotfy, W. Nasif, I. El-Kady, and M. Al-Badrawy, "Elevated serum level of interleukin (IL)-18, interferon (IFN)-γ and soluble fas in patients with pulmonary complications in tuberculosis," *Acta Microbiologica et Immunologica Hungarica*, vol. 54, no. 1, pp. 65–67, 2007.

[14] K. Nakanishi, T. Yoshimoto, H. Tsutsui, and H. Okamura, "Interleukin-18 regulates both Th1 and Th2 responses," *Annual Review of Immunology*, vol. 19, no. 1, pp. 423–474, 2001.

[15] N. A. Turner, "Effects of interleukin-1 on cardiac fibroblast function: relevance to post-myocardial infarction remodeling," *Vascular Pharmacology*, vol. 60, no. 1, pp. 1–7, 2014.

[16] C. Duque, L. Arroyo, H. Ortega et al., "Different responses of human mononuclear phagocyte populations to *Mycobacterium tuberculosis*," *Tuberculosis*, vol. 94, no. 2, pp. 111–122, 2014.

[17] G. Lopez-Castejon and D. Brough, "Understanding the mechanism of IL-1β secretion," *Cytokine & Growth Factor Reviews*, vol. 22, no. 4, pp. 189–195, 2011.

[18] L. D. Church, G. P. Cook, and M. F. McDermott, "Primer: inflammasomes and interleukin 1β in inflammatory disorders," *Nature Clinical Practice Rheumatology*, vol. 4, no. 1, pp. 34–42, 2008.

[19] M. Ricote, I. García-Tuñón, F. R. Bethencourt, B. Fraile, R. Paniagua, and M. Royuela, "Interleukin-1 (IL-1alpha and IL-1beta) and its receptors (IL-1RI, IL-1RII, and IL-1Ra) in prostate carcinoma," *Cancer*, vol. 100, no. 7, pp. 1388–1396, 2004.

[20] F. L. van de Veerdonk, M. G. Netea, C. A. Dinarello, and L. A. B. Joosten, "Inflammasome activation and IL-1β and IL-18 processing during infection," *Trends in Immunology*, vol. 32, no. 3, pp. 110–116, 2011.

[21] M. G. Netea, A. Simon, F. van de Veerdonk, B.-J. Kullberg, J. W. M. Van der Meer, and L. A. B. Joosten, "IL-1β processing in host defense: beyond the inflammasomes," *PLoS One*, vol. 6, no. 2, p. e10000661, 2010.

[22] A. Halle, V. Hornung, G. C. Petzold et al., "The NALP3 inflammasome is involved in the innate immune response to amyloid-beta," *Nature Immunology*, vol. 9, no. 8, pp. 857–865, 2008.

[23] H. Yamada, S. Mizumo, R. Horai, Y. Iwakura, and I. Sugawara, "Protective role of interleukin-1 in mycobacterial infection in IL-1 alpha/beta double-knockout mice," *Laboratory Investigation*, vol. 80, no. 5, pp. 759–767, 2000.

[24] H. Guo, J. B. Callaway, and J. P. Ting, "Inflammasomes: mechanism of action, role in disease, and therapeutics," *Nature Medicine*, vol. 21, no. 7, pp. 677–687, 2015.

[25] G. dos Santos, M. A. Kutuzov, and K. M. Ridge, "The inflammasome in lung diseases," *American Journal of Physiology-Lung Cellular and Molecular Physiology*, vol. 303, no. 8, pp. 627–633, 2012.

[26] X. Liu and J. Lieberman, "A mechanistic understanding of pyroptosis: the fiery death triggered by invasive infection," *Advances in Immunology*, vol. 135, pp. 81–117, 2017.

[27] D. R. McIlwain, T. Berger, and T. W. Mak, "Caspase functions in cell death and disease," *Cold Spring Harbor Perspectives in Biology*, vol. 5, no. 4, p. a008656, 2013.

[28] F. Martinon, K. Burns, and J. Tschopp, "The inflammasome: a molecular platform triggering activation of inflammatory caspases and processing of proIL-beta," *Molecular Cell*, vol. 10, no. 2, pp. 417–426, 2002.

[29] A. J. S. Choi and S. W. Ryter, "Inflammasomes: molecular regulation and implications for metabolic and cognitive diseases," *Molecules and Cells*, vol. 37, no. 6, pp. 441–448, 2014.

[30] B. K. Davis, H. Wen, and J. P. Ting, "The inflammasome NLRs in immunity, inflammation, and associated diseases," *Annual Review of Immunology*, vol. 29, no. 1, pp. 707–735, 2011.

[31] J. P. Ting, R. C. Lovering, E. S. Alnemri et al., "The NLR gene family: a standard nomenclature," *Immunity*, vol. 28, no. 3, pp. 285–287, 2008.

[32] Y. K. Kim, J. S. Shin, and M. H. Nahm, "NOD-like receptors in infection, immunity, and diseases," *Yonsei Medical Journal*, vol. 57, no. 1, pp. 5–14, 2016.

[33] J. Bertin, W. J. Nir, C. M. Fischer et al., "Human CARD4 protein is a novel CED-4/Apaf-1 cell death family member that activates NF-kB," *Journal of Biological Chemistry*, vol. 274, no. 19, pp. 12955–12958, 1999.

[34] N. Roy, M. S. Mahadevan, M. McLean et al., "The gene for neuronal apoptosis inhibitory protein is partially deleted in individuals with spinal muscular atrophy," *Cell*, vol. 80, no. 1, pp. 167–178, 1995.

[35] K. Schroder and J. Tschopp, "The inflammasomes," *Cell*, vol. 140, no. 6, pp. 821–832, 2010.

[36] B. Faustin, L. Lartigue, J. M. Bruey et al., "Reconstituted NALP1 inflammasome reveals two-step mechanism of caspase-1 activation," *Molecular Cell*, vol. 25, no. 5, pp. 713–724, 2007.

[37] J. Chavarría-Smith and R. E. F. Vance, "The NLRP1 inflammasomes," *Immunology Reviews*, vol. 265, no. 1, pp. 33-34, 2015.

[38] J. L. Poyet, S. M. Srinivasula, M. Tnani, M. Razmara, T. Fernandes-Alnemri, and E. S. Alnemri, "Identification of Ipaf, a human caspase-1-activating protein related to Apaf-1," *Journal of Biological Chemistry*, vol. 276, no. 30, pp. 28309–28313, 2001.

[39] J. A. Cridland, E. Z. Curley, M. N. Wykes et al., "The mammalian PYHIN gene family: phylogeny, evolution and expression," *BMC Evolutionary Biology*, vol. 12, no. 1, pp. 140–156, 2012.

[40] J.-W. Yu, J. Wu, Z. Zhang et al., "Cryopyrin and pyrin activate caspase-1, but not NF-κβ, via ASC oligomerization," *Cell Death and Differentiation*, vol. 13, no. 2, pp. 236–249, 2006.

[41] C. de Torre-Minguela, P. M. de Castillo, and P. Pelegrin, "The NLRP3 and pyrin inflammasomes: implications in the pathophysiology of autoinflammatory diseases," *Frontiers in Immunology*, vol. 8, p. 43, 2017.

[42] K. D. Mayer-Barber, D. L. Barber, K. Shenderov et al., "Cutting edge: caspase-1 independent IL-1β production is critical for host resistance to *Mycobacterium tuberculosis* and does not require TLR signaling *in vivo*," *Journal of Immunology*, vol. 184, no. 7, pp. 3326–3330, 2010.

[43] I. Sugawara, H. Yamada, H. Kaneko, S. Mizuno, K. Takeda, and S. Akira, "Role of interleukin-18 (IL-18) in mycobacterial infection in IL-18-gene-disrupted mice," *Infection and Immunity*, vol. 67, no. 5, pp. 2585–2589, 1999.

[44] I. Sugawara, H. Yamada, S. Hua, and S. Mizuno, "Role of interleukin (IL)-1 type 1 receptor in mycobacterial infection," *Microbiology and Immunology*, vol. 45, no. 11, pp. 743–750, 2001.

[45] C. M. Fremond, D. Togbe, E. Doz et al., "IL-1 receptor-mediated signal is an essential component of MyD88-dependent innate response to *Mycobacterium tuberculosis* infection," *Journal of Immunology*, vol. 179, no. 2, pp. 1178–1189, 2007.

[46] B. E. Schneider, D. Korbel, K. Hagens et al., "A role for IL-18 in protective immunity against *Mycobacterium tuberculosis*," *European Journal of Immunology*, vol. 40, no. 2, pp. 396–405, 2010.

[47] V. Briken, S. E. Ahlbrand, and S. Shah, "*Mycobacterium tuberculosis* and the host cell inflammasome: a complex relationship," *Frontiers in Cellular and Infection Microbiology*, vol. 9, no. 3, p. 62, 2013.

[48] R. Wassermann, M. F. Gulen, C. Sala et al., "*Mycobacterium tuberculosis* differentially activates cGAS- and inflammasome-dependent intracellular immune responses through ESX-1," *Cell Host Microbe*, vol. 17, no. 6, pp. 799–810, 2015.

[49] O. Gross, H. Poeck, M. Bscheider et al., "Syk kinase signalling couples to the Nlrp3 inflammasome for anti-fungal host defence," *Nature*, vol. 459, no. 7245, pp. 433–436, 2009.

[50] J. A. Duncan, X. Gao, M. T. Huang et al., "*Neisseria gonorrhoeae* activates the proteinase cathepsin B to mediate the signaling activities of the NLRP3 and ASC-containing inflammasome," *Journal of Immunology*, vol. 182, no. 10, pp. 6460–6469, 2009.

[51] S. Mariathasan, D. S. Weiss, K. Newton et al., "Cryopyrin activates the inflammasome in response to toxins and ATP," *Nature*, vol. 440, no. 7081, pp. 228–232, 2006.

[52] K. Yamasaki, J. Muto, K. R. Taylor et al., "NLRP3/cryopyrin is necessary for interleukin-1beta (IL-1beta) release in response to hyaluronan, an endogenous trigger of inflammation in response to injury," *Journal of Biological Chemistry*, vol. 284, no. 19, pp. 12762–12771, 2009.

[53] H. Watanabe, O. Gaide, V. Pétrilli et al., "Activation of the IL-1beta-processing inflammasome is involved in contact hypersensitivity," *Journal of Investigative Dermatology*, vol. 127, no. 8, pp. 1956–1963, 2007.

[54] D. Eklund, A. Welin, H. Andersson et al., "Human gene variants linked to enhanced NLRP3 activity limit intra-macrophage growth of *Mycobacterium tuberculosis*," *Journal of Infectious Diseases*, vol. 209, no. 5, pp. 749–753, 2014.

[55] P. J. Shaw, M. F. McDermott, and T. D. Kanneganti, "Inflammasomes and autoimmunity," *Trends in Molecular Medicine*, vol. 17, no. 2, pp. 57–64, 2011.

[56] V. Pétrilli, S. Papin, C. Dostert, A. Mayor, F. Martinon, and J. Tschopp, "Activation of the NALP3 inflammasome is triggered by low intracellular potassium concentration," *Cell Death and Differentiation*, vol. 14, no. 9, pp. 1583–1589, 2007.

[57] R. Muñoz-Planillo, L. Franchi, L. S. Miller, and G. Núñez, "A critical role for hemolysins and bacterial lipoproteins in *Staphylococcus aureus*-induced activation of the Nlrp3 inflammasome," *Journal of Immunology*, vol. 183, no. 6, pp. 3942–3948, 2009.

[58] Y. He, M. Y. Zeng, D. Yang, B. Motro, and G. Núñez, "NEK7 is an essential mediator of NLRP3 activation downstream of potassium efflux," *Nature*, vol. 530, no. 7590, pp. 354–369, 2016.

[59] V. Hornung, F. Bauernfeind, and A. Halle, "Silica crystals and aluminum salts activate the NALP3 inflammasome through phagosomal destabilization," *Nature Immunology*, vol. 9, no. 8, pp. 847–856, 2008.

[60] M. E. Heid, P. A. Keyel, C. Kamga et al., "Mitochondrial reactive oxygen species induces NLRP3-dependent lysosomal damage and inflammasome activation," *Journal of Immunology*, vol. 191, no. 10, pp. 5230–5238, 2013.

[61] M. T. Sorbara and S. E. Girardin, "Mitochondrial ROS fuel the inflammasome," *Cell Research*, vol. 21, no. 4, pp. 558–560, 2011.

[62] R. Zhou, A. S. Yazdi, P. Menu, and J. Tschopp, "A role for mitochondria in NLRP3 inflammasome activation," *Nature*, vol. 469, no. 7329, pp. 221–225, 2011.

[63] K. Nakahira, J. A. Haspel, V. A. Rathinam et al., "Autophagy proteins regulate innate immune responses by inhibiting the release of mitochondrial DNA mediated by the NALP3 inflammasome," *Nature Immunology*, vol. 12, no. 3, pp. 222–230, 2011.

[64] H. M. Lee, J. J. Kim, H. J. Kim et al., "Upregulated NLRP3 inflammasome activation in patients with type 2 diabetes," *Diabetes*, vol. 62, no. 1, pp. 194–204, 2013.

[65] C. Juliana, T. Fernandes-Alnemri, S. Kang, A. Farias, F. Qin, and E. S. Alnemri, "Non transcriptional priming and deubiquitination regulate NLRP3 inflammasome activation," *Journal of Biological Chemistry*, vol. 287, no. 43, pp. 36617–36622, 2012.

[66] V. Hornung, A. Ablasser, M. Charrel-Dennis et al., "AIM2 recognizes cytosolic dsDNA and forms a caspase-1-activating inflammasome with ASC," *Nature*, vol. 458, no. 7237, pp. 514–518, 2009.

[67] T. Fernandes-Alnemri, J. W. Yu, P. Datta, J. Wu, and E. S. Alnemri, "AIM2 activates the inflammasome and cell death in response to cytoplasmic DNA," *Nature*, vol. 458, no. 7237, pp. 509–513, 2009.

[68] H. Saiga, S. Kitada, Y. Shimada et al., "Critical role of AIM2 in *Mycobacterium tuberculosis* infection," *International Immunology*, vol. 24, no. 10, pp. 637–644, 2012.

[69] V. A. K. Rathinam, Z. Jiang, S. N. Waggoner et al., "The AIM2 inflammasome is essential for host-defense against cytosolic bacteria and DNA viruses," *Nature Immunology*, vol. 11, no. 5, pp. 395–402, 2010.

[70] J.-D. Sauer, C. E. Witte, J. Zemansky, B. Hanson, P. Lauer, and D. A. Portnoy, "*Listeria monocytogenes* triggers AIM2-mediated pyroptosis upon infrequent bacteriolysis in the macrophage cytosol," *Cell Host & Microbe*, vol. 7, no. 5, pp. 412–419, 2010.

[71] T. L. Roberts, A. Idris, J. A. Dunn et al., "HIN-200 proteins regulate caspase activation in response to foreign cytoplasmic DNA," *Science*, vol. 323, no. 5917, pp. 1057–1060, 2009.

[72] T. Jin, A. Perry, J. Jiang et al., "Structures of the HIN domain: DNA complexes reveal ligand binding and activation mechanisms of the AIM2 inflammasome and IFI16 receptor," *Immunity*, vol. 36, no. 4, pp. 561–571, 2012.

[73] T. Jin, A. Perry, P. Smith, J. Jiang, and T. S. Xiao, "Structure of the absent in melanoma 2 (AIM2) pyrin domain provides insights into the mechanisms of AIM2 autoinhibition and inflammasome assembly," *Journal of Biological Chemistry*, vol. 288, no. 19, pp. 13225–13235, 2013.

[74] S. M. Man, R. Kark, and T. D. Kanneganti, "AIM2 inflammasome in infection, cancer, and autoimmunity: role in DNA sensing, inflammation, and innate immunity," *European Journal of Immunology*, vol. 46, no. 2, pp. 269–280, 2016.

[75] R. P. Lai, G. Meintjes, K. A. Wilkinson et al., "HIV-tuberculosis-associated immune reconstitution inflammatory syndrome is characterized by Toll-like receptor and inflammasome signaling," *Nature Communications*, vol. 6, p. 8451, 2015.

[76] W. C. Chao, C. L. Yen, and Y. H. Wu, "Increased resistin may suppress reactive oxygen species production and inflammasome activation in type 2 diabetic patients with pulmonary tuberculosis infection," *Microbes and Infection*, vol. 17, no. 3, pp. 195–204, 2015.

[77] M. Galle, P. Schotte, M. Haegman et al., "The *Pseudomonas aeruginosa* type III secretion system plays a dual role in the regulation of caspase-1 mediated IL-1beta maturation," *Journal of Cellular and Molecular Medicine*, vol. 12, no. 5, pp. 1767–1776, 2008.

[78] I. E. Brodsky, N. W. Palm, S. Sadanand et al., "A *Yersinia* effector protein promotes virulence by preventing inflammasome recognition of the type III secretion system," *Cell Host & Microbe*, vol. 7, no. 5, pp. 376–387, 2010.

[79] S. S. Master, S. K. Rampini, A. S. Davis et al., "*Mycobacterium tuberculosis* prevents inflammasome activation," *Cell Host & Microbe*, vol. 3, no. 4, pp. 224–232, 2008.

[80] J. Wang, P. Ge, L. Qiang et al., "The mycobacterial phosphatase PtpA regulates the expression of host genes and promotes cell proliferation," *Nature Communications*, vol. 8, no. 1, p. 244, 2017.

[81] T. D. Kanneganti, M. Lamkanfi, and Y. G. Kim, "Pannexin-1-mediated recognition of bacterial molecules activates the cryopyrin inflammasome independent of Toll-like receptor signalling," *Immunity*, vol. 26, no. 4, pp. 433–443, 2007.

[82] J. W. Jones, N. Kayagaki, P. Broz et al., "Absent in melanoma 2 is required for innate immune recognition of *Francisella tularensis*," *Proceedings of the National Academy of Sciences of the United States of America*, vol. 107, no. 21, pp. 9771–9776, 2010.

[83] K. Tsuchiya, H. Hara, I. Kawamura et al., "Involvement of absent in melanoma 2 in inflammasome activation in macrophages infected with *Listeria monocytogenes*," *Journal of Immunology*, vol. 185, no. 2, pp. 1186–1195, 2010.

[84] S. Shah, A. Bohsali, S. E. Ahlbrand et al., "Cutting edge: *Mycobacterium tuberculosis* but not nonvirulent mycobacteria inhibits IFN-β and AIM2 inflammasome-dependent IL-1β production via its ESX-1 secretion system," *Journal of Immunology*, vol. 191, no. 7, pp. 3514–3518, 2013.

[85] K. D. Mayer-Barber, B. B. Andrade, D. L. Barber et al., "Innate and adaptive interferons suppress IL-1α and IL-1β production by distinct pulmonary myeloid subsets during *Mycobacterium tuberculosis* infection," *Immunity*, vol. 35, no. 6, pp. 1023–1034, 2011.

[86] A. Novikov, M. Cardone, R. Thompson et al., "*Mycobacterium tuberculosis* triggers host type I IFN signaling to regulate IL-1β production in human macrophages," *Journal of Immunology*, vol. 187, no. 5, pp. 2540–2537, 2011.

[87] H. B. Huante, S. Gupta, V. C. Calderon et al., "Differential inflammasome activation signatures following intracellular infection of human macrophages with *Mycobacterium bovis* BCG or *Trypanosoma cruzi*," *Tuberculosis*, vol. 110, pp. S35–S44, 2016.

[88] A. Dorhoi, G. Nouailles, S. Jörg et al., "Activation of the NLRP3 inflammasome by *Mycobacterium tuberculosis* is uncoupled from susceptibility to active tuberculosis," *European Journal of Immunology*, vol. 42, no. 2, pp. 374–384, 2012.

[89] T. Bergsbaken, S. L. Fink, and B. T. Cookson, "Pyroptosis: host cell death and inflammation," *Nature Reviews Microbiology*, vol. 7, no. 2, pp. 99–109, 2009.

[90] L. Sborgi, S. Rühl, E. Mulvihill et al., "GSDMD membrane pore formation constitutes the mechanism of pyroptotic cell death," *EMBO Journal*, vol. 35, no. 16, pp. 1766–1778, 2016.

[91] M. M. Gaidt and V. Hornung, "Pore formation by GSDMD is the effector mechanism of pyroptosis," *EMBO Journal*, vol. 35, no. 20, pp. 2167–2169, 2016.

[92] T. L. M. Thurston, S. A. Matthews, E. Jennings et al., "Growth inhibition of cytosolic *Salmonella* by caspase-1 and caspase-11 precedes host death," *Nature Communications*, vol. 7, p. 13292, 2016.

[93] J. Lukens, V. D. Dixit, and T.-D. Kanneganti, "Inflammasome activation in obesity-related inflammatory diseases and autoimmunity," *Discovery Medicine*, vol. 12, no. 62, pp. 65–74, 2014.

[94] P. Gurung and T.-D. Kanneganti, "Autoinflammatory skin disorders: the inflammasome in focus," *Trends in Molecular Medicine*, vol. 22, no. 7, pp. 545–564, 2016.

[95] D. De Nardo, C. M. De Nardo, and E. Latz, "New insights into mechanisms controlling the NLRP3 inflammasome and its role in lung disease," *American Journal of Pathology*, vol. 184, no. 1, pp. 42–54, 2014.

[96] G. Szabo and T. Csak, "Inflammasomes in liver diseases," *Journal of Hepatology*, vol. 57, no. 3, pp. 642–654, 2012.

[97] H. J. Anders and D. A. Muruve, "The inflammasomes in kidney disease," *Journal of the American Society of Nephrology*, vol. 22, no. 6, pp. 1007–1018, 2011.

[98] A. P. Demidowich, A. I. Davis, N. Dedhia, and J. A. Yanovski, "Colchicine to decrease NLRP3-activated inflammation and improve obesity-related metabolic dysregulation," *Medical Hypotheses*, vol. 92, pp. 67–73, 2016.

[99] G. Nuki, "Colchicine: its mechanism of action and efficacy in crystal-induced inflammation," *Current Rheumatology Reports*, vol. 10, no. 3, pp. 218–227, 2008.

[100] A. A. Jesus and R. Goldbach-Mansky, "IL-1 blockade in autoinflammatory syndromes," *Annual Review of Medicine*, vol. 65, no. 1, pp. 223–244, 2014.

Permissions

List of Contributors

Rousseau Djouaka, Razack Adeoti, Innocent Djegbe and Manuele Tamo
AgroEcoHealth Platform, International Institute of Tropical Agriculture (IITA), 08 Tri-Postal, Cotonou, Benin

Francis Zeukeng
AgroEcoHealth Platform, International Institute of Tropical Agriculture (IITA), Tri-Postal, Cotonou, Benin
Faculty of Science, Department of Biochemistry, University of Yaoundé I, Yaoundé, Cameroon

Genevieve Tchigossou and Romaric Akoton
AgroEcoHealth Platform, International Institute of Tropical Agriculture (IITA), Tri-Postal, Cotonou, Benin
Faculty of Science and Techniques, University of Abomey-Calavi, Abomey-Calavi, Benin

Jude Daiga Bigoga, Clavella Nantcho Nguepdjo and Wilfred Fon Mbacham
Faculty of Science, Department of Biochemistry, University of Yaoundé I, Yaoundé, Cameroon

David N'golo Coulibaly, Sylla Aboubacar and Solange E. Kakou-Ngazoa
Department of Technics and Technology, Platform of Molecular Biology, Pasteur Institute Abidjan, Abidjan 01, Abidjan, Côte d'Ivoire

Sodjinin Jean-Eudes Tchebe
Faculty of Science and Techniques, University of Abomey-Calavi, Abomey-Calavi, Benin

Anthony Ablordey
Department of Bacteriology, Noguchi Memorial Institute for Medical Research, University of Ghana, Legon, Accra, Ghana

María Noel Bianco, Felipe Schelotto and Gustavo Varela
Bacteriology and Virology Department, Hygiene Institute, Medicine Faculty, Universidad de la República, Uruguay

Vivian Peirano
Bacteriology and Virology Department, Hygiene Institute, Medicine Faculty, Universidad de la República, Uruguay
Mercedes Hospital Laboratory, State Health Services Administration (ASSE), Uruguay

Armando Navarro
Public Health Department, Medicine Faculty, UNAM (Universidad Nacional Aut´onoma de Mexico), Mexico City, Mexico

Igor Dumic
Mayo Clinic College of Medicine and Science, Rochester, MN, USA
Division of Hospital Medicine, Mayo Clinic Health System, Eau Claire, WI, USA

Edson Severnini
Carnegie Mellon University, Heinz College, 4800 Forbes Ave., Pittsburgh, PA, USA

Keila Isaac-Olivé, Pablo Moreno Pérez and Ninfa Ramírez Durán
Facultad deMedicina, Universidad Autónoma del Estado de México, Paseo Tollocan/Jesús Carranza s/n, 50180 Toluca, MEX,Mexico

Adrian Zaragoza Bastida
Facultad deMedicina, Universidad Autónoma del Estado de México, Paseo Tollocan/Jesús Carranza s/n, 50180 Toluca, MEX, Mexico
Área Académica de Medicina Veterinaria y Zootecnia, Instituto de Ciencias Agropecuaria, Universidad Autónoma del Estado de Hidalgo, Av. Universidad Km 1, Ex-Hda. de Aquetzalpa, 43600 Tulancingo, HGO, Mexico

Nallely Rivero Pérez
Área Académica de Medicina Veterinaria y Zootecnia, Instituto de Ciencias Agropecuaria, Universidad Autónoma del Estado de Hidalgo, Av. Universidad Km 1, Ex-Hda. de Aquetzalpa, 43600 Tulancingo, HGO, Mexico

Benjamín Valladares Carranza
Centro de Investigacíon y Estudios Avanzados en Salud Animal, Facultad de Medicina Veterinaria y Zootecnia, Universidad Autónoma del Estado de México, Km 15.5 Carretera Panamericana Toluca Atlacomulco, 50200 Toluca, MEX, Mexico

Horacio Sandoval Trujillo
Departamento de Sistemas Biol´ogicos, Universidad Autónoma Metropolitana-Xochimilco, Calzada del Hueso 1100, 04960 Ciudad de México, Mexico

Saeed Banawas, Mohammed Alaidarous, Bader Alshehri, Abdul Aziz Bin Dukhyil and Mohammed Alsaweed
Department of Medical Laboratory Sciences, College of Applied Medical Sciences, Majmaah University, Majmaah 11952, Saudi Arabia

Ahmed Abdel-Hadi
Department of Medical Laboratory Sciences, College of Applied Medical Sciences, Majmaah University, Majmaah 11952, Saudi Arabia
Department of Botany and Microbiology, Faculty of Science, Al-Azhar University, Assuit Branch, Cairo, Egypt

Mohamed Aboamer
Department of Medical Equipment Technology, College of Applied Medical Sciences, Majmaah University, Majmaah 11952, Saudi Arabia

Chongyang Wu, Chaoqing Lin, Qiyu Bao and Yunliang Hu
The Second Affiliated Hospital and Yuying Children's Hospital, Wenzhou Medical University, Wenzhou 325027, China
School of Laboratory Medicine and Life Science, Institute of Biomedical Informatics, Wenzhou Medical University, Wenzhou 325035, China

Qingli Chang
The Second Affiliated Hospital and Yuying Children's Hospital, Wenzhou Medical University, Wenzhou 325027, China
School of Laboratory Medicine and Life Science, Institute of Biomedical Informatics, Wenzhou Medical University, Wenzhou 325035, China
Department of Clinical Laboratory, The First Affiliated Hospital of Xinxiang Medical University, Xinxiang 453100, China

Kaibo Zhang, Junwan Lu, Cong Cheng and Shunfei Lu
School of Medicine and Health, Lishui University, Lishui 323000, China

Peizhen Li, Lei Xu, Yabo Liu and Jinsong Li
School of Laboratory Medicine and Life Science, Institute of Biomedical Informatics, Wenzhou Medical University, Wenzhou 325035, China

Thawatchai Kitti
Faculty of Oriental Medicine, Chiang Rai College, Chiang Rai, Thailand

Rathanin Seng, Natnaree Saiprom and Narisara Chantratita
Department of Microbiology and Immunology, Faculty of Tropical Medicine, Mahidol University, Bangkok, Thailand

Rapee Thummeepak
Department of Microbiology and Parasitology, Faculty of Medical Sciences, Naresuan University, Phitsanulok, Thailand

Sutthirat Sitthisak
Department of Microbiology and Parasitology, Faculty of Medical Sciences, Naresuan University, Phitsanulok, Thailand
Centre of Excellence in Medical Biotechnology, Faculty of Medical Science, Naresuan University, Phitsanulok, Thailand

Chalermchai Boonlao
Chiangrai Prachanukroh Hospital, Amphoe Meuang, Chiangrai, Thailand

Xue-min Wu, Qiu-yong Chen, Ru-jing Chen, Yong-liang Che, Long-bai Wang, Chen-yan Wang, Shan Yan, Yu-tao Liu and Lun-jiang Zhou
Institute of Animal Husbandry and Veterinary Medicine, Fujian Academy of Agriculture Sciences/ Fujian Animal Disease Control Technology Development Center, Fuzhou 350013, China

Jin-sheng Xiu
College of Animal Sciences, Fujian Agricultural and Forestry University, Fuzhou, Fujian 350002, China

Lijuan Lu, Huaqing Zhong, Liyun Su, Lingfeng Cao, Menghua Xu, Niuniu Dong and Jin Xu
Department of Clinical Laboratory, Children's Hospital of Fudan University, Shanghai 201102, China

Qingbin Liu, Wei Jing and Wei Wang
Department of Pediatric, Affiliated Hospital of Changchun University of Traditional Chinese Medicine, Changchun 130021, China

Mengistu Abayneh
School of Medical Laboratory Sciences, Mizan-Tepi University, Mizan Aman, Ethiopia

Getnet Tesfaw and Alemseged Abdissa
School of Medical Laboratory Sciences, Institute of Health Sciences, Jimma University, Jimma, Ethiopia

Isabel Soares-Silva
i3S-Instituto de Investigaçãoe Inovaçãoem Saúde, Universidade do Porto, Porto, Portugal

INEB-Instituto de Engenharia Biomédica, Universidade do Porto, Rua Alfredo Allen 208, 4200-180 Porto, Portugal

Liliana Simões-Silva
i3S-Instituto de Investigação e Inovação em Saúde, Universidade do Porto, Porto, Portugal
INEB-Instituto de Engenharia Biomédica, Universidade do Porto, Rua Alfredo Allen 208, 4200-180 Porto, Portugal
Faculty of Medicine, University of Porto, Porto, Portugal

Benedita Sampaio-Maia
i3S-Instituto de Investigação e Inovação em Saúde, Universidade do Porto, Porto, Portugal
INEB-Instituto de Engenharia Biomédica, Universidade do Porto, Rua Alfredo Allen 208, 4200-180 Porto, Portugal
Faculty of Dental Medicine, University of Porto, Porto, Portugal

Manuel Pestana
i3S-Instituto de Investigação e Inovação em Saúde, Universidade do Porto, Porto, Portugal
INEB-Instituto de Engenharia Biomédica, Universidade do Porto, Rua Alfredo Allen 208, 4200-180 Porto, Portugal
Department of Nephrology, São João Hospital Center, EPE, Porto, Portugal
Department of Renal, Urological and Infectious Diseases, Faculty of Medicine, University of Porto, Porto, Portugal

Ricardo Araujo
i3S-Instituto de Investigação e Inovação em Saúde, Universidade do Porto, Porto, Portugal
Ipatimup, Institute of Molecular Pathology and Immunology of the University of Porto, Porto, Portugal
Department of Medical Biotechnology, School of Medicine, Flinders University, Adelaide, SA 5042, Australia

Sara Silva and Joana Sousa
Faculty of Dental Medicine, University of Porto, Porto, Portugal

Carla Santos-Araujo
Department of Nephrology, São João Hospital Center, EPE, Porto, Portugal
Department of Physiology and Cardiothoracic Surgery, Cardiovascular R&D Center, Faculty of Medicine, University of Porto, Porto, Portugal

Mirela C. M. Prates, Edwin Tamashiro, Tamara H. Saturno, Guilherme P. Buzatto, Marcos G. Jacob, Lucas R. Carenzi, Ricardo C. Demarco, Eduardo T. Massuda, Fabiana C. P. Valera and Wilma T. Anselmo-Lima
Department of Ophthalmology, Otorhinolaryngology, Head and Neck Surgery, Ribeirao Preto Medical School, University of São Paulo, Ribeirao Preto, SP 14049-900, Brazil

Miriã F. Criado, Anibal S. Oliveira and Bruna L. S. Jesus
Department of Cell Biology, Ribeirao Preto Medical School, University of São Paulo, Ribeirao Preto, SP 14049-900, Brazil

Eurico Arruda
Department of Cell Biology, Ribeirao Preto Medical School, University of São Paulo, Ribeirao Preto, SP 14049-900, Brazil
Virology Research Center, Ribeirao Preto Medical School, University of São Paulo, Ribeirao Preto, SP 14049-900, Brazil

José L. Proenca-Modena
Department of Cell Biology, Ribeirao Preto Medical School, University of São Paulo, Ribeirao Preto, SP 14049-900, Brazil
Virology Research Center, Ribeirao Preto Medical School, University of São Paulo, Ribeirao Preto, SP 14049-900, Brazil
Department of Genetics, Evolution and Bioagents, Institute of Biology, University of Campinas, Campinas, SP 13083-970, Brazil

Davi Aragon
Department of Pediatrics, Ribeirao Preto Medical School, University of São Paulo, Ribeirao Preto, SP 14049-900, Brazil

Markos Negash and Demeke Geremew
Department of Immunology and Molecular Biology, School of Biomedical and Laboratory Sciences, College of Medicine and Health Sciences, University of Gondar, Gondar, Ethiopia

Habtamu Wondifraw Baynes
Department of Clinical Chemistry, School of Biomedical and Laboratory Sciences, College of Medicine and Health Sciences, University of Gondar, Gondar, Ethiopia

Omar Ariel Espinosa
Post Graduation Program in Health Science, Faculty of Medicine, Federal University of Mato Grosso (UFMT), Cuiaba, Mato Grosso, Brazil

Department of Medicine, Faculty of Health Sciences, State University of Mato Grosso (UNEMAT), Caceres, Mato Grosso, Brazil

Silvana Margarida Benevides Ferreira
Cuiabá University (UNIC), Cuiaba, Mato Grosso, Brazil
Post Graduation Program in Nursing, Faculty of Nursing, Federal University of Mato Grosso (UFMT), Cuiaba, Mato Grosso, Brazil

Fabiana Gulin Longhi Palacio
The Brazilian Centre for Evidence-based Healthcare: A Joanna Briggs Institute Centre of Excellence, Sao Paulo, Brazil

Denise da Costa Boamorte Cortela
Department of Medicine, Faculty of Health Sciences, State University of Mato Grosso (UNEMAT), Caceres, Mato Grosso, Brazil

Eliane Ignotti
Department of Immunology and Molecular Biology, School of Biomedical and Laboratory Sciences, College of Medicine and Health Sciences, University of Gondar, Gondar, Ethiopia
Department of Nursing, Faculty of Health Sciences, State University of Mato Grosso (UNEMAT), Caceres, Mato Grosso, Brazil

Kalash Neupane and Pradeep Kumar Shah
Department of Microbiology, Trichandra Multiple Campus, Tribhuvan University, Kathmandu, Nepal

Dipendra Shrestha
National College, Tribhuvan University, Khusibu, Kathmandu, Nepal

Binod Rayamajhee and Binod G C
National College, Tribhuvan University, Khusibu, Kathmandu, Nepal
Department of Infectious Diseases and Immunology, Kathmandu Research Institute for Biological Sciences, Lalitpur, Nepal

Jyoti Acharya and Nisha Rijal
Department of Bacteriology, National Public Health Laboratory, Teku, Kathmandu, Nepal

Mahesh Raj Pant
Department of Microbiology, Kathmandu College of Science and Technology, Kamalpokhari, Kathmandu, Nepal

David B. Huang
Motif BioSciences, New York, NY, USA
Rutgers New Jersey Medical School, Trenton, NY, USA

Stephen Hawser
IHMA Europe Sàrl, Route de l'Ile-au-Bois 1A, 1870 Monthey, Valais, Switzerland

Curtis G. Gemmell
Department of Bacteriology, University of Glasgow Medical School, Glasgow, UK

Daniel F. Sahm
IHMA, Schaumburg, IL, USA

Lucie Bardet and Jean-Marc Rolain
Aix-Marseille Université, IRD, AP-HM, MEPHI, IHU-Méditerranée Infection, Marseille, France

Marie-Claude Letellier
Université Laval, Quebec City, Canada

Vladimir Gilca and Chantal Sauvageau
Université Laval, Quebec City, Canada
Institut National de Santé Publique du Québec, Quebec City, Canada
Centre Hospitalier Universitaire de Québec — Université Laval, Quebec City, Canada

Rachid Amini and Gisele Trudeau
Institut National de Santé Publique du Québec, Quebec City, Canada

Samuel Asamoah Sakyi and Linda Ahenkorah Fondjo
Department of Molecular Medicine, School of Medical Sciences, Kwame Nkrumah University of Science and Technology (KNUST), Kumasi, Ghana

Kwabena Owusu Danquah and Venus Frimpong
Department of Medical Laboratory Technology, Faculty of Allied Health Sciences, Kwame Nkrumah University of Science and Technology (KNUST), Kumasi, Ghana

Richard Dadzie Ephraim
Department of Medical Laboratory Technology, School of Allied Health Sciences, University of Cape Coast (UCC), Cape Coast, Ghana

Anthony Enimil
Department of Child Health, School of Medical Sciences, Kwame Nkrumah University of Science and Technology (KNUST), Kumasi, Ghana

Esther Love Darkoh
Department of -eoretical and Applied Biology, College of Science, Kwame Nkrumah University of Science and Technology (KNUST), Kumasi, Ghana

Stefano Busani, Erika Roat, Giulia Serafini, Elena Mantovani, Emanuela Biagioni and Massimo Girardis
Intensive Care Unit, Modena University Hospital, L.go del Pozzo 71, 41100 Modena, Italy

Sebastian Wawrocki and Magdalena Druszczynska
Division of Cell Immunology, Department of Immunology and Infectious Biology, Institute of Microbiology, Biotechnology and Immunology, Faculty of Biology and Environmental Protection, University of Lodz, Banacha 12/16, 90-237 Lodz, Poland

Index